Praise for *ROAR*

"Dr. Stacy Sims is a singular voice and an epic intellectual talent in the health and fitness world. As former professional athletes turned fitness entrepreneurs, we have found that her insights into the unique interworkings of the female athletic body were a total game changer. *ROAR* will help athletes everywhere become faster, stronger, and healthier."

—Juliet and Kelly Starrett, *New York Times* bestselling authors and cofounders of San Francisco CrossFit and MobilityWOD

"Dr. Sims has taken her years of experience as an endurance athlete and scientist to create the ultimate guide to nutrition and performance for female athletes. No matter what your sport of choice is, *ROAR* is a book that no athlete should be without."

—Shaluinn Fullove, two-time U.S. Olympic marathon trials qualifier

"Having completed over fifty-six Ironmans, I can say with certainty learning how your body reacts to high-endurance training and racing never stops. It's discouraging to prepare for a race and have it derailed, not because you didn't do the work, but because your body didn't respond on that particular day. Dr. Sims will show you how you can take the steps to toe the start line with the best chance of delivering your maximum potential!"

—Meredith B. Kessler, professional triathlete

"Dr. Sims helped me recover from hip surgery to win a World Championship bronze medal. Her personalized approach to training, recovery, and nutrition can unlock an athlete's potential to achieve next level goals. Now all active women have access to the same groundbreaking information that made a significant impact on my career."

—Lea Davison, professional mountain bike racer and Olympian

"An enlightening guide [for women] to fueling and strengthening themselves for peak fitness. . . . This book is a must for female athletes."

—*Publishers Weekly*

ROAR

RO

AR

REVISED EDITION

MATCH YOUR FOOD AND FITNESS TO YOUR UNIQUE FEMALE PHYSIOLOGY FOR OPTIMUM PERFORMANCE, GREAT HEALTH, AND A STRONG BODY FOR LIFE

STACY T. SIMS, PHD, WITH
SELENE YEAGER

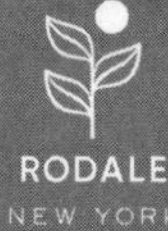

RODALE
NEW YORK

Published in the United States by Rodale Books, an imprint of Random House,
a division of Penguin Random House LLC, New York.
rodalebooks.com | RandomHouseBooks.com

RODALE and the Plant colophon are registered trademarks of Penguin Random House LLC.

Originally published in different form in the United States by Rodale Books, an imprint of Random House,
a division of Penguin Random House LLC, in 2016.

Grateful acknowledgment is made to the following for permission to reprint previously published material:

BMJ Publishing Group Ltd: Infographic on pg. 32 from "IOC Consensus Statement on Relative Energy Deficiency in Sport (RED-S): 2018 update" by Margo Mountjoy, Jorunn Kaiander Sundgot-Borgen, Louise M. Burke, Kathryn E. Ackerman, Cheri Blauwet, Naama Constantini, Constance Lebrun, Bronwen Lundy, Anna Katarina Melin, Nanna L. Meyer, Roberta T. Sherman, Adam S. Tenforde, Monica Klungland Torstveit, and Richard Budgett, reproduced from *British Journal of Sports Medicine*, vol 52, issue 11, copyright © 2018, with permission from BMJ Publishing Group Ltd.

Hannah Grant: Recipes on pages 330–334 from *The Grand Tour* Cookbook by Hannah Grant, published by Musette Publishing ApS, June 5, 2015. (English Edition.) Reprinted by permission.

Kelly Starrett: "Brace Yourself" by Kelly Starrett, originally published in *Becoming a Supple Leopard* by Kelly Starrett and Glen Cordoza, Victory Belt Publishing, Las Vegas, NV in 2013. Reprinted by permission.

Library of Congress Cataloging-in-Publication Data
Names: Sims, Stacy T., author.
Title: Roar: match your food and fitness to your unique female physiology for optimum performance, great health, and a strong body for life
Stacy T. Sims.
Identifiers: LCCN 2023036792 | ISBN 9780593581926 (paperback) | ISBN 9780593797112 (ebook)
Subjects: LCSH: Women athletes—Health and hygiene. | Women—Health and hygiene. | Women athletes—Physiology. | Women athletes—Nutrition.
Classification: LCC RC1218.W65 S56 2024 | DDC 613.7/11082—dc23/eng/20230906
LC record available at https://lccn.loc.gov/2023036792

ISBN 978-0-593-58192-6
Ebook ISBN 978-0-593-79711-2

Printed in the United States of America

Cover design by Irene Ng
Cover photograph by Mitch Mandel
Illustrations by Paige Vickers

1st Printing

First Revised Edition

CONTENTS

INTRODUCTION

YOU ARE NOT A SMALL MAN.
STOP EATING AND TRAINING LIKE ONE.

Long before I was a nutrition scientist and exercise physiologist, I was an athlete. I ran. I raced bikes. I competed in triathlons, including the Ironman World Championships in Kona, Hawaii, and XTerra Worlds in Maui, Hawaii. I wish I'd known then what I know now.

See, back then, I trained and fueled myself like a man because that's what everyone did. Sure, I took in fewer calories because I was smaller. But I followed the same progressive training plans, ate the same bars and gels, and raced like a guy. And I suffered because of it. Some races I would feel great. But others, especially those that were in the week or so before my period started, were awful. I wouldn't be able to handle the heat (even though I prepped for it). I got dehydrated. I lost power. I had gastrointestinal issues.

Being a scientific person by nature, I started taking notes on all my races in an attempt to spot trends and get to the bottom of my uneven performance. My initial suspicion was that it was something in my training plan, that I didn't taper right or I didn't have the right level of fitness going into each race.

It never occurred to me that it was actually my physiology working against me. Or more specifically, I was not working properly with my physiology. The breaking point was ending up in the medical tent at Ironman Kona after becoming hyponatremic (low sodium levels in the blood). I distinctly remember riding out to Hawi, the halfway point of the 112-mile bike portion of the course, in winds so intense that I saw a woman about my size get picked up by the wind and dumped into the ditch on the side of the road. Yes, I was freaking out and probably not 100 percent on top of my fueling needs, but I noticed on the way back that I had a low-grade headache and was getting swollen. I knew those were early signs of hyponatremia, so I pulled a couple of Gastrolyte tablets (a glucose and electrolyte combination) out of my pocket and ate them ASAP. Within a few minutes, I had to pee like a racehorse. I then spent the remaining time of the race wondering if and why any of my fellow teammates from New Zealand had similar issues. When the race was said and done, I asked the other Kiwi women how they found the race. What was incredibly interesting was that those of us in the high hormone phase (a few days out from getting our periods) had borderline hyponatremic issues; two ended up in the medical tent with clinically low blood sodium and on IV drips. My friends who were in the low-hormone phase (day 1 through 14 of your menstrual cycle, starting with the first day of your period) had great races and didn't have any fluid or heat issues, even though we all did the same heat-acclimation protocols and followed the same nutrition protocols! This prompted me to change my PhD topic from altitude to heat and to try to figure out why those of us in the high-hormone phase had experienced such problems.

That's when I decided to become a biohacker for the female race. I was already living in New Zealand and studying for my PhD in environmental exercise physiology, nutrition science at the University of Otago, where I had access to a lab, state-of-the-art data analysis systems, and lots of active friends, teammates, and colleagues. With full access to an environmental chamber; core temperature monitoring systems; blood analysis equipment for things such as hemoglobin, hematocrit, fluid balance, and other hormones; a refractometer for urinalysis; and fully supportive PhD supervisors (who are wicked smart!) and lab managers, I went to work researching how hormones impact thermoregulation, macronutrient usage, hydration, performance, and recovery. Right out of the gate, it was apparent that sex differences extend far beyond ponytails and sports bras.

I soon developed what has become my mantra today: *Women are not small men.*

That may seem blatantly obvious, but for ages, that's how most sports-nutrition manufacturers treated us. They simply formulated products that had fewer calories and put them in pretty packages, maybe tossing in extra calcium or a bit of soy protein, and labeled them women's specific. For many years, women got the nutritional equivalent of "shrink it and pink it." That's a huge disservice, and it's time to acknowledge, treat, train, and fuel women as the different physiological beings we are.

HORMONE POWER

Hormones are your body's messengers; they course through your veins delivering orders from your organs to your brain (and vice versa) to perform nearly everything you do. Hormones tell your body when to eat, sleep, and even when to grow. They give us our appetite and sex drive. They help us have babies. They make us happy, sad, and giddy in love. In men, these hormones are pretty stable day in and day out (though they certainly change over a lifetime). In women, however, it's another story. And that story centers on the menstrual cycle.

The menstrual cycle not only has a profound effect on your fertility and moods (and chocolate cravings), it also can significantly affect your training and performance. Yet very few coaches and trainers take it into consideration with their athletes—even those in the most elite competitive spheres!

Case in point, marathon world-record holder Paula Radcliffe made headlines around the world when she dared to speak about periods and performance. Calling out coaches and sports doctors who intervene in ways that make things worse, the legendary endurance runner plainly proclaimed, "They are men and just don't understand." Radcliffe recalled a time in 2013 where British Athletics medics gave fellow runner Jessica Judd norethisterone (synthetic progesterone, a female hormone produced in the ovaries and adrenal glands that helps the body prepare for conception and pregnancy and regulates the menstrual cycle) to delay her period at the 2013 World Championships. Judd lost. Radcliffe, who had been given synthetic progesterone herself in the past and found it made things a hundred times worse, wasn't surprised. In fact, Radcliffe told the BBC that she broke the world record at the 2002 Chicago Marathon while suffering from menstrual cramps. She wants the public to know this because everyone finds it so surprising.

In 2015, former British number one female tennis player Annabel Croft told the BBC that the impact of sportswomen's menstrual cycles on performance is "the last taboo" and that women "suffer in silence."

In good news, women are being less silent. In 2016, Chinese Olympic swimmer Fu Yuanhui made headlines in *The Guardian* and around the world after she fell short in her leg of the 4 x 100 medley relay and her team came in fourth, saying, "It's because my period came yesterday, so I felt particularly tired—but this isn't an excuse, I still didn't swim well enough."

In August 2022, Great Britain sprinter Dina Asher-Smith missed gold in her 100m finals at the European Athletic Championships, which she later blamed on cramps related to her period. As she told BBC Sport, "It's something I think more people need to actually research from a sports science perspective . . . and I feel that if it was a men's issue, we'd have a million different ways to combat things."

And in 2022, Lydia Ko (who later that year became Golf's world number one), was praised by women around the world for being honest about her period during a broadcast interview. During the final round of a tournament, her physical therapist was working on her back. When a reporter asked her what was up, she said, "It's that time of the month . . . when that happens, my back gets really tight, and I'm all twisted." She left the reporter speechless, according to the report in CNN. But the rest of us cheered . . . and have plenty to say about how it's about time periods are spoken about openly and plainly.

So we've made progress over the past decade, but as these examples show, we still have a ways to go. And it is certainly frustrating that it's 2023 and so many people are still stumbling around in the dark about what is a fairly straightforward hormonal phenomenon that occurs like clockwork in half the population.

You'll find a detailed discussion of how the menstrual cycle influences performance in Chapter 2, but to boil it down, women have two main hormone phases each month: low and high. During the low-hormone phase, we are physiologically more like men in our carbohydrate metabolism and recovery. When our hormones rise during the other half of the month, however, it's a different story.

High estrogen makes us spare glycogen (stored glucose/carbohydrates your body uses for fuel, especially during high-intensity exercise) and increases the amount of fat we use for fuel—not exactly what you're looking for when racing or doing threshold intervals. Progesterone's main job is to provide building blocks for the uterine lining, so it shuttles carbohydrates right to the lining to create a lush glycogen-rich tissue. It also increases muscle breakdown (while also hindering our ability to synthesize muscle because we can't access the building blocks of protein, amino acids, as well). Not only this, but progesterone increases your resting body temperature by promoting heat conservation (which also comes with a delayed sweat response and a change in our thirst sensation). The one-two punch of high estrogen and progesterone after ovulation as your hormones ramp up leading to your period causes fluid shifts (hello, bloat), decreases your blood plasma volume, and makes you more predisposed to central nervous system fatigue, which makes exercise feel harder than usual.

All that can really stink when you've been training for months, even years, and your A-race falls right before your period when hormones are sky-high. That's why I tell my athletes that it's not their fitness; it's their physiology. In order to succeed, you need to work with—not against—your natural physiology.

FEMALE PHYSIOLOGY IN ACTION

Menstruation is just the tip of the iceberg of the physiological differences between male and female athletes, and it's time for women to understand that. This book is about empowering women with the fitness and nutrition knowledge they need to compete on the same even playing field as men.

We'll start by taking an in-depth look at your female physiology in action: how we as women are built to be naturally good at endurance; where we carry our muscle and our power; how we sweat differently from men; and all the other ways our physiology makes us unique. Because your physiology changes over time, you'll also find entire chapters devoted to your menstrual cycle, pregnancy, and menopause (which, until very recently, nobody ever talked about!).

From there, we'll give you the expert training and nutrition advice you need to build a rock-solid fitness foundation. This is what I call getting fit to get fit, the phase where you train your body to optimally adapt to exercise. This includes determining—and reaching—your high-performance body composition (which may or may not be your dream number on the scale); making lean muscle where you need it most; building strong bones; and boosting power and endurance.

Oh, and say goodbye to wild mood swings and uncontrollable chocolate cravings. What you as a woman may think—and have been told for decades—is all in your head is actually all in your gut or, more specifically, what's not in your gut. In our fast-moving lives, we are often overtired, overstressed, undernourished (although overfed), and immune compromised. This combination reaches far beyond that wanting-to-sleep-at-work feeling and extends to the interruption of our symbiosis with our gut bacteria. What does that have to do with your moods and cravings? Turns out, everything.

You'll learn all about these essential colonies of bacteria in your gut in Chapter 8, but as a preview: The human intestines contain more than 100 trillion microbes (10 times more than any other cells in the body). These enormous microscopic armies manipulate our eating behaviors and moods for their own survival—often at the expense of our overall health. But news flash: You don't have to be at the mercy of your bacterial microbiome. You'll learn to master your gut, your moods, and your cravings and improve your overall health.

Finally, we'll pull it all together in your plan for peak performance. Women not only need different fuel before and during exercise, but we also have unique recovery needs. Our recovery window is a lot shorter than men's; it's harder to hold on to our valuable muscle tissue; and we are susceptible to performance difficulties in the heat. Worse, some of the products sold to us to offset the disadvantages of our physiology (looking at you, soy protein) can actually make matters worse.

This final section of the book will arm you with the knowledge you need to hack into your personal female physiology, decipher what you find, and take action to be in the healthiest, fittest, strongest shape of your life. Now, that's something worth roaring about!

A NOTE ABOUT THE RESEARCH SCOPE OF *ROAR*

Our goal is to present women with knowledge about their unique physiology as it pertains to training and performance. There are limitations in that science. Existing training, nutrition, and performance science has been conducted largely on people of the female and/or male sex who are not using masculinizing and/or feminizing hormone therapy. There is a need for sports nutrition and performance research on trans women and trans men who may have a puberty trajectory that has been modified with the use of exogenous hormone therapy, as well as on adults who have started using gender affirming therapies later in life. Currently, the majority of transgender research is on the health and medical impacts of those therapies. We will be watching the research landscape for future revisions to include as much performance information for as many women as possible.

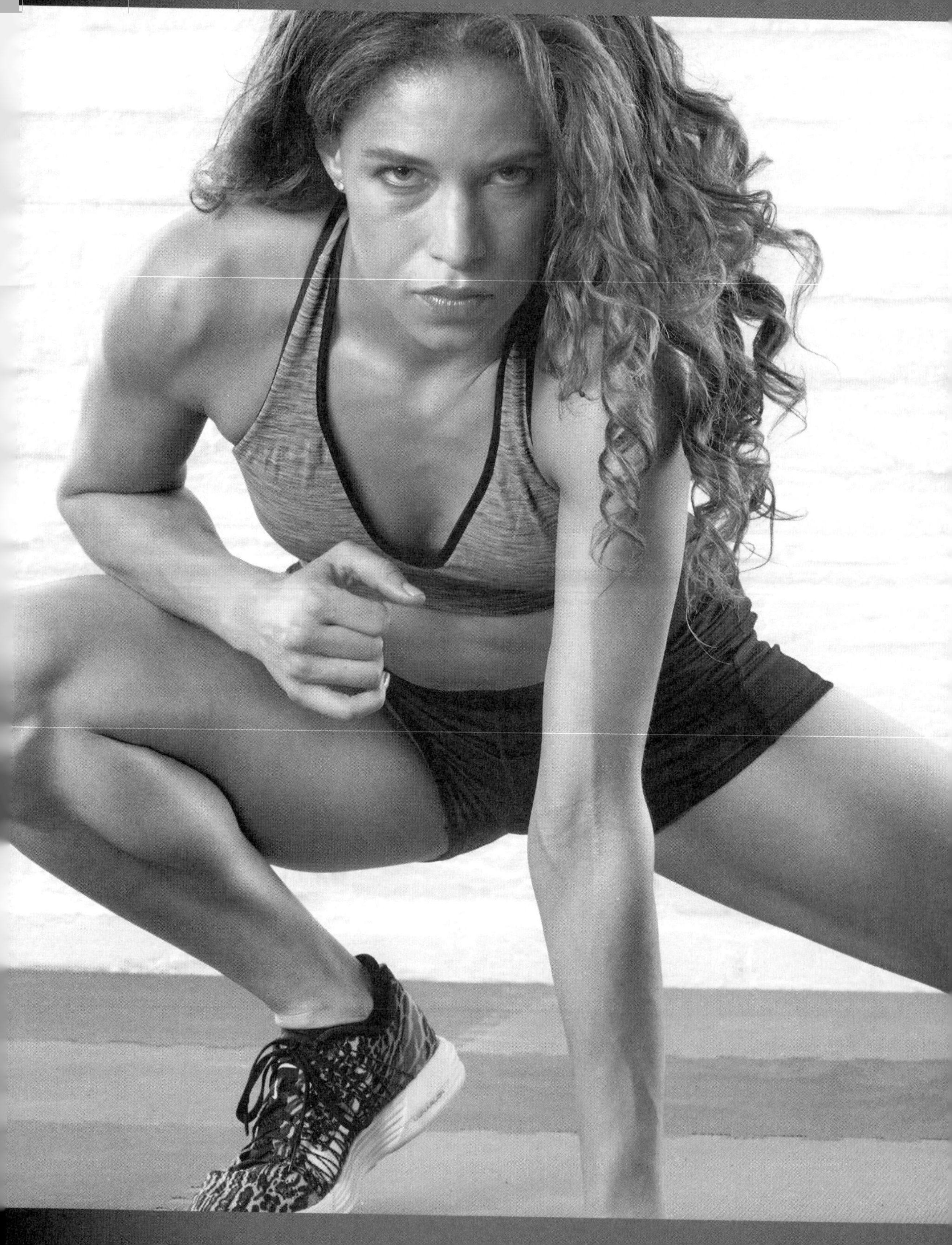

PART I

YOUR FEMALE PHYSIOLOGY

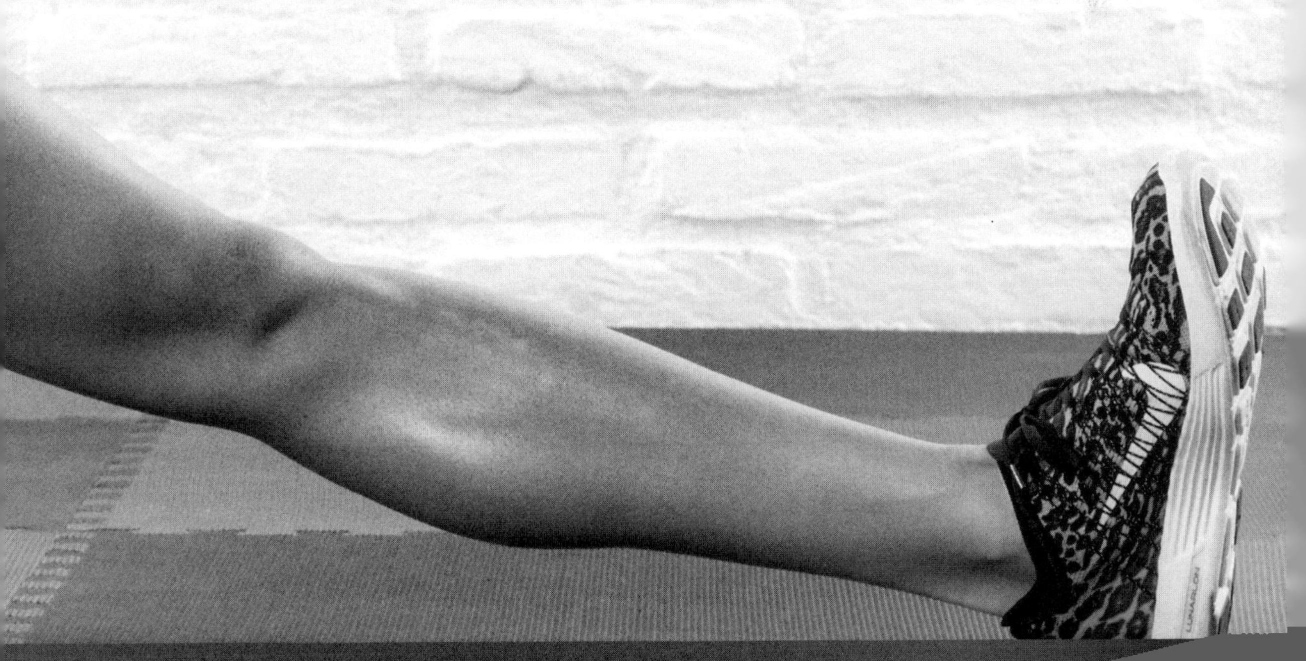

1

WHAT IT MEANS TO BE "LIKE A GIRL"

ALL THE PHYSIOLOGICAL STUFF THAT MAKES FEMALES UNIQUE

You "throw like a girl." You "run like a girl." The "like a girl" insult has been so ubiquitous, such a strong underlying current in our culture, that in 2015, Always, one of the biggest makers of feminine hygiene products, stole the show during the Super Bowl with a 60-second ad spot that challenged the culture to dismantle the phrase with its #LikeAGirl campaign, which turns the insult into an inspirational compliment. You saw what it can mean to compete like a girl in the introduction—how women can dominate their sport.

Look, I'm not one to sugarcoat anything, so I'll give it to you straight. Yes, in head-to-head objective physical performance comparisons, females may have some disadvantages compared to males. We also have some distinct advantages, but you never hear about those. So let's set the stage here with a complete look at your female physiology in action.

SUGAR AND SPICE AND EVERYTHING NICE: WHAT WE'RE REALLY MADE OF

No surprise: Women tend to be smaller and lighter and have a higher portion of body fat (hello breasts, hips, and all things childbearing!) than men. But dig a little deeper, and the comparisons become more interesting and revealing.

First, let's talk about body mass and how it's distributed. Our mass is the stuff we're made of, which everyone commonly refers to as weight—the number you see on the scale. That's not exactly accurate. For one, technically, weight is determined by gravitational pull, so you'd weigh less on the moon and far more on Jupiter, but that's being picky. The more important factor is that the number you see on the scale—your weight—fluctuates widely depending on fluid intake, what you've eaten during the day, salt intake, and how much glycogen you're storing in your muscles. (For every 1 gram of glycogen, you store 3 grams of water; as you get fitter, you become better at glycogen storage. So before a big event, you can gain 5 or more pounds that you will blow through during your event—but you haven't gained or lost any fat.) Body mass, by contrast, is the actual stuff you're made of—bone, muscle, fat, and organs—that requires tissue loss or gain and is harder to change.

We'll cover bones in Chapter 9, because a strong skeleton is essential for vibrant living, and women's bones are vulnerable to getting brittle. For now, however, let's focus on muscle and fat.

When researchers take core needles and pull out a column of muscle tissue from the designated muscle of interest (usually the shoulder, biceps, or quadriceps) of men and women, the findings might surprise you: There's not much difference. Men and women generally have the same muscle composition as far as the percentage of type I endurance (aerobic) fibers and type II power (anaerobic) fibers. What is different is that the largest fibers in women's bodies tend to be type I endurance fibers, while in men the type II power fibers take up the lion's share of real estate.

That fiber type difference makes a difference when you're looking at pure strength between the sexes. In head-to-head strength comparisons, women fall a bit short. Studies show that, generally, the strength of women is typically reported in the range of 40 to 75 percent of that of men, with women about 52 percent as strong as men in their upper bodies and 66 percent as strong as men in their lower bodies. In well-muscled women, those strength differences evaporate a bit. When you look at sheer strength relative to lean body mass, a trained woman's strength shoots up to 70 and 80 percent as strong as men in the arms and legs respectively. Still less powerful, but definitely closer. We also tend to carry more of our lean muscle tissue below the waist, with much of our power coming from our hips and legs.

Then there's fat, which many athletes I work with still consider a four-letter word, even though you can't train, race, or even live without it. Most of us have been conditioned to think of any fat under our skin as unwanted. But that's far from the truth. That's our storage fat. Those are energy reserves we accumulate. That fat also acts as padding and generates key hormones such as adiponectin that regulate insulin (the hormone that helps your body use and store blood sugar). We need some storage fat to perform our best. Most of the fat you don't see in the mirror is essential body fat, which is in your nerves, bone marrow, and organs. Essential fat in men is about 4 percent, but in women, it is about 12 percent (because we are designed to reproduce!). As a woman, your breasts are also largely fatty tissue.

How much fat either men or women carry depends largely on lifestyle, but you can't dismiss the fact that there are also very distinct body types. For instance, there are people who are endomorphs. They tend to be larger, and they carry more body fat. On the other end of the scale are the ectomorphs, who are naturally slimmer. And in the middle are mesomorphs, who tend to be medium built and naturally muscular. You can also be a blend of the two; for example, a mesomorph with endomorph tendencies. How active you are and the type of activity you do can impact the dominance of one body type over another. Your physical activity directly affects your body fat levels and distribution.

We'll delve into the topic of body composition in great depth in Chapter 5, but generally speaking, healthy body fat ranges span from 12 to 30 percent in women and 5 to 25 percent in men.

In the athletic world, muscle is usually prized, while fat is shunned. As I see it, however, what you're made of is important, but more important is the impact of what you're made of on what you do and/or want to do. Take two cyclists, for instance. A man may have big pectorals (pecs) and biceps, but those heavy upper-body muscles will only weigh him down when faced with a 10 percent climb. A woman who is lighter in the torso but still powerful in the hips and legs will have a far easier time pedaling her way up the mountain.

Likewise, women often dominate in the sport of open-water swimming. When you look at the records, female swimmers often perform on par with or better than their male counterparts, especially as the swims get longer. Research investigating the sex difference in performance for successful women and men crossing the Catalina Channel—an arduous 20-mile swim from the Southern California coast to Catalina Island—reports that the fastest woman ever was about 22 minutes faster than the fastest man ever. The three fastest women ever were about 20 minutes faster than the three fastest men ever. Though the overall difference in performance didn't reach statistical significance, women appear to be continuously narrowing the performance gap.

And let's not forget that in 2013 Diana Nyad became the first person ever to swim the 110.86 miles between Cuba and Florida without the use of a shark cage for protection in a mind-boggling 52 hours and 54 minutes. Fat is more buoyant than muscle, so that extra padding may be a distinct advantage in the open water.

WOMEN ON THE RUN: OUR CAPACITY FOR CARDIO AND ENDURANCE

Whether you run marathons, cycle Gran Fondos, compete in triathlons, or just exercise to stay fit and healthy, training works similarly for both sexes. As you train longer and harder, you get fitter. Your body can deliver and use more oxygen (that's your max VO_2); you can push the pace to a higher point before your muscles beg for mercy (that's your lactate threshold talking); you become stronger and better at burning fat; and your performance improves.

But that open-water swimming example aside, pound for pound, men still generally outrun, outwalk, and outcycle us. Research published in 2022 reported that the performance gap was relatively small at very short distances, but widened as the events got longer (to a point; we'll discuss ultraendurance in a bit). So women were 8.6 percent slower in the 60 meter, 9.6 percent slower in the 100 meter,

11 percent slower in the 200 meter, and 11.7 percent slower in the 400 meter. After that point, there's a relatively consistent 10 to 12 percent discrepancy in endurance performance.

Why? Well, for the same reason that a Prius will have to pull some wily moves if it wants to race against a Mustang—we start with a smaller engine. As a woman, you have a smaller heart (26 percent lighter than the male heart), smaller heart volume, smaller lungs (10 to 12 percent less volume than men), and lower diastolic pressure (the pressure in the arteries when the heart is resting between beats and the ventricles fill with blood), which predisposes us to have lower maximum heart rates and greater problems with dehydration in the heat. This also means we pump out less oxygenated blood with every beat—about 20 percent less cardiac output than men.

Less oxygenated blood means we have to breathe more often, and as a consequence, our respiratory muscles—such as the diaphragm and intercostals between our ribs—need to work harder and use a lot of energy. Like other skeletal muscles, the contracting respiratory muscles require enough blood flow to meet oxygen demand. If you have a greater oxygen cost of breathing, you also likely dedicate a greater amount of blood flow toward your respiratory muscles during maximal exercise. When you push the pace and breathe hard, it can be difficult to race against the guys because less blood flow is going to your legs.

Testosterone also gives men a bit of an edge because the male sex hormone increases the production of red blood cells, which absorb and carry oxygen to working muscles. On average, men have higher red blood cell counts (41 to 50 percent versus 35 to 45 percent in women) and 10 to 15 percent more hemoglobin (which is the molecule in red blood cells that carries the oxygen) concentration than women.

Our combined smaller heart and lungs and lower oxygen-carrying capacity means we have a lower max VO_2 (the maximum amount of oxygen your body can use to make fuel) than men, about 15 to 25 percent lower on average, as shown in the chart. So if two athletes are doing the same amount of work, the woman will have a higher heart rate and need more oxygen to get the job done.

Because of our hormones, we also use energy differently during aerobic exercise. We'll get into this in much greater detail in the following chapters, but in general, because of our estrogen and different proteins in our muscle mitochondria,

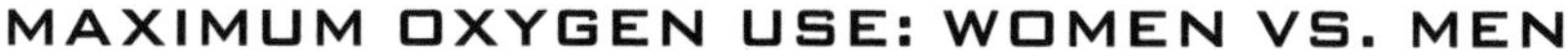

MAXIMUM OXYGEN USE: WOMEN VS. MEN

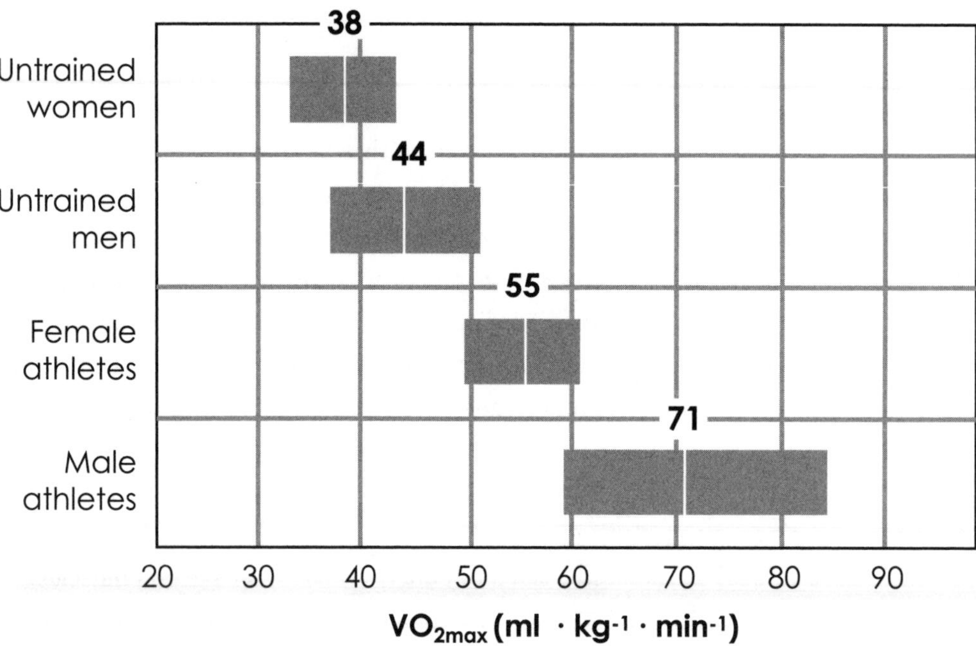

we rely less on carbs and more on fat than our male counterparts. That sounds like a good thing, and in some ways, it is, since fat is the main fuel for aerobic exercise. But it's not such a good thing when we need to go really hard, because that tendency to spare glycogen (which is really strong during the high-hormone phase of your menstrual cycle right before your period) can make it harder to hit high intensities. We really need those carbs to fuel the anaerobic energy system when we push past our threshold. If you're running low on carbs in your bloodstream, it may mean slamming on the brakes instead of hitting the gas, because your body just can't get the glycogen stores it needs to make the energy you want.

Speaking of energy, because men have bigger type II fibers and the energy-producing enzymes that go with them, they have a higher glycolytic capacity than women, which is a fancy way of saying that they can burn through more glucose in the absence of oxygen. That helps them outperform us in short, intense bursts of effort, but it also means they accumulate more lactate (a chemical your body makes and uses for energy during very high-intensity efforts; accumulating more than you can use leads to muscle acidity or "the burn" and forces you to slow down) and need longer recovery time for all-out efforts.

Women, on the other hand, have a greater advantage in the endurance world, as our type I fibers are much more efficient at using fat as fuel and sparing glucose. Compared to men, women may use a greater relative proportion of the carbohydrates consumed during endurance exercise, which, in turn, spares more glycogen and fatty acids usually used as fuel (so eating carbohydrates during exercise can be particularly beneficial). Fatigue outcomes generally support the idea that women have a higher capacity to maintain endurance performance with a faster recovery following challenges that elicit significant muscle work.

With all that in mind, let's go back to that wily Prius for a moment. Sure, that Mustang is going to beat her in a drag race. Maybe even in a race across New Jersey. But that smaller, efficient vehicle will hum along much longer on less fuel and may even beat the high-horsepower vehicle in the long run, which is why you see female ultrarunners like Courtney Dauwalter racking up first place overall (men and women) finishes in races over 100 miles like the Moab 240 and Big's Backyard Ultra,

HORMONES AT A GLANCE

Hormones play a huge role in every physical function of living. You see that very clearly in the sphere of athletics. Here, at a glance, are the major impacts of male and female hormones.

Testosterone (the primary male hormone) leads to:

- Bone formation, larger bones
- Protein synthesis (the biological muscle-building process), larger muscles
- Erythropoietin (EPO) secretion, increased red blood cell production

Estrogen (the primary female hormone) leads to:

- Fat deposition (lipoprotein lipase—the enzyme responsible for taking fatty acids from the blood and putting them into fat tissue; estrogen increases this process)
- Increased muscle cell synthesis, strength of muscle contraction
- Faster, more brief bone growth
- Shorter stature, lower total body mass

where she completed a record 68 laps and accumulated 283.33 miles to win the event in 2022.

Pulling it all together, on the pointy end of most non-ultraendurance events, the fastest woman probably won't ever break the tape in front of the fastest man because they are too close in body size (top marathoners—male and female—often weigh within 5 pounds of each other). But for the rest of us, hanging with and passing men in endurance competition is very much in the realm of possibility, so long as we know and work with our unique physiology. In this case, it's a matter of building up your plasma (the watery part of your blood) volume through training and feeding your body what it needs to keep your metabolism humming, which we'll cover in great depth in the chapters to come.

FAST WOMEN: OUR STRENGTH, SPEED, AND POWER

Okay, CrossFit athletes and sprinters, this one's for you. As you saw in the section on body composition, your biggest fibers are your type I fibers, which can help you run a fast 10-K but don't necessarily chip in much for kipping pullups or shuttle runs on the soccer field. But that's not to say you can't build your type II fibers through strength training. You most certainly can.

With training, you can honestly get nearly as strong as a man, relatively speaking. For example, when researchers pitted 52 young men against 50 young women in max power tests on a stationary bike, the men frankly smoked the women—generating about 50 percent greater peak power. But the men were significantly heavier. When the researchers looked at how much power they could produce per kilogram of body weight, the difference dropped dramatically to 15 percent. Taking that one step further, when power outputs were adjusted for fat-free mass, the values plummeted to a 2.5 percent difference, or not statistically different—a pretty even match.

Just as is the case in the cardio realm, the strongest, most powerful woman will not out bench press or win a 100-yard dash against the strongest, most powerful man. But there are certainly plenty of women who can outperform and who are stronger than plenty of men. We are every bit as trainable. Even if we get less absolute hypertrophy (muscle growth and an increase in the size of muscle cells) through training than men, research shows that when women and men train equally, their relative strength and hypertrophy gains are pretty much the same.

Which brings me to a question that I get asked less than I used to, but which still concerns a fair number of women: Can women get "bulky" from strength training? Everyone says no, but then you read plenty of articles in women's magazines that caution against too much muscle-building activity so you don't "get fat" (never mind the fact that muscle isn't fat). Case in point, there was a spate of articles several years ago about spinning (aka indoor studio cycling) "making you fat" and "bulking your thighs." One such piece in *Harper's Bazaar* titled "Is Spinning Making You Fat?" quotes a celebrity trainer who forbids his fashion-model clients to ride at all, lest their lower bodies get too big. Sigh.

So what's the truth? Yes, heavy resistance training in the gym or on a spin bike can make your muscles bigger. Have you seen track racers? Their quads are not small. They are powerful and, yes, often large. That's from heavy, hard work in the gym and pushing a monster gear on the bike. It's the same for CrossFit enthusiasts, rowers, sprinters, and everyone else who trains for maximum strength. These women are generally not one bit bothered by the size of their muscles because those muscles enable them to do the work and compete at the level they want.

Hypertrophy is what gives you muscle tone. That said, if you're truly averse to larger muscles, you can still train to get strong without gaining unwanted mass. And in fact, as a woman, you might have an advantage there. Neural mechanisms (mind-muscle connections) are actually more important for women's adaptations to strength training than they are for men's. So by doing power moves and low-rep, high-weight strength training, you enhance the number of fibers recruited for a contraction but don't really grow the size of your muscles very much. The short of it is that you end up with a stronger, more powerful contraction with less muscle "bulk."

As you'll see in Chapter 6, there are many ways to get the strength and power you want and need without gaining mass. But *please*, don't be afraid of muscle. Strong is far preferable for health and performance than skinny. It's also plain smart, because as you get older and start losing precious lean muscle tissue, you'll be happy for all you kept in reserve!

HOW WOMEN RECOVER

When it comes to reaping all the benefits of your hard work in the gym or on the court, field, bike, or trail, the quality of your training must be matched by the quality of your recovery if you hope to see measurable improvement. In short: Train hard, recover harder. And here is where I break the news to you that it is, in fact, somewhat harder for women to recover.

For one, our capacity for muscle glycogen turnover (accessing and using stored carbs) is generally lower, especially during times when our estrogen levels are high. That slows our recovery time because our bodies need available carbs not only to prevent us from eating into our muscles during exercise, but also to help us recover quickly when we're done.

Although we mobilize more fat during exercise, the opposite is true during recovery. At this point women tend to burn an increased proportion of carbs, whereas men burn an increased proportion of fat. What's more, women's fat-burning postexercise metabolism drops back to normal about 3 hours after they've showered and gone about their day, while men's levels remain elevated up to 18 hours later. Progesterone also increases muscle breakdown (catabolism), and with the catabolic responses during exercise, getting a good dose of protein postexercise becomes critical for us to rebuild our muscles and reduce the signaling to store body fat. So if you've ever wondered why the men you may train with seem to lose body fat more quickly than you do, physiology is a major factor.

WOMEN IN THE WORLD: HOW WOMEN RESPOND TO HEAT, COLD, AND ALTITUDE

As a woman, your size, blood volume, and metabolism impact how you respond to your environment, especially when you're out working up a sweat (or trying to stay warm). And, you guessed it, how you react to any given environment is likely a bit different from how your male counterparts do.

Let's start with the main one: thermoregulation, your body's ability to maintain a consistent core temperature—about 98 degrees—regardless of how blazing hot or freezing cold it is.

Hormones definitely play a role in the ability to keep your cool when the going gets hot—core temp rises along with those hormones—but estrogen and progesterone aside, research shows that women generally start sweating later into a workout (if you exercise with guys, you've likely seen this phenomenon firsthand—they're pouring rivers and you've barely begun to glisten), and we sweat less. So if you take two nonacclimated folks and have them run a 5-K in Florida, the woman will generally struggle more with the heat than the man.

That said, and this will be a recurring theme throughout the book, it's trainable. Given time to acclimate (which can take up to 2 weeks), exercise heat-tolerance time for women actually increases more than men's, which makes that sex difference evaporate like a bead of sweat in the Arizona sun.

After you've completed a particularly steamy workout is another story. Women do have a more difficult time offloading the heat they built up during exercise, particularly when hormones are high. A few extra cooling measures such as a dip in the pool, drinking an ice-cold recovery drink, or running the hose over your head can accelerate the process.

How about the opposite extreme? It's a bit less clear. Some research indicates that women have a slightly higher average core temperature than men (97.8 versus 97.4). But their hand temperatures are much cooler by comparison (87.2 versus 90). This is also one reason Raynaud's syndrome (where your blood flow reduces dramatically in response to cold or emotional stress, causing pain and discoloration in your fingers, toes, and sometimes other areas) is considered a woman's disease. When your hands feel cold, you feel cold. So you might need thicker mittens or some heating packs in your gloves to exercise in the same relative comfort as the man next to you when the temperatures dip. (You'll learn about dealing with extreme conditions in Chapter 13.)

How about when we go up into the thin air of high altitude? In one study, researchers examined a group of men and women at sea level and then again while they acclimated to high altitude at Pikes Peak in Colorado (14,109 feet of elevation). They found that while men tend to use more carbohydrates as exercise fuel at high altitude compared to sea level, women burned even more fat than they did in the lower elevations. Since women have more fat stores at their disposal and fat is a less limited source of energy than carbs, we may have an advantage in the high mountains.

EQUAL BUT DIFFERENT

The best way to sum up the whole question of how women compare to men in exercise performance is that we are really pretty equal, even if we have different physiological needs. In absolute terms, we may not be able to match a similarly sized man in strength, speed, and absolute endurance. But we're not that far off.

And—I'll say it again—we're very trainable. Once you throw training into the equation, the sex-difference gap shrinks considerably. If you look at records from the Olympics, the average difference between the gold-medal performances by men and women is about 10 percent across all events. In events such as shooting and equestrian competitions, where success lies not just in physical prowess but balance and mental concentration, the outcomes for women are often on par with the men.

I contend that many of the differences we perceive in ability are just that, perceptions. Society still has different athletic expectations for women than it does for men. Oftentimes as women, we have different expectations for ourselves than we do for men. We have the power to change much of that. We just have to be willing to learn and try. So let's keep roaring on.

STRUCTURAL DIFFERENCES

Women have wider hips than men for a reason: We need them if we choose to give birth to babies. The problem is, the same wide hips that make delivery easier can make other physical tasks, such as running and jumping, trickier for us than they are for our male peers. Wide hips increase what's known as our Q-angle—the angle between our quadriceps muscle and the patellar tendon that helps our knee track properly.

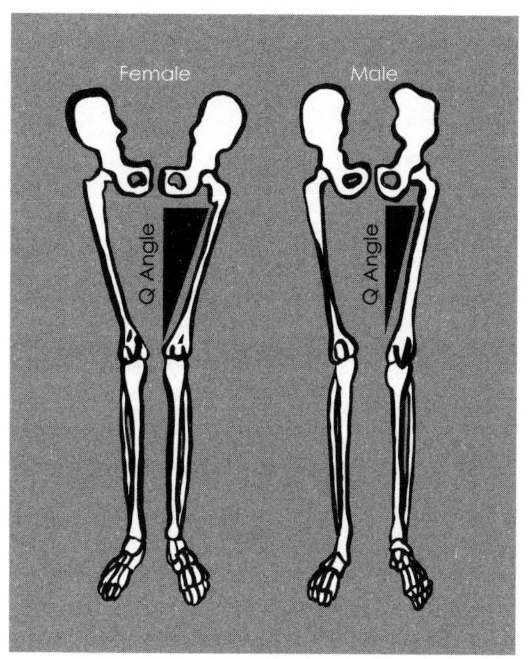

In one study of 100 men and women, the average Q-angle for women was 15.8 degrees compared to 11.2 degrees among the men. That's a significant difference and one that makes us more vulnerable to having knock-knees and pronated feet. Research shows we also have greater peak hip adduction and hip internal rotation (aka more nonsagittal plane movement) than men when we run. Female joints (and tissues including collagen, the main building block) also tend to be hypermobile, which is great for gymnastics but maybe less so for overall stability, so areas such as the patella of the knee are particularly vulnerable for slipping out of place, causing pain and injury.

These structural differences are also why women are more susceptible to chronic exercise-related knee issues, such as chondromalacia and anterior knee pain, because their knees aren't tracking properly. Over time we can damage the cartilage underneath without even realizing it. We're also more prone to acute knee trauma such as anterior cruciate ligament (ACL) tears and blowouts. In fact, girls and women are up to six times more likely to tear their ACL, the key stabilizing ligament in the knee, than the boys and men on the field. That's because when they land from a jump, their knees collapse inward.

These imbalances and their consequences can be easily evaluated (even by yourself) and corrected so you have more solid, stable biomechanics. It's mostly a matter of strengthening those stabilizers in your core and hips so your knees can fall in line no matter how you run, cut, jump, and land. We'll get into the details of that in Chapter 6.

ROAR ▶▶▶ SOUND BITES

▶ As a woman, you have more essential fat, carry most of your lean mass in your lower body, and have a greater distribution and proportion of type I endurance (also called slow-twitch) muscle fibers than men.

▶ Women are naturally good fat-burners. That's great for endurance, but when you want to hit those high intensities, carb is queen.

▶ Pound for pound, a well-trained woman is darn near as powerful as her male counterpart.

▶ Men lose fat more easily than women. Pumping up your protein intake can help if that's your goal.

▶ The top female athletes will likely never catch the top men, but they've gotten pretty close (within 10 percent nearly across the board). And plenty of strong, trained women can best the average guy.

2

DEMYSTIFYING AND MASTERING YOUR MENSTRUAL CYCLE

YOUR PERIOD DOESN'T HAVE TO BE A CURSE WHEN IT COMES TO YOUR PERFORMANCE

Women have a long history of being shamed into silence about their periods. Even if it's not directly stated, the underlying message is it's not something you talk about. You just deal with it. In the sports sector, matters related to menstruation have historically been sidestepped and ignored. Some women even worry that their periods may be viewed as a sign of weakness. In fact, even well into the last century, women were warned against taking part in sports during menstruation because of concerns it would harm their health.

If you are led to believe that menstruation is to be ignored, you are most likely not going to talk about it with your coach or even consider it yourself when trying to perform at your best. Even when we do speak up, we're often more or less dismissed. While I was at Purdue working on my undergraduate degree and participating in metabolism labs, I asked my professor why I was getting different results between two experimental sessions when I was diligent about standardizing everything from one trial to the next (I later realized it was due to the phase of my cycle). The response I got was very typical: "Oh, it just is an anomaly; we'll just use the guys' data." Later, when I wanted to pursue research in sex differences, my advising professor actually cautioned me against it, warning me that women are too difficult to understand, since the changing levels of estrogen and progesterone across a menstrual cycle can skew results.

But the physiological impact is real. There are sex differences from birth, which become most apparent at the onset of puberty, when testosterone rises in boys (stimulating muscle mass development) and the menstrual cycle begins in girls. Once that cycle is set in motion, it will have a profound impact on a woman for the rest of her reproductive life. It's the natural rhythm of life that we work with. We owe it to ourselves to stop being blind to the impact of our menstrual cycle, no matter how profound or slight it may be for you. You don't have to suffer in silence. You can manage—and actually master—it through nutrition and smart exercise programming so that migraines, nausea, bloating, and cramps don't derail your fitness goals.

Things have significantly improved since my university days, but we still have a *long* way to go. I still hear from athletes whose coaches tell them losing your period is "normal" when you train. I still hear from women who want to take hormones to stop their periods so they don't have to worry about them. I still see many women who don't know what's actually happening internally during their menstrual cycle (because, as we'll talk about in a moment, we were never really taught!), let alone how to train with it. There's plenty of progress still to be made, and I'm here for it.

DEMYSTIFYING YOUR PHASES

You likely learned all of this in junior-high health class, but unless you've had a refresher course, you may not remember all the technicalities of the menstrual cycle. Truth be told, many women never really got them the first time around. So let's start with a little review.

The average menstrual cycle is 28 days long (though it can range between 21 and 40 days and doesn't always run like clockwork) and is broken down into several phases. The cycle begins with the first day of menstruation (cycle day 1) and can be

YOUR CYCLE AT A GLANCE

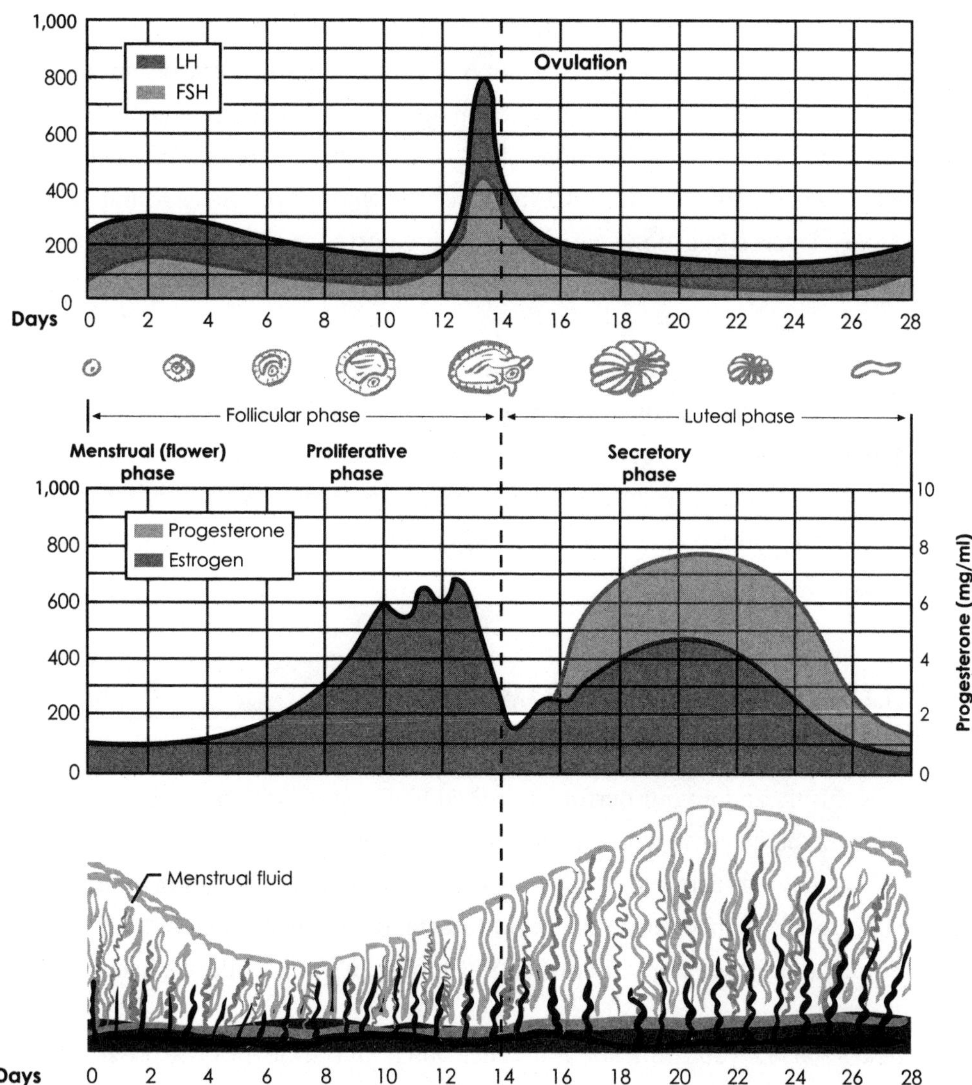

divided into three consecutive phases associated with specific changes in ovarian function: (1) the follicular phase (from the onset of menses to ovulation); (2) the ovulatory phase; and (3) the luteal phase (from ovulation to the onset of the next cycle). The follicular phase is widely variable (which is why the menstrual cycle length varies), whereas the luteal phase is relatively constant and averages 13 to 15 days in most women. The ovulatory phase is shortest and lasts only 24 to 48 hours. Rising and falling hormone levels trigger all of it.

After your period ends—about day 5 or 6 of your cycle—your ovaries gradually start ramping up their production of estrogen during the follicular phase. Through the rise in follicle-stimulating hormone (FSH) during the first days of the cycle, a few ovarian follicles are stimulated to "mature" the eggs for release. Around day 12, your estrogen levels surge along with a luteinizing hormone (LH), which causes ovulation, and an egg is released from your fallopian tubes. Estrogen levels dip at this point but will soon rise again as the body goes into nesting mode in case that egg is fertilized. During this stretch—the luteal phase—your hormones kick into high gear. Progesterone levels rise, surpassing estrogen, to prepare the lining of the uterus for egg implantation. Both estrogen and progesterone reach peak levels about 3 to 5 days before menstruation. This is where premenstrual syndrome (PMS) symptoms can rear up. If a fertilized egg isn't implanted, progesterone levels fall and you shed the lining and are back to day 1.

PERIODS AND PERFORMANCE: MASTERING YOUR CYCLE

What does this mean for your performance? I'd like to start with a fact that surprises many women. You can stop worrying about having your period on race day. Everyone worries about having their period for a big event, but in reality, your hormones are favorable for performance once your period starts. Remember Paula Radcliffe broke the world record for the fastest marathon in Chicago in 2002 while she had menstrual cramps!

It makes sense if you think about it. Once you're in the clear of the possibility of pregnancy, the body goes into a more relaxed mode and all those energy systems used in the high-hormone phase are at your disposal for exertion. There is also a shift in the immune system during this phase of your cycle that lowers inflammation and increases immune-cell activity, which can make you more resilient to stress and able to absorb higher, harder training loads.

Same goes for the low-hormone phase that follows your period. This can be a time you feel stronger, too. In one study of 20 active females, researchers found that the women could make greater strength gains and produce more force when they strength trained during their low-hormone phase compared to training in the high-hormone phase. You're also likely to feel less pain and recover faster.

So, whether you're working out, training, or racing, it may feel easier when you're in the low-hormone phase of your cycle, which starts the first day of menstrual bleeding. Your performance *may* be stronger as well. Though there are very few specific studies on performance throughout the menstrual cycle, one study conducted on swimmers found that the women clocked their fastest times during menstruation and their slowest during the premenstrual period. However, I want you to bear in mind that our own experiences and how we feel again can supersede some of the physiological aspects, and there are many elements that go into how we feel beyond the menstrual cycle.

I'm also obviously painting with a broad brush here, as one must in a book as opposed to an individual consultation. Every woman's cycle is unique, so I always encourage each woman to track her cycle along with her performance to determine her own patterns and power days. For instance, if you're one of the 35 percent of women who sometimes have heavy menstrual bleeding, that will definitely affect your power during your period—the good news is that there is help for that, as we address on page 27. (See "Why You Should Track Your Menstrual Cycle" on page 27, for a deep dive on how to track all this!)

Also, I always want to clearly emphasize that you are *not* doomed if a key event lands on a high-hormone day. Research shows that key performance indicators such as max VO_2 and lactate threshold (the point at which your muscles start to burn) remain constant throughout your cycle, so you can still score a personal best even with PMS in endurance sports. However, if you play stick-and-ball sports, such as soccer and lacrosse, you may notice a downtick in performance during this time. Several studies have found reduced reaction time, neuromuscular coordination, and manual dexterity during the premenstrual and menstrual phases. There is also evidence that blood sugar levels, breathing rates, and thermoregulation are negatively impacted during this time of the month, which may well account for the slight decreases in aerobic capacity and strength. Importantly, however, from a physiological standpoint, there is never a "bad" day in your cycle to hit that PR. By tracking and knowing your own patterns, you can mitigate any of these hormonal influences;

remember that you've put in the work, are mentally on your game, and are prepared for these influences.

That being said, exercise can feel a bit harder for women during those high-hormone days before your period. And there's no doubt that it can mess with your performance. Case in point, British tennis sensation Heather Watson caused a stir when she blamed "girl things" on her unexpected defeat in the first round of the Australian Open in 2015. It's a fact that the cyclical rise and fall of your hormones affects more than your menstruation. The natural fluctuations of these powerful biochemical messengers impact your exercise metabolism, the fuels that you burn and spare, your plasma volume levels (which are needed to sweat), how well you tolerate heat, moods, and much more. Here are some of the "girl things" that can happen, especially as those hormone levels rise, and how best to control them:

It's harder to make muscle. Everyone credits testosterone for giving folks their muscle mass. However, that's not the full story. Our high levels of female hormones play a huge role in the equation. The upsurge in estrogen and progesterone in women has a profound effect on muscle-cell turnover and protein synthesis. What I mean by this is that estrogen is the female anabolic or growing capacity hormone, specific to muscle, and progesterone turns up the catabolism or breakdown of muscle tissue, using those amino acids to build the endometrium instead of muscle. As a result, you have higher rates of muscle breakdown during hard efforts at this time. It's simply harder for us to make and maintain muscle when these hormones are high.

That's why it's particularly important for women to take in protein that's high in leucine (the muscle-building amino acid) within 30 minutes after exercise. Whey protein is rich in leucine and particularly good at this time. Lots of athletes swear by chocolate milk because it's rich in whey protein as well as carbs (sugar) to restock your glycogen stores, and of course it's tasty. It's okay as 10 ounces (300 milliliters) of low-fat organic chocolate milk has about 200 calories, 10 grams of protein, 30 grams of carbohydrate, and 4 grams of fat—hitting the protein:carbohydrate ratio of 1:3—but women need more protein, in particular leucine, than chocolate milk provides to trigger muscle repair and growth factors. Consider adding an ounce (28 grams) of pumpkin seeds (0.7 gram leucine) or 2 tablespoons of spirulina (0.7 gram leucine) or eating a hardboiled egg with your chocolate milk to get what you need. (For even more specific nutrition recommendations and examples of high-leucine foods, see Chapter 10.)

Metabolism and cravings change. Where's the chocolate? Actually, pass the chips and anything else that's sweet and starchy while you're at it. Many women crave sweets and carbs during this time of their cycle. Why? For one, estrogen and progesterone work to shift your reliance on carbohydrates, likely to help you save those limited glycogen stores in case of pregnancy, famine, and emergency, while it increases fat burning and fatty acid availability. This is great for endurance activities, but you'll need to eat more carbs for high-intensity activity, especially since your body is also building your uterine lining, which uses carbohydrates and raises your metabolic rate (aka how many calories you're burning at rest). Your body also does not use or store carbohydrates as effectively in the luteal phase as in the follicular phase.

So, you need to put more carbs into your system during the premenstrual part of your cycle, especially if you're doing long bouts of intense exercise. We'll go into great detail in Chapter 10, but in general aim for a combination of 10 to 15 grams of protein and 30 grams of carbohydrates (about 180 calories) before any workout longer than 90 minutes, and 30 grams of carbohydrates combined with protein and fat (real food, not straight carbs from gels!) per hour while you're out there.

Again, you burn more calories overall during the premenstrual period. Studies show a 5 to 10 percent uptick in metabolism in the days before you start bleeding. That translates into about 100 to 300 additional calories. (That's one small chocolate bar or a snack bag of chips. Coincidence?)

You may be bloated. Your clothes may feel a bit tight in the days before your period because high estrogen and progesterone affect the hormones that regulate the fluid in your body. Estrogen increases the expression of a hormone called vasopressin (also known as arginine vasopressin or AVP), which is responsible for retaining water and constricting blood vessels. With more AVP going to the hypothalamus of your brain, your body retains water and constricts your blood vessels a bit, which in turn increases your blood pressure enough to signal a drop in your plasma volume by as much as 8 percent. Meanwhile, progesterone competes for the same receptor site as another fluid regulatory hormone called aldosterone (responsible for retaining sodium), which means less aldosterone is released. This sets off another chain of events that ultimately leads to a reduction in blood volume (due to less total-body sodium retention) and therefore a reduction in cardiac output and blood pressure.

All these hormone interplays come across to the average woman as bloating, along with that drop in plasma volume. This isn't just a problem for squeezing into our jeans; it's an exercise performance problem as well. Plasma volume is the volume of fluid in our blood. When it's low, our blood is thicker, less blood is pumped out with every heartbeat, and all of this makes exercise feel harder.

Heat feels hotter. Progesterone elevates your core temperature, so you'll feel hotter to begin with. On top of that, threshold shifts during the high-hormone days means it takes longer for your body to start sweating and cool itself. Progesterone also makes you shed more sodium, which increases your risk of heat stress as well as hyponatremia (dangerously low blood-sodium levels) during endurance events such as running a marathon in the heat.

To compensate for the shift in core temperature and body water, it's important to do some PMS pregaming and start drinking before you begin your workout—especially if you're exercising in the heat. The night before, preload on sodium with a high-sodium broth such as chicken soup. This works to increase both the sodium and fluid in your body, giving you a bit more to draw on when you hit those efforts. There are "hyperhydration" products in the sports nutrition market that you can use; but the basic concept is to increase the amount of water in your blood (plasma); you need both sodium and water together. When you are out in the heat, think about drinking a low-carbohydrate, sodium-containing beverage (e.g., no more than 7 to 8 grams of carbohydrates with 180 to 190 milligrams sodium per 8 ounces for high-sweat activities).

Prepare for cramping. The lining of your uterus doesn't just shed itself. The process is driven by the release of hormone-like chemicals called prostaglandins, which make your uterus contract and expel its lining. This can be an uncomfortable if not downright painful process. Fifty percent of polled athletes in a 2014 *ESPN The Magazine* survey reported that menstrual cramps affected their game at some point. The best way to mitigate this is to do some preplanning. In the 5 to 7 days before your period starts, you can reduce the effect of cramp-causing chemicals (specifically PE-2, an estrogen-mediated prostaglandin) by taking magnesium, omega-3 fatty acids, and low-dose 80-milligram aspirin. Yes, it has to be aspirin if it is not contraindicated for you, not ibuprofen or another nonsteroidal anti-inflammatory drug (NSAID), because aspirin suppresses the production of prostaglandins irreversibly, unlike the other NSAIDs, which are reversible.

Headaches can happen. Some women suffer menstrual headaches, particularly migraines, when estrogen levels shift. Unlike other premenstrual symptoms that are related to rising hormones, however, headaches tend to happen when levels drop right before the start of your menstrual flow. They're generally brought on by a change of blood pressure and the sudden dilation and constriction of your blood vessels. The best way to head off these headaches is to stay hydrated and eat more nitric oxide (NO)—rich foods, such as beets, pomegranate, watermelon, and spinach in the days leading up to the start of your period. The NO-rich foods will promote dilation and help reduce the severity of the shift.

Playing the field is trickier. Spatial cognition, which you use to locate teammates on the field or to identify and hit your target in sports such as golf or tennis, is strongest during menstruation and lowest during the midluteal or high-hormone phase. Testosterone has a strong positive influence on this ability.

GI issues may occur. Many women report having GI issues such as gas and diarrhea when their periods start. This has less to do with estrogen and progesterone (though progesterone, and to a small effect estrogen, slows the contractility of the smooth muscle of the digestive tract) and more with the prostaglandins that cause the uterine contractions and shedding. If you make more than you need, they can float around your body and trigger other smooth muscles (like your bowels) to react similarly—hence the unpleasant GI distress. In extreme cases, they can also cause nausea and vomiting. You can head off the effect of prostaglandins by following the same anticramping strategies mentioned earlier.

May notice mood swings and lost mojo. My coauthor, Selene Yeager, told me that when she was premenopausal, she wanted to burn down the house about one day a month. Another client talks about how she feels like her world is crashing in. During a recent ride with a pro sprinter, she confided that the day or two before her period, "I feel like a newbie on my bike. Head's foggy. Body is bloated and unresponsive. It's really great, let me tell you."

As we've all experienced, hormones impact moods. We know that estrogen increases serotonin and the number of serotonin receptors in the brain. It also modifies the production of endorphins and other feel-good chemicals in your gray matter. That should have a positive effect on mood, but it's not quite that simple.

It comes down to how your hormones affect different regions of your brain. Estrogen and progesterone affect the hypothalamus—the regulator of fatigue, among other functions. Since the hypothalamus is highly interconnected with the central nervous system, anything that affects the hypothalamus can have a direct effect on the limbic system (center for emotion and emotional control) and autonomous nervous system (heart rate, breathing rate, digestion). This can also increase fatigue, lethargy, and low mood.

Getting more leucine (with your other essential amino acids) can help mitigate some of these unpleasant effects. Leucine crosses the blood-brain barrier, slows down the effect of serotonin, and helps fend off central nervous system fatigue.

Obviously no remedy is 100 percent effective all of the time. And a woman's performance is likely to be diminished to some extent if she is experiencing any or all of these symptoms, but it is worth remembering that personality, state of mind, and attitude can negate or exaggerate this effect.

This brings up the question of whether you should try to tinker with your cycle if you're training for a big event. We all know someone (and maybe that's you) who has tried to manipulate her cycle for a major event such as a marathon or bike trip. It can work, but you have to really understand what you're taking and how it will affect you. Going back to Paula Radcliffe and Jessica Judd, they both took the drug norethisterone, a synthetic progesterone, to delay menstruation. Both experienced negative results, which isn't surprising when you consider all the exercise-hindering side effects of high levels of progesterone.

Other athletes use oral contraceptives to better synchronize their cycles with their training and competitions. According to a 2015 article in the British publication the *Globe and Mail*, Dr. Greg Wells, a researcher and sports scientist at the University of Toronto and the Hospital for Sick Children, synced up the cycles of the whole synchronized swimming team he was coaching. He told the paper, "We actually planned out [and altered, with birth control] when the team would hit parts of their cycle 12 months in advance of the Olympics."

According to the article, Radcliffe adopted a similar approach, taking birth control pills for 3 weeks at the start of each season to synchronize her cycle with priority races. That obviously won't work for everyone. If you play a sport such as tennis that demands peak performance for weeks at a time or follows a more sporadic schedule, it would be impossible to perfectly manipulate your cycle. I personally don't believe it's a good idea to manipulate your cycle with the Pill because of potential blunted adaptations to training, and it masks any changes in endocrine function so we cannot tell if a woman using oral contraceptives is in low energy availability (LEA) or in full relative energy deficiency in sport (REDs). It's better to mitigate your menstrual symptoms naturally using the advice in this chapter. Or, if you really want to control the timing of your cycle, use an intrauterine device (IUD), vaginal ring, or other localized hormone product.

Some women experience heavy bleeding. If you have heavy periods, you're at higher risk of becoming anemic because your body may not be able to pump up your blood-iron stores fast enough to keep pace with your blood loss. Your risk is even greater if you are an athletic woman, since you have more muscle stress, damage, and inflammation following hard efforts. When there is increased inflammation, your liver pumps out more of the hormone hepcidin, which has a negative impact on iron absorption. We know that exercise acutely increases hepcidin levels, peaking around 3 to 6 hours after exercise completion; and baseline hepcidin is elevated in the luteal phase, making it difficult for many women to get above the low end of normal. Anemia can cause fatigue as well as shortness of breath, light-headedness, and heart palpitations during exercise. If you have any of these—especially if you also have heavy periods—get checked out by your doctor and consider taking an iron supplement.

WHY YOU SHOULD TRACK YOUR MENSTRUAL CYCLE

These days my clients are all about tracking every little move. They have activity trackers and sleep monitors and apps that help them analyze every morsel they put into their mouths. Yet I'm surprised how few women make note of their menstrual cycle and how they feel during it. I highly recommend that every menstruating woman start now. Why?

- **It's an indicator of health.** Irregularities in your menstrual cycle frequency and/or length can be the first sign that something is amiss, whether your body is not recovering from stress (of training or life!), you're getting sick, or you're underfueling and in low energy availability.
- **Understanding your response to stress.** When you track over time, you can see how your body responds to large blocks of stress through work, life, travel, and training. For instance, women often see that high levels of stress may shorten cycles and periods of relaxation like vacations can lengthen it.
- **No more second-guessing yourself.** If you track for a few cycles and you see that on day 23 you always feel flat and tired, you won't be second-guessing yourself wondering what you

did "wrong" when you feel flat and tired on day 23. (You can also take some of the advice in this book to relieve that fatigue and boost your energy!)

- **It's psychologically empowering.** Knowing yourself and being able to really tap into your unique physiology is empowering. You can also plan some hard training days on the times you know you're going to be on fire.

Once you start tracking, you can also use it as a training guide. And I'm strictly talking about training here. Some people misconstrue this to mean that I'm saying you should plan your event calendar around your cycle. That is NOT the case. As I mentioned earlier, performance is different from training. You can hit a personal record anytime in your cycle, even if you don't always feel your best. This is why the literature doesn't always reflect differences in performance during different phases of the menstrual cycle (which some argue means we should just ignore the cycle during training). The psychological elements of performance supersede the physiological—you're going to get the job done even if it feels hard because of where you are in your cycle.

The benefit of using tracking for training is that you can give your body that stimulus it needs when it is most primed to absorb that training. That takes your strength and fitness to new heights!

So when you know you're in the low-hormone phase and you're going to be more resilient and recover well, you can plan a particularly hard block and really go for it. If you always feel bulletproof 2 days after ovulation, you can plan to go for a PR. On days you know aren't the ones you feel the best, you can schedule a mobility session or build in more recovery time. All of this leads to better chronic, long-term training adaptations.

You can also use what you're learning through tracking during training for performance benefits. You might look at the calendar and see you might have a flat day on the day of your race. Instead of fretting, you'll have a concrete plan of action, like taking some branched-chain amino acids or increasing your hydration and carbs to boost your clarity and energy.

For details on "Menstrual Cycle Tracking," see page 319.

THE CONTRACEPTIVE CONUNDRUM

As I mentioned earlier, I don't recommend using oral contraceptives like the Pill to manipulate your cycles for training and performance purposes, because it can potentially blunt training adaptations and make it difficult to detect changes in endocrine function due to underfueling or full-blown REDs.

Of course, many women aren't taking the Pill for athletic performance purposes. They're taking it to not get pregnant. Hormonal contraceptives contain estrogen and/or progesterone and work by preventing ovulation as well as changing the lining of the uterus, making it harder for an egg to be fertilized and implanted if one should sneak through. Common forms of hormonal contraceptives are pills, arm implants or shots, and vaginally inserted devices such as the IUD and the NuvaRing. Let's take a look at how these hormonal contraceptives may or may not impact your training and performance—and what to do if they have a negative impact.

The Pill: One of the most common forms of hormonal contraception is "the Pill," the oral birth control pill you take that is a combination of estrogen in the form of estradiol and progesterone in the form of progestins, synthetic forms of progesterone that interact with progesterone receptors in your body to produce progesterone-like effects. Brand names include Microgynon 30 or 30 ED, Levlen, Norimin, Yaz, Yasmin, and Ginette. If you're on the Pill, check the estradiol dose. Is it a 30-, 20-, or 10-microgram dose? With higher doses, you may notice an increase in muscle mass gain (though not necessarily an equal increase in strength). Also, note what generation of progestin it contains. First and second generations of progestin are more androgenic, so they have more of a testosterone-type effect. New generations of progestin have more of an antiandrogenic effect. First-generation progestins include norethindrone, norethindrone acetate, and ethynodiol. Second-generation progestins include levonorgestrel and norgestrel. Third generations include desogestrel and norgestimate. Fourth generations include drospirenone. If you're not sure, check with your doctor. There are also progestin-only pills, called the mini pill, such as Noriday and Cerazette. (Their impact on your training and recovery is not quite as pronounced as it is with combined oral contraceptives.) No matter what you're taking, it's good to know the potential side effects so you can track and account for them.

With combined oral contraceptives, though you bleed, you don't ovulate or have the same native cycle and hormonal response. With an oral contraceptive, you have active pills and a placebo week. The first few days of taking the active pill, you have pregnancy protection (provided you've followed the directions; when you first start taking the Pill, you may not be protected for up to 7 days, depending on when you begin), but the hormones have not built up enough to affect your training metrics. During the second and third week, the hormones accumulate and reduce your heart rate variability (HRV, an indication of how resilient your body is to stress, which we'll cover in depth in Chapter 17), your respiratory rate, and your ability to recover. During the week that you take the sugar/placebo pills, the hormones drop but take a few days to leave your system, so there are still some lingering impacts on your recovery and sleep. Once they drop, you have your withdrawal bleed, and your recovery metrics and ability to train hard increase.

So when you're on combined oral contraceptives, there are two areas in the cycle where your body can hit it hard and respond to intense training and recover really well: the first 5 days of the active Pill and the last 5 days of the sugar pill. That's a 10-day block of really high-intensity training on either side of the Pill cycle, which is different from our natural cycle, as well as progestin-only oral contraceptives, which are somewhat closer to our natural cycle in this regard.

It's important to note that the Pill also impacts your hormones on a day-to-day basis. You have a spike in hormones when you take the Pill, which taper off over a 24-hour period until you take your next Pill. This spike can attenuate your training response. So it can be advantageous to take the Pill in the evening if you train in the morning and vice versa.

Implants and injections: Other popular progestin-only hormonal contraception products are implants, which are little rods that are implanted in the upper arm, like Jadelle and Nexplanon, the most popular implant in the United States. Jadelle (not available in the US) contains levonorgestrel (also used in Plan B emergency contraception), which is an older, more androgenic-type progestin; and Nexplanon contains etonogestrel, which is a newer generation that has less androgenic effects. Depo-Provera (medroxyprogesterone acetate) is a contraceptive injection that creates an amenorrheic effect (aka stopping menstruation) in 70 percent of women. Like the Pill, implants and injections suppress ovulation, but there has not been much research done on any performance effects of these types of birth control. Note: longer-term use shows a greater degradation of bone using injections than hormonal IUDs, implants, and oral contraceptives, especially in adolescents.

IUD: IUDs are another type of progestin-only contraception. Common brand names are Mirena, Skyla, and Kyleena. It's a fit and forget. It gets inserted, and it's good for five years, sometimes longer depending on the brand. Though women might initially have bleeding and cramping, it helps with heavy menstrual bleeding and is also prescribed for polycystic ovary syndrome (PCOS) and menstrual cycle irregularities. It makes bleeding very light (some women have no periods at all; the uterine lining becomes so thin) and reduces cramping. There are also nonhormonal IUDs, such as the copper IUD. It does not interfere with the native menstrual cycle but does create heavier, more painful periods in a lot of women.

Unlike the other forms of birth control, many women who use a hormonal IUD will continue to ovulate. So you can use a basal body thermometer and ovulation kit to pinpoint ovulation and track your menstrual cycle accordingly to dial in your phases using an IUD.

THE MYTH OF MISSING PERIODS

It's an all-too-common scenario these days. A client will come to me because she has missed a few periods, and her family doctor or ob-gyn has warned her that she is too lean and is falling into the female athlete triad, a condition that has been traditionally identified in the medical community in somewhat limited terms.

In the past, the female triad was defined as a perfect storm of disordered eating and a drop in estrogen and other hormones that in turn led to irregular periods and low bone density. Experts believed that active women were on a spectrum that ranged from a healthy athlete with optimal energy availability (adequate nutrition), regular periods, and healthy bones to the opposite end of the spectrum where active women had poor nutrition, missed periods, and thinning bones.

Often doctors would prescribe oral contraceptives or suggest a reduction in exercise (which they zeroed in on instead of adequate nutrition) to stimulate weight gain. The concern is understandable, because the true female triad is a serious condition. But the high percentage of active women who experience menstrual dysfunction are not all extremely lean and/or excessive in their exercise. And this phenomenon is becoming common across the fitness spectrum. So what is going on? After looking a bit deeper into some of the other outlying causes that can contribute to menstrual dysfunction, it became clear that it's not exactly a perfect storm of three factors; rather, it's a cascade of hormonal disruption that results from one main factor: inadequate nutrition. These women aren't feeding themselves enough to meet their physical demands, and their physiology is in upheaval. I'm happy to report that I'm not alone in this revelation.

In 2014, the International Olympic Committee (IOC) issued a statement that the triad is really a syndrome that is the result of "relative energy deficiency that affects many aspects of physiological function including metabolic rate, menstrual function, bone health, immunity, protein synthesis, cardiovascular and psychological health." The triad is still under that umbrella, but it's certainly more than a triad! And although they have different symptoms, it also affects men. The IOC then issued a name change to reflect this new understanding: relative energy deficiency in sport (REDs). (The IOC updated this consensus paper in 2018 and again in 2023. The chart that follows gives a picture of what REDs looks like and where the triad fits in.)

HEALTH CONSEQUENCES OF RELATIVE ENERGY DEFICIENCY IN SPORT (REDS)

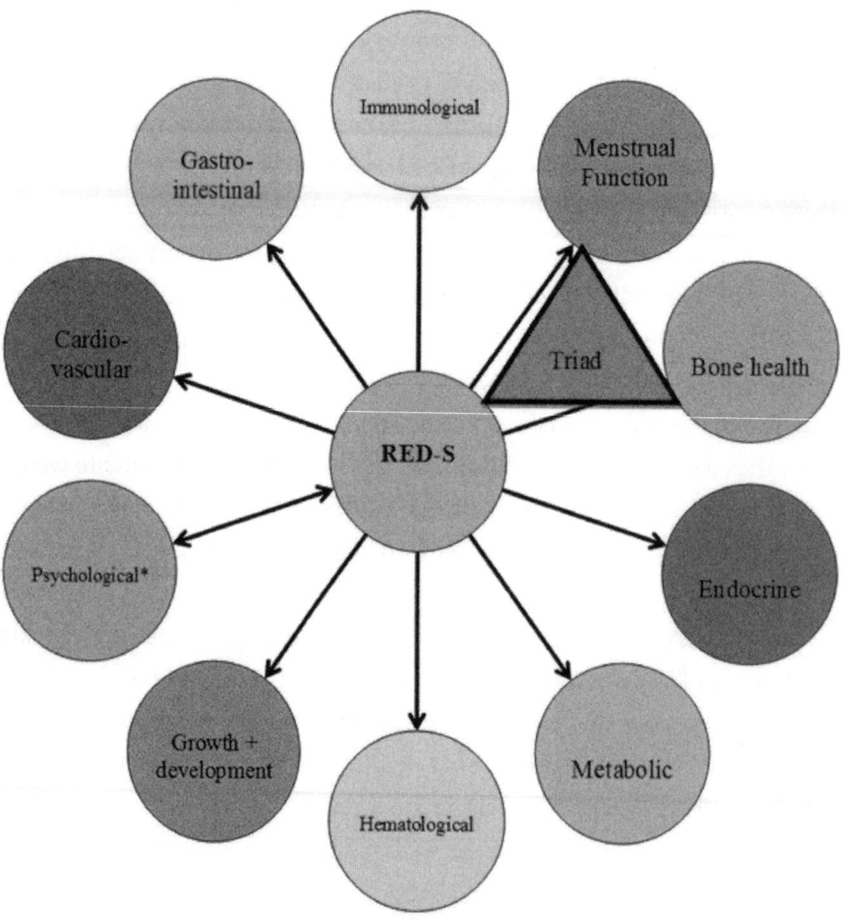

Psychological consequences can either precede REDs or be the result of REDs.

This makes a lot more sense to me, and it also explains the uptick in triad or REDs cases I've seen. The diet trends among active (and even inactive) people are leaving them insufficiently fueled or in a state of low energy availability (LEA), which paves the way for REDs. Specifically, the big trend in the endurance and CrossFit worlds right now is low-carbohydrate, higher-fat and/or higher-protein diets. Whether you call them metabolic efficiency, paleo, keto, or intermittent fasting, they all have similar goals: to reduce overall calories from carbohydrates and increase fat and protein intake.

Overall, there is some merit in being more cognizant of the kind of carbohydrates you eat. Remember those 1980s low-fat, high-carb diets? It was a disaster for our metabolic health. Reducing our carbs from those high-carb, low-fat days is wise. But here's the catch: As women, we respond differently from our male counterparts. You know how a man can nonchalantly follow the same diet as his female partner and drop weight faster than a one-rep max fail, yet she will struggle to lose 1 or 2 pounds? There's a reason for that: physiology.

When women drop too low in carbohydrates (the grams are individual, as each woman is different; calculate your personal carb intake with the formula on page 189), it causes the hypothalamus to perceive that there is not enough nutrition coming in to support all the systems in the body, let alone carrying a pregnancy to term. So there is a downregulation of the endocrine system, specifically a drop in luteinizing hormone, which shuts off the signals for ovulation and estradiol production. This reduction of estradiol also comes with rises in estrone (one of the three estrogen hormones that fat tissue secretes, which signals your body to store more fat) and the stress hormone cortisol (which also signals fat storage under long periods of high stress).

Translation: We become more masculinized in our reproductive status and conserve fat. From a survival standpoint, your body is thinking *famine*, and in a widespread famine, the last thing that is needed is new babies. But in men, the low-carbohydrate–famine mechanism is to become fight ready: Lean up, increase anabolic activities, and increase testosterone.

It makes sense from an evolutionary standpoint—women needed to not reproduce and men needed to fight to get food when resources were low. Even if you are 25 to 30 percent body fat—well above what experts typically consider amenorrhea territory—you can experience menstrual dysfunction: With a hypocaloric, high-stress state, the hormonal changes signal a stop in reproduction.

This alteration in reproductive hormones is why so many women struggle on intermittent fasting, keto, and low-carb, high-fat diets while men tend to thrive on them. Women are *not* small men. Keep this in mind before jumping onto the latest diet bandwagon.

Frankly, it's also important to be aware that if you stop getting your period during training, it's something you need to address. In a survey of more than 300 ultramarathoners (who are at a relatively high risk of REDs because they're burning through thousands of calories on a regular basis), 92.5 percent of the runners had never heard of the female triad (let alone the current name, REDs). More disturbingly, one-third of these athletes had some form of disordered eating while half restricted calories—which of course puts them at a high risk of REDs. Worse, while up to 40 percent of female athletes have menstrual cycle disorders, 22 to 31 percent (depending upon the sport) said they would not seek help for unexplained amenorrhea. Many still think it's "normal"! It's important that we denormalize losing your period. The health consequences are too steep, and we can perform at our best while still having our period. Menstruation is a sign of healthy, functioning female physiology. We'll get into a full discussion of LEA and REDs and how to avoid them in Chapter 10.

ACTION PLAN FOR POWER IN THE HIGH-HORMONE PHASE

There's a lot to digest here. To make it easier to put this information into action, here is an action plan I devised for a mother-daughter mountain biking duo who are both rising to the top of their game.

Peak performance during PMS: Take 250 milligrams of magnesium, 45 milligrams of zinc, 1 gram of omega-3 fatty acids (flaxseed and fish oil), and if there are no contraindications, 80 milligrams of aspirin (baby aspirin) each night for the 7 days before your period starts.

Why does this PMS cocktail work? The biggest issue here is inflammation. Often women hear they should just take an over-the-counter NSAID, which can help reduce pain and heavy bleeding but does not address prostaglandins' effects on other organs, like the kidneys. When your sex hormones drop, it triggers the release of inflammatory compounds like prostaglandins and the enzyme cyclooxygenase (specifically COX-1 and COX-2), which interact with your kidneys to play a key role in fluid balance in the body and are the main reasons for the fluid shifts and bloating of PMS. Newer NSAIDs do not work as well as aspirin to inhibit both COX-1 and COX-2. So I recommend low-dose aspirin along with omega-3 fatty acids, which not only inhibit COX-2 but also stimulate COX-2 to trigger antiinflammatory mechanisms. Your body uses more magnesium and zinc during the luteal phase as part of the uterine lining buildup. Increasing magnesium can decrease vascular endothelial growth factor (VEGF), which can reduce the severity of bleeding. And zinc can help reduce the severity of pain, cramping, and bleeding.

Pretraining: Take 3 to 5 grams of essential amino acid supplement (EAAs) to fight the lack of mojo. These amino acids cross the blood-brain barrier, decrease central nervous system fatigue, and supply a bit of extra fuel for the hard work at hand.

In training: Consume a few more carbohydrates per hour. The ideal recommendation for the amount of carbohydrates per hour during activity for women is 30 to 60 grams (rate limited due to slower gastric emptying for women as compared to men). In this high-hormone phase, aim for 50 to 60 grams per hour; in the low-hormone phase, aim for 30 to 45 grams per hour.

Post-training: Recovery is critical. Progesterone is extremely catabolic (breaks muscle down) and inhibits recovery. Aim to consume 25 to 30 grams of protein within 30 minutes of finishing your session. Overall you should aim to get 0.9 to 1 gram of protein per pound (1.8 to 2.2 grams per kilogram) per day (a 135-pound woman needs about 122 to 135 grams of protein per day; see the "Roar Daily Diet Cheat Sheet for Athletes" on pages 188 to 190 for more information).

HEAR HER ROAR

THE MARTIAL ARTIST WHO BEAT HER BLOAT

It may not be nice to fool Mother Nature, but there are definitely times when you need to trick her a little. Take Amanda Tortorici, RD, CSCS, and PhD student, for example. Amanda, 33, competes in Brazilian jujitsu, which requires her to make weight to be placed in a particular weight division so she can compete against other women of similar size.

"The divisions vary by whichever federation is hosting the tournament," she explains. "If I'm training regularly (not in school), then my normal body weight is around 120. If I'm in school and not able to train as often, it's around 125. Most of the time I just compete in the division where I sit at my normal body weight. But for bigger competitions a few times per year, I go down to 115."

Because Amanda is already lean—just 16 percent body fat according to lab tests—trains regularly, and as a dietitian knows how to eat healthy, shaving those final 5 pounds is a challenge. "If I'm 'lucky' enough to compete near the time I have my period, it feels exponentially harder to lose the weight. I've never checked to see exactly how much weight I gain during preperiod bloat, but I'm sure it packs on at least a few extra pounds."

So when a big competition fell right before her period, Amanda came to me looking for a way she could avoid the bloat and still make weight. I told her the best way to mitigate this was with some preplanning. I had her follow the first step of the peak performance during PMS protocol on page 34. She followed her usual precompetition training and nutrition schedule.

"It worked!" says Amanda, who e-mailed me a picture of her six-pack abs and sculpted torso. "I was able to get down to 118 from 127 (I ate a lot this summer, haha!!) in 2 weeks—something I normally wouldn't do, but my coach found out about the tournament last minute and I really wanted to do it," she says. "I made my weight class, no problem! I also won my division and got promoted to blue belt afterward!"

ROAR ▸▸▸ SOUND BITES

▸ The typical menstrual cycle is 21 to 40 days long with several phases. The cycle begins with the first day of menstruation (day 1) and can be divided into three consecutive phases:

- ▸ Phase 1: the follicular phase (from the start of your period to ovulation)
- ▸ Phase 2: the ovulatory phase (ovulation)
- ▸ Phase 3: the luteal phase (from ovulation to the onset of the next cycle).
- ▸ Ironically, you are most like a man when it comes to exercise, fueling, and thermoregulation during your period and the follicular phase.

▸ Your blood plasma can drop up to 8 percent during the high-hormone luteal phase of your period. This can impact your hydration and cooling strategies especially since women tend to store more heat than men during exercise.

▸ The follicular phase is widely variable (which is why the menstrual cycle length varies), whereas the luteal phase is relatively constant and averages 13 to 15 days in most women. The ovulatory phase is shortest and lasts only 24 to 48 hours.

▸ It's harder to hit high intensities and recover from hard exercise during the high-hormone phase (like PMS time).

▸ You can offset many of the unwanted side effects of high hormones with dietary interventions, specifically timing your carbohydrates, protein, and hydration correctly.

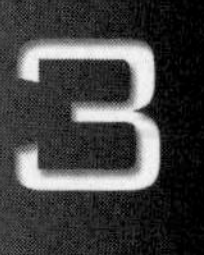

MOVING THROUGH MENOPAUSE

THE END OF YOUR PERIODS ISN'T THE END OF THE LINE

Menopause, the point in life when you're no longer menstruating, was long regarded as simply "the change," which implies just one change—the end of your menstrual periods and in turn your reproductive life. However, it's really a series of changes that occur over the course of years—sometimes a decade—and lead to not just one singular change but rather to diverse physical and psychological changes that impact everything you do for the rest of your life.

After all these profound changes, some women I work with actually feel like they don't need women-specific training and nutrition advice because they're no longer menstruating or having babies. Take Claire Lange, a 67-year-old Ironman athlete, for example.

"I didn't think fueling properly for women applied to me since I'm older and postmenopausal, but boy, was I wrong!" Claire was trying to sustain her training on a steady diet of fructose-based drinks, gels, and bars. Little did she realize that postmenopausal women have an even harder time metabolizing fructose (fruit sugar) than those still in their reproductive years.

That finding actually isn't new. In the 1960s, British researchers made the connection when they noticed that postmenopausal women had more fatty acids in their blood after drinking fructose-loaded beverages than they did after consuming glucose-based drinks. Premenopausal women didn't have this problem. More recently, Swiss researchers publishing in *Diabetes Care* reported further fructose problems for postmenopausal women. While premenopausal women could store the excess energy from fructose as subcutaneous fat stores (i.e., hips and thighs), postmenopausal women were not able to do so and ended up with more fatty acids circulating in their bloodstream, where they wreaked metabolic havoc, including high triglyceride levels and insulin resistance.

For postmenopausal athletes this means less fructose is converted to glucose and available for energy. "I was fueling with foods and sports drinks that were literally hampering my performance and leaving me wrung out and tired at the end of long workouts and bike rides," Claire recalls. "I also had lots of GI issues, cramping, and bloating." Her training and race fueling were typical of an endurance athlete: heavy on the gels, Powerade, Gatorade, and other carbohydrate-heavy sports nutrition products. First I explained that all those carbohydrates weren't being absorbed and were just sitting in her gut, pulling water from her blood into her intestines, contributing to GI distress. Second, she wasn't actually getting the proper hydration or fuel, which contributed to poor recovery and lingering fatigue.

We changed her carbohydrates to avoid fructose and switched her diet to pump up the protein (see "Hear Her Roar"), and the impact was immediate. "The right ingredients made all the difference in the world! I have so much durability now for training and workouts. I can do harder efforts, and I don't fade at the end of a long, tough workout. Instead I have lots of energy left to keep giving a strong effort all the way through the finish," says Claire.

Menopause doesn't have to mean slowing down and suffering, or worse, stopping. With some simple nutritional and training adjustments, women like Claire are training and racing strong well into their sixties and beyond! In fact, at the last triathlon, my coauthor, Selene Yeager, did, she spied three ladies with numbers in their eighties written on their calves. (For those who haven't done triathlon, they typically write your age on your calf with a Sharpie so you know who is in your age group—or not—when they pass you or you try to pass them.) One was 80, one was 81, and one was 83. "As I sat there pulling on my swim cap, I thought, 'I want to be them one day—still out there in great shape, being competitive.'" I'm sure Selene will be, because it's clear to me that there is no age limit to endurance sports (or any sports for that matter) if you fuel and train properly. Here's more of how these changes affect you and what you as an athlete can do to actually make the most of them.

(NOTE: After *ROAR* was published in 2016, the demand for more information on performing through and beyond the menopause transition was so high that we created an entire book on menopause training, nutrition, performance, therapies, and more called *Next Level*. This updated chapter is designed to cover the basics more broadly.)

HEAR HER ROAR

THE 60-SOMETHING IRONMAN TRIATHLETE

With age, women become more sensitive to carbohydrates and have greater issues digesting them, and insulin resistance to carbohydrates outside of training and competition increases. I sketched out the following daily nutrition plan that cut down Claire's high-glycemic carbohydrate choices and replaced them with fruit, veggies, and whole grains. The plan also increased her overall protein intake to about 130 grams per day, increased her overall fat intake, and strategically implemented branched-chain amino acids (BCAAs) or whole protein before and after each training session.

During exercise, Claire separated her fueling from hydration so that she could take in the appropriate calories from foods that were low in fructose to minimize GI issues and maximize training. "Now I'm still riding strong at the end of a 70-mile bike ride with energy left over!" she says.

CLAIRE'S DAILY FOOD PLAN TO OPTIMIZE BODY COMPOSITION AND RECOVERY

The emphasis is not on weight change but on improving overall body composition and recovery and ensuring that Claire's food choices maximize her nutrition while minimizing GI issues. Based on Claire's body composition, height, and ideal weight (around 123 pounds), we focused on the quality of protein (higher leucine content) as well as lower-glycemic carbohydrate intake. Also, adding more power-based work to training helped delay the hormone-triggered change in body composition. With a focus on recovery, strength, endurance, and performance, this was the best power-to-weight ratio for Claire.

Grams of carbohydrate per day: 170–195
Calories: 680–780

Grams of protein per day: 120–130
Calories: 480–520

Grams of fat per day: 75–80
Calories: 675–720

Baseline calories per day: 1,835–2,020
(40% carbohydrate, 25% protein, 35% fat)

Keep in mind that this caloric intake is a recommended baseline, and it is specific to Claire's plan. The lower end of the spectrum is for rest and recovery days; the upper end of the spectrum is for long training days and does not include calories from training food. When the volume and intensity of exercise increase, the body's caloric and nutrient needs will change.

MEAL PLAN

This meal plan is specific to triathlon training, but the concepts are adaptable to other forms of exercise. Carbohydrate choices are essential—choose nutrient-dense, complex carbs. Try to eat more veggies and fruit for your carbohydrate choices outside of training. (See Chapter 10 for daily nutrition recommendations.) Incorporate 75 to 80 grams of fat into your diet each day.

Specific Nutrition for 70.3-Mile Triathlon (1.2-Mile Swim, 56-Mile Bike Ride, and 13.1-Mile Run):

RACE PREP: As you taper 2 to 3 weeks before competition, stick to your usual recovery food after every training session. Even though your training volume and intensity are lower, replenish protein within 30 minutes after exercise and glycogen within 2 hours. Then, 2 to 3 hours postworkout, consume another 20 to 25 grams of protein. During these final weeks, fuel up on essential-to-racing electrolytes by adding 150 milligrams of magnesium, 500 milligrams of calcium, 300 milligrams of potassium, and 1,000 milligrams of sodium to your diet daily. You can do this with foods or supplements.

SAMPLE PRERACE MEAL PLAN FOR A RACE ON SUNDAY

TIME	
TAPER WEEK	Focus on increasing total carbohydrate intake, especially after training, for the 7 days before competition. Aim for 2.7 to 3.6 g carbohydrate per lb of body weight (6 to 8 g per kg) per day. (For reference: 1 lb = 0.45 kg.) Snack on these throughout the week: almonds, oatmeal, yogurt, apples, bananas, oranges, potatoes, bread, almond and/or peanut butter, jam, and almond milk.
FRIDAY NIGHT	Eat dinner as you normally would.
SATURDAY NIGHT	Eat dinner around 5:00 p.m. Quinoa mixed with rice; lean, palm-size protein such as chicken or fish and veggies; and a cup of miso soup. Have a snack such as a protein bar before bed.
SUNDAY MORNING	Low-fiber toast with peanut butter, honey, and sliced banana or oatmeal with almond milk and a tablespoon of nut butter stirred in. Sip on water as desired. Take 1 Tums to prevent GI issues.

TIME	
SUNDAY MORNING PRERACE	Drink 0.15 oz per lb (4.5 ml per kg) of body weight of a hyperhydration drink about 20 minutes before the start of the race. Consume water to thirst. Top off your nutrition with ½ bar (Picky Bar is a good option) or have ½ low-fiber bagel with jam.

AT TRANSITION 1 (SWIM TO BIKE): After you've been swimming for roughly 30 minutes, glycogen levels will be a bit low, as will your hydration. At the transition, have a bottle of low-carbohydrate, functional hydration. Take a few gulps and grab solid food (bar, protein bites, sandwich) to eat on the first 3 miles of the bike ride. This will front-load you for the second half of the bike ride.

FLUID INTAKE GOAL PER HOUR ON BIKE: Low end is 0.10 to 0.12 ounce per pound (6 to 6.5 milliliters per kilogram) and high end is 0.15 to 0.18 ounce per pound (11 to 11.5 milliliters per kilogram) per hour (when racing in the heat, shoot for the high end). Based on Claire's weight, this translates to 12 to 22 ounces (330 to 650 milliliters) per hour.

CALORIE INTAKE GOAL PER HOUR ON BIKE: 1.3 to 1.6 food calories per pound (3 to 3.5 food calories per kilogram) per hour. The idea is to front-load calories to fuel the bike ride and to have reserves for the run. For Claire, this translates to 160 to 195 calories per hour.

AT TRANSITION 2 (BIKE TO RUN): Keep Tums in your pocket for any stomach upset. Take a few glucose tablets (chewable sugar tablets you can buy at the drugstore) or a few bites of a soft pretzel (carbs, salt, and change for the palate). If you are going to use caffeine, have ½ dose here and the other ½ dose around 9 miles into the run.

FLUID INTAKE GOAL PER HOUR ON THE RUN: Similar as for the bike but on the lower end to avoid gastric distress. Based on Claire's weight, this translates to 12 to 15 ounces (330 to 440 milliliters) per hour; using an alarm to remind her to sip along the way.

CALORIE INTAKE GOAL PER HOUR ON THE RUN: 0.9 to 1.13 food calories per pound (2 to 2.5 food calories per kilograms) per hour. For Claire, this translates to 110 to 140 calories per hour. The goal is to maintain a steady intake to keep blood glucose levels up; when it is too hard to eat, glucose tablets work well.

BODY COMPOSITION SHIFTS AS FEMALE HORMONES DROP

The number one complaint I hear from women as they enter menopause is that they feel as though their body has taken on a new shape of its own no matter what they do. They lose muscle, gain fat, and it's harder to maintain their body composition—despite the fact that they haven't changed their eating or exercise habits. Case in point: Tracy Paxton, a vegan triathlete who came to me distressed over her ever-diminishing muscle and strength.

"I have been active my entire life and doing triathlons for the last 15 years, but I was slowly losing muscle mass," Tracy recalls. "It was frustrating because I was eating a whole-foods, plant-based diet with no junk food or foods laden with preservatives or chemicals, but I was still not seeing the fitness gains I wanted or expected, especially with the amount of training I was doing. I had tried a lot of different techniques, such as increasing my weight lifting and doing HIIT [high-intensity interval training], and still saw no real improvements in body composition."

Tracy decided that enough was enough when she turned 50. "My body was changing, and I was not ready to accept that my loss of muscle mass and growing thickness were just age-related catabolism."

Tracy was correct; it wasn't just age-related muscle loss. It was her body reacting to the profound hormonal shift called perimenopause that occurs in the 5 to 10 years before menopause. The end result of this shift eventually becomes your new normal once you reach menopause, generally between the ages of 48 and 55.

Estrogen levels fluctuate and ultimately decline as you progress through your forties. Estrogen is responsible for regulating reproductive functions, but it also plays a starring role in metabolism, specifically in relation to how we store fat and how we respond to and recover from exercise. As estrogen levels drop over time, your body composition changes. There's a tendency to accumulate fat in your belly (which increases your risk of fatty liver and cardiovascular disease) rather than your hips and thighs.

So what's the deal with the muscle loss? If estrogen levels are declining and your body fat is shifting to resemble patterns we typically see in men—think apple shape instead of pear shape—shouldn't you have proportionately more testosterone and be better able to make and maintain muscle?

Well, it's complicated. Testosterone helps build and maintain muscle mass. Although your testosterone levels peak in your twenties and slowly decline throughout adulthood, your ovaries and adrenal glands continue to produce some testosterone even after your estrogen production stops at menopause. But there's more to the story. It comes down to protein synthesis (turning the protein you eat into the lean muscle tissue you use to lift, run, and jump) and breakdown (where your body breaks down your muscles to get protein for energy). With age, the balanced ratio of synthesis to breakdown shifts.

At first glance, the shift seems favorable to muscle making. With declining ovulatory cycles, women have more estrogen and less progesterone, which seems like a favorable balance for increasing the ability to build and conserve lean mass.

Great, but why do postmenopausal women have such difficulty building and maintaining muscle? Because the high protein-synthesis rates in postmenopausal women are counteracted by an even higher uptick in protein breakdown, and the ratio is no longer balanced. Making matters more difficult, as estrogen drops, postmenopausal women become less reactive to the muscle-making stimulus from resistance training and eating protein.

In one study, young women and young men had the same rate of protein synthesis after both resistance training and eating protein, but postmenopausal women lagged behind on both fronts when compared to men of the same age.

This is a problem for a few reasons. If you can't maintain muscle, you can't produce power, and you're bound to slow down, especially if you're also gaining body fat. Even if you're not a competitive athlete, the cycle of gaining weight and slowing down can drain your quality of life.

Even if you maintain your body composition, menopause can create some permanent changes in your nutrient metabolism that are capable of throwing your training and racing for a loop if you don't adjust for them.

At the same time it becomes more difficult for your body to synthesize the protein you eat into the muscle you need, you also burn less fat than you used to. In fact, when researchers had 41 women ranging from premenopausal to postmenopausal pedal stationary bikes for 45 minutes in what would typically be considered a "fat-burning" or aerobic intensity, the postmenopausal women burned 33 percent less fat. When the researchers adjusted those figures based on total lean body mass (the younger women had more), the menopausal women still burned 23 percent less. That means the menopausal and postmenopausal women have to rely more heavily on their limited carbohydrate stores.

Here's the kicker: Estrogen (especially estradiol) also increases your insulin sensitivity, so it requires less insulin to pull sugar out of your bloodstream and into your cells after eating. As you lose estrogen, you become more insulin resistant, so your body pumps out more insulin, which in turn triggers more fat storage. This puts you on the blood-sugar roller coaster of surges and drops that can leave you fatigued and hungry all the time.

Another aspect of hormonal change and metabolism that is often overlooked is the decline in dehydroepiandrosterone (DHEA), a hormone produced by the adrenal glands and a precursor for testosterone and estrogen. DHEA limits the effects of cortisol by encouraging glucose to be burned as fuel. As the levels of DHEA drop with age, you become more sensitive to glucose and therefore more likely to store it as belly fat. This phenomenon isn't unique to perimenopause and menopause; it also occurs with high stress, so if you're stressed out, the effects are even worse.

Are we hopelessly screwed? Of course not. Just as is true for women in the reproductive stages of their lives, women who are entering and past menopause need to work with their physiology to support their changing needs. For example, Tracy was fueling herself and working out the same way as she had for decades, and nothing was working because she wasn't the same person in terms of her physiology.

Together, Tracy and I altered her carbohydrate intake to sit lower on the

SKELETAL STRENGTH

You're only as strong as the frame that holds you up. At no other time in your life is the importance of skeletal health more urgent than menopause, when your bone density can begin a precipitous decline. Left unchecked, a woman's bone density can decline up to 20 percent during the 5 to 7 years following menopause. That sets the stage for osteoporosis—a skeletal condition marked by brittle bones. Approximately one in two women over age 50 will break a bone because of osteoporosis, according to the National Osteoporosis Foundation. I don't want you to be one of them. If you haven't already, get a baseline bone-density scan done. Then turn to Chapter 9 to learn how to keep that skeleton strong.

glycemic index (more veggies and fruit; less grains, breads, and pastas, which are not off the table during menopause, just best used around exercise and training) and included more fat and nonanimal protein in her training and racing food. Overall, she increased the quality and quantity of her protein and carbohydrate intake across the board to maximize lean-mass development and body fat loss.

"I noticed a change within the first week of starting the program: I was experiencing better sleep quality and not feeling thick," says Tracy. "By the second week, the quality of my workouts was becoming more consistent. I was experiencing a quicker recovery time from day-to-day training, which, over several more weeks, eventually became quicker recovery between double workouts on the same day. As a result, I had higher-quality training sessions, which led to better times with less effort. While I have not lost a significant amount of weight (which was not my main priority), my body composition has certainly changed (I can now see muscles that I haven't seen in a while), I've lost inches, and my strength has increased exponentially."

You'll find more complete nutrition programming in the chapters that follow, but this exemplifies that you don't have to change everything you eat, but you can simply make adjustments to what your body now needs for optimal performance.

SOUND SLEEP CAN BE FLEETING

There's a saying among athletes that the race is won in bed. Hard training and good nutrition are essential, but sleep is where your body recovers, repairs, and gets ready for peak performance. Unfortunately, this is where a lot of women in the various stages of menopause struggle. More than 60 percent of postmenopausal women complain of problems with insomnia, according to the National Sleep Foundation.

Again, it's hormonal. Progesterone, the antianxiety hormone, has direct sedative effects and is a respiratory stimulant. As levels of progesterone drop during menopause, sleep disturbances rise. Estrogen increases REM (deep dream) sleep, assists serotonin (a relaxing hormone) metabolism, and has been shown to decrease sleep latency (how long it takes you to fall asleep). Furthermore, estrogen decreases the number of times you wake in the night and increases total sleep time and quality. It also helps regulate your body temperature, which is essential for restful sleep. Lastly, estrogen regulates cortisol to help stabilize sleep. As it declines, you're more susceptible to nighttime cortisol spikes even from mild stress such as noise and light.

HEAR HER ROAR

CRUSHING IT AS A 50-YEAR-OLD VEGAN

When Tracy came to see me, she was at the end of her rope. A perimenopausal Olympic and 70.3-mile triathlon competitor, she was losing muscle and gaining fat, particularly in her waistline, and her body had stopped responding to her former diet and training regimen.

Being a vegan, Tracy relied on only plant sources for protein. Although from a mathematical point of view she was getting enough protein to meet her age guidelines, from a functional point of view she was falling short. Tracy lacked the amino acids needed to maximize recovery and stimulate protein synthesis and body fat loss because so much of her protein was coming from soy.

Let me explain. We have heard time and time again that soy protein is great for perimenopausal and menopausal women because of the moderate beneficial effects the isoflavones (plant estrogens with estrogen-like actions in the human body) have on hot flashes and other menopausal symptoms. But the truth of the matter is that soy protein is not a good source of protein to increase protein synthesis and encourage lean mass development. Why? It has to do with the amino acid profile of the protein: It takes 40 grams of soy protein to match the biological effect of 25 grams of whey protein.

Whey is better for making muscle because it's higher in the amino acid leucine. High-intensity exercise, changes in protein synthesis, and postexercise recovery all change the amino acid and protein metabolism in your muscles and ultimately increase the metabolism of leucine. Specifically, the damage in the muscle tissue stimulates the breakdown of branched-chain amino acids (BCAAs) and total muscle-cell breakdown. To recover, you need to take in high enough amounts of leucine to shut down the breakdown processes. The more leucine you get into your system, the faster the tissue levels rise and the more quickly your muscles get the signal to repair and grow.

Generally speaking, if you consume 35 to 40 grams of whole protein in any given meal, the leucine content should be 3 to 3.5 grams.

With Tracy's vegan diet, she was lacking adequate leucine to trigger the postexercise muscle-mending response needed to stimulate lean mass development and less fat accumulation. We addressed this issue by topping off her diet with BCAAs before and after each exercise session. With an increase of circulating amino acids, the level of leucine in her muscle tissues remained at an optimal physiological state.

"It has only been about 5 months since I've been following Stacy's plan, but I have made significant gains in this short time frame, including improved body composition, improved pacing, increased strength, better sleep quality, consistent training sessions, and better race experiences. I am happy to know that I can stave off age-related catabolism for many more years!"

TRACY'S DAILY FUEL PLAN TO OPTIMIZE BODY COMPOSITION AND RECOVERY

The timing of protein is critical. For vegan athletes, it is important to combat the decreased ability to lose body fat and maintain lean mass. Focus on food quality to increase the leucine content of your muscles, which will improve recovery and training adaptations.

The emphasis is not specifically on weight change but on improving overall body composition and recovery and ensuring that Tracy's vegan choices maximize her nutrition. Based on Tracy's body composition, height, and ideal weight (around 125 pounds), she needed to focus on quality of protein (higher leucine content) and lower glycemic carbohydrate intake. Additionally, adding more power-based work to training helped delay the hormone-mediated change in body composition. With focus on recovery, strength, and performance, this was the best power-to-weight ratio for Tracy.

Grams of carbohydrate per day: 300–375
Calories: 1,200–1,500
Grams of protein per day: 120–140
Calories: 480–560

Grams of fat per day: 90–100
Calories: 810–900
Baseline calories per day: 2,490–2,960
(48% carbohydrate, 21% protein, 31% fat)

Keep in mind that this caloric intake is a recommended baseline, and it is specific to Tracy's plan. The lower end of the spectrum is for rest and recovery days; the upper end of the spectrum is for long training days and does not include calories from training food. When the volume and intensity of exercise increase, the body's caloric and nutrient needs will change.

MEAL PLAN

This meal plan includes morning training sessions. Carbohydrate choices are essential—choose nutrient-dense, complex carbs. Try to eat more veggies and fruit for your carbohydrate choices outside of training. (See Chapter 10 for daily nutrition recommendations.) Incorporate 90 to 100 grams of fat into your diet each day.

SAMPLE MEAL PLAN WITH A MORNING TRAINING SESSION

TIME	
WAKE UP: 7:00 A.M. 7:30 A.M. BREAKFAST	Quinoa Bowl (see recipe on page 329) OR Green Goddess Smoothie (see recipe on page 329) with 2 pieces sprouted whole grain toast with 2 tsp almond or other nut butter OR Protein pancakes (use flapjack mix or a protein powder–based recipe)
9:00–11:00 A.M. SWIM WITH SHORT RUN	On the pool deck: one 24-oz bottle functional hydration beverage Transition between swim and run: 4 oz protein recovery drink (composed of ½ scoop [10 g] protein powder mixed in water or unsweetened rice milk)
11:30 A.M. Recovery (within 30 minutes of finishing session)	1½ scoops pea protein isolate protein powder (30 g) mixed in 6 oz (180 ml) almond or rice milk, with 6 oz (180 ml) water and 1 Tbsp almond or other nut butter stirred in
1:00 P.M. LUNCH	2 slices sprouted whole grain bread, 2 Tbsp hummus, tomato, avocado, grated carrots, and ½ cup quinoa or barley (and 1 hard-cooked organic egg, if you choose to add egg into your diet) 1 piece fresh fruit: apple, orange, kiwifruit, or banana OR 4 oz meat substitute (such as tempeh) in a mixed green salad with spinach, chopped apple, walnuts, flaxseeds, peppers, cucumbers, artichokes, or other veggies (A rice bowl can be similar to this—just increase the protein and veggies and decrease the brown rice.)
3:00 P.M. SNACK	Protein Peanut Butter Banana: 1 Tbsp nut butter, mixed with ½ oz vanilla protein powder and enough water to make a spread. Serve on ½ banana. OR 1 piece sprouted grain toast with 2 tsp Toasted Almond Spread with Cinnamon (see recipe on page 331)

TIME	
5:00 P.M. DINNER	2 cups stir-fry mixed veggies (e.g., cauliflower, broccoli, snap peas, carrot strips, peppers) over 1–1½ cups cooked quinoa Small side salad of mixed greens with ½ cup cubed tempeh and olive oil vinaigrette OR Quinoa, Broccoli, Apple, and Pomegranate Salad with Lime Vinaigrette over 1½ cups mixed spinach and arugula greens (see recipe on page 330). Save some for lunches!

MEAL PLAN FOR A WEEKEND DAY WITH MORE INTENSE TRAINING

TIME	
WAKE UP: 7:30 A.M. 8:00 A.M. BREAKFAST	Coffee with splash of almond or oat milk 2 slices toasted sprouted whole grain bread with 2 Tbsp almond or other nut butter and honey 6 oz protein drink (e.g., 1 scoop protein powder mixed in 6 oz [180 ml] sweetened milk alternative) OR Oatmeal with Blueberries and Chia Seeds (see recipe on page 331)
9:00 A.M.– 12:00 P.M. TRAINING	On the bike: Hydration: 0.10–0.12 oz per lb (6 to 6.5 ml per kg) per hour hydration beverage. Drink this beverage with food about 60 minutes into your ride (assuming you ate breakfast). Calorie intake on the bike should be 1.3–1.6 food calories per lb (3 to 3.5 food calories per kg) per hour. 1 nut butter sandwich (2 slices low-fiber bread with 1 Tbsp almond or other nut butter and 1 tsp jam), Date Brownie (see recipe on page 332), 5 small new potatoes (cooked and salted), 3–4 Salty Balls (see page 212 for recipe) On the run: Calorie intake should be 0.9–1.13 food calories per lb per hour. If run is more than 60 minutes, try using glucose tablets for the last 30–45 minutes, one every 5–7 minutes.
12:30 P.M. RECOVERY	2 scoops protein powder (40 g) in 12 oz (350 ml) fluid with 1 Tbsp almond or other nut butter

TIME	
1:30 P.M. **LUNCH** **(SNACK)**	2–3 whole grain waffles topped with 20 dry-roasted almonds, ¼ cup fresh blueberries, and 1 Tbsp pure maple syrup OR Green Goddess Smoothie (see recipe on page 329) plus 2 pieces sprouted whole grain toast with 1 Tbsp almond or other nut butter OR 4 oz (115 g) meat substitute (such as tempeh) in a mixed green salad with spinach, chopped apple, walnuts, flaxseeds, peppers, cucumbers, artichokes, or other veggies. Sprinkle with hemp oil and sea salt.
3:30 P.M. **SNACK**	15 veggie sticks (carrots, celery, snow peas) and 2–3 Tbsp hummus and a smoothie with 15 g protein
6:00 P.M. **DINNER** **(Okay to have beer or wine but moderate intake: 1–2 servings max)**	1 cup steamed veggies of your choice 2 cups mixed green salad with ¼ cup berries, ½ chopped apple, ½ grapefruit, 10 cherry tomatoes, and black beans or chickpeas, topped with crumbled grain tempeh or Quorn, sea salt, and pepper (no dressing) OR 2 cups stir-fry veggies of your choice with 4–6 oz lean protein (palm size) over 1–1½ cups cooked purple or red rice or quinoa Mixed green salad with spinach, apple, berries, grapefruit, tomato, light balsamic vinaigrette, and 2 Tbsp pumpkin or sunflower seeds OR Caramelized Cauliflower and Almond Salad with Cider Vinegar Vinaigrette (see recipe on page 332)

Then there's the melatonin factor. Melatonin is a key hormone for regulating sleep. In menstruating women, increased melatonin production during the low-hormone phase helps lower body temperature in the evening hours to encourage sleep, but in the high-hormone phase, progesterone interferes with melatonin release and effectiveness, resulting in higher core body temperature and more disrupted sleep.

A number of factors wreak havoc on core body temperature and sleep during peri- and postmenopause. Estrogen withdrawal prompts increased bursts of a hormone called gonadotropin-releasing hormone (GnRH), which increases vasodilation (the dilation of blood vessels and the resulting decrease in blood pressure), so you dump too much heat and start shivering to warm up. You also have higher norepinephrine levels in your brain, which hampers your ability to handle temperature changes. If that isn't enough, you also produce less melatonin, so your body doesn't readily cool down enough to trigger optimal sleep. Even those who aren't suffering from insomnia often experience hot flashes—the sudden feeling of heat rising up in your body and accompanying night sweats, which are extremely disruptive to sleep.

Lack of quality sleep is detrimental to performance and recovery and has adverse effects on overall well-being. What can be done to improve sleep and sleep quality?

From a behavioral standpoint, establish a regular bedtime, eliminate light and screens (phones, tablets, TVs) from your bedroom, and keep the room temperature cool. On the nutritional front, try to avoid alcohol and caffeine to help mitigate the onset of hot flashes and anxiety. Also consider the following alternative sleep aids.

Melatonin: A hormone produced in the pineal gland of the brain, it is critical for your natural sleep-wake cycle. Often I am asked if taking melatonin will help with overall sleep issues, but melatonin's role in sleep is a bit complex. As mentioned earlier, your hormones impact melatonin production. Should you take melatonin? I would recommend using valerian and tart cherry juice (below) first, as these have been shown to naturally increase the body's production of melatonin and do not have the melatonin hangover side effect that is common when taking straight melatonin. If temperature-related sleep issues still continue, try the smallest effective dose of melatonin: 0.3 to 1.0 milligram 30 minutes before bed.

Montmorency tart cherry juice concentrate: Tart cherry juice is high in the sleep-promoting chemical melatonin and also has anti-inflammatory properties (inflammation can disrupt sleep). Research shows that older women (and men) slept better and for longer when they drank it before bed. For the best results, drink an ice-cold glass 30 minutes before bed to help your core temperature drop and send you into slumber.

Valerian root (tea or capsules): In one natural sleeping aid study, volunteers given 400 milligrams of valerian extract before bed experienced improved sleep, including better sleep quality, than those taking a placebo. The results of another study that used the same valerian extract dose suggest that valerian extract also helps you fall asleep faster.

If you do choose to use a melatonin supplement, valerian can be a perfect complement. Melatonin enhances deep sleep, whereas valerian helps you fall asleep much faster.

HOT IN HERE: THERMOREGULATION

Hot flashes don't just happen at night. They can happen anytime, anywhere and are disruptive no matter when or where they occur. Estrogen is a key regulator of your autonomic nervous system (ANS), which is responsible for pumping out fight-or-flight hormones such as epinephrine, norepinephrine, and adrenaline. Estrogen also helps regulate a group of cells in the brain's hypothalamus region called KNDy neurons, which help control your body's thermostat. Without estrogen to modulate these neurons and govern the ANS, it goes a little haywire, causing you to break out in a hot sweat and feel panicked.

Not surprisingly, this hormonal havoc can make it harder for menopausal athletes to perform in the heat, since they are quicker to heat up and less able to cool down than their younger peers. The biological safeguards that protect us from overheating can be a little sluggish to kick in. Case in point, one recent study compared the sweat rate, sweat volume, sweat sodium content, and level of thirst among three groups of women ranging from premenopausal (average age 22) to postmenopausal (average age 52) as they exercised on a treadmill. They found that after menopause, women sweat less and feel less thirst, which makes sense. Problem is, they are also likely to have a higher core temperature than younger women, so ideally they should begin to sweat earlier and get cues to drink sooner.

SHOULD YOU TRY MENOPAUSAL HORMONE THERAPY?

The million-dollar question is, if estrogen is so great for you and protects you in all these wonderful ways, why wouldn't every menopausal woman go on menopausal hormone therapy (MHT, sometimes also referred to as hormone replacement therapy) to put it back? Well, for a while it seemed like everyone did. But in 2002, a large, decade-long study revealed that women taking MHT had higher rates of breast cancer, heart attacks, strokes, dementia, and other health problems compared to those taking dummy pills. Prescriptions plummeted, and we've been scared away from MHT ever since. That is, until recently.

It's become clear that the risks of hormone therapy were overblown. Today more researchers, scientists, and doctors are reexamining the role of MHT in a woman's life. The 2022 NAMS Position Statement on hormone therapy states: "For women aged younger than 60 years or who are within 10 years of menopause onset and have no contraindications, the benefit-risk ratio is favorable for treatment of bothersome VMS and prevention of bone loss. For women who initiate hormone therapy more than 10 years from menopause onset or who are aged older than 60 years, the benefit-risk ratio appears less favorable because of the greater absolute risks of coronary heart disease, stroke, venous thromboembolism, and dementia. Longer durations of therapy should be for documented indications such as persistent VMS, with shared decision-making and periodic reevaluation."

Generally, I tell women that MHT is a *therapy* to be used in conjunction with specific nutrition and exercise changes if your symptoms are interfering with daily life. It should not be used for body composition changes, as these changes are more involved than just supplying exogenous hormones. (There are changes in hormone-receptor sensitivity and the gut microbiome during perimenopause, thus exogenous hormones are not metabolized or do not stimulate the receptors quite the same as your endogenous hormones.) The general consensus is that if you and your doctor agree on the hormone therapy route, you should have regular checkups to make sure the dose and formulation are right for your body to help you get through this transition. Be sure to work with your doctor to determine your individual needs and formulations, as well as how long you may need to use it.

There are other therapies you can use during menopause, depending on what you're experiencing, including new pharmaceutical interventions like fezolinetant, which works by interacting with KNDy neuron pathways to moderate neuronal activity in the thermoregulatory center of the brain to reduce hot flashes and night sweats. Some women also use selective serotonin reuptake inhibitors (SSRIs) and serotonin and norepinephrine reuptake inhibitors (SNRIs) and other therapies successfully.

The solution? Precooling for training and hydrating are nonnegotiable. Precooling is as easy as drinking an icy, low-sugar electrolyte drink to reduce core temperature. (See Chapter 13 for additional precooling techniques.) Hydrating is as simple as adding ¹⁄₁₆ teaspoon of salt to 20 ounces (600 ml) of water (spoiler alert: plain water doesn't hydrate—see Chapter 12 for more information on hydration) or using a low-carbohydrate electrolyte drink. You should also rely on watery fruits, vegetables, protein drinks, tea, and mineral waters as means of hydrating throughout the day.

BLOATING AND GI ISSUES

Generally speaking, women are more prone to bloating and GI issues than men. But there are phases of our lives, particularly perimenopause and menopause, when this is all the more true. Wildly fluctuating hormones during these years can send your digestive functions into a tailspin, leading to diarrhea, vomiting, constipation, and abdominal cramps or pain. High levels of cortisol—also common during menopause—slow down digestion and make matters worse.

Sex hormones help control the amount of water your body reabsorbs as it filters through your kidneys, according to a recent study published in the *American Journal of Physiology—Renal Physiology.* When estrogen levels are high, you reabsorb water and urinate more often. When they fall, you retain more water, which leads to bloating.

It goes beyond salt and water. You have to consider your overall diet and nutrition to reduce overall inflammation. Peri- and postmenopausal women often tell me that when they start eating a more whole food and less ultraprocessed food diet, they lose 6 to 8 pounds in the first week and their clothes fit better. It isn't fat loss but excess water loss because they have less inflammation and water redistribution to the blood. The other significant contributors to bloat are sugar substitutes and sugar alcohols such as xylitol, mannitol, and sorbitol.

PAIN DOWN UNDER

Many women experience some level of genitourinary syndrome of menopause (GSM) (formerly known as vaginal atrophy) as estrogen levels decline toward menopause. The thinning, drying, and shrinking of the tissues in and around your vagina can not only make sex more painful, it can also interfere with other physical activities, such as bicycling and even running, because the exposed skin gets rubbed raw. If pain is preventing you from exercising and being active, you need to take action. Lubricants can help mild cases. But better choices are vaginal moisturizers like Revaree and Replens, which contain ingredients like hyaluronic acid and polycarbophil, which promote intracellular water absorption. A topical estrogen treatment such as a cream, tablet, or ring can provide relief for more severe or persistent cases.

MEMORY AND MOJO COME AND GO

Can't remember your coworker's name even though you walk by her desk ten times a day? Where are your keys? Don't feel like going to the gym? And what is the point of working out, anyway? If any of this sounds even vaguely familiar, don't worry. You're not alone. Mood and memory disturbances are extremely common during menopause, especially in the years leading into it and the years immediately following your last period. In the landmark Study of Women's Health Across the Nation (SWAN), which included more than 12,400 women between the ages of 40 and 55, results found 31 percent of premenopausal, 44 percent of early or late perimenopausal, and 42 percent of menopausal women experienced spells of forgetfulness. Other research finds that women were also more likely to suffer from depression during this phase of life, particularly the perimenopausal period. In fact, perimenopausal women are three times more likely than premenopausal women to report symptoms of depression.

There's an important connection here. Estrogen increases the concentration of neurotransmitters for feel-good chemicals such as serotonin and dopamine, which have a calming effect on the brain and help boost both mood and memory. Estrogen also inhibits the stress (fight-or-flight) hormone cortisol. Progesterone is also connected to mental health, as it can prevent panic symptoms.

As these hormone levels plummet, you're extremely vulnerable to anxiety, depression, and brain fog. It doesn't take a neuroscientist to tell you that these symptoms, combined with poor sleep, can kill your motivation pretty quickly.

The transitional years seem the worst, until your brain adjusts to its new hormonal milieu. But you don't have to just sit there and stew. In the meantime, use strategically placed branched-chain amino acids, or BCAAs (before and after training, as they cross the blood-brain barrier and support central nervous system actions), try tart cherry juice and valerian to improve your sleep, and recover well from hard training sessions to support your changing physiology and moods.

MENOPAUSE AND EXERCISE: JUST THE FACTS

As more and more women are staying highly active into their late forties and beyond, there are a few specific changes for postmenopausal athletes. Here are some common shifts that occur in menopause and some possible solutions:

1. Blood vessels are less compliant (meaning blood pressure changes are slower).
   Solution: Consider using a beta-alanine supplement as a vasodilator to enhance blood circulation during exercise.
2. There is less core-temperature flux tolerance (meaning you can't handle heat very well).
   Solution: Cooling postexercise is a great way to facilitate blood flow for recovery. Use cool towels or cool-water immersion to get a bit of skin constriction and to push the blood back into central circulation. During exercise, consume cool foods and fluids. See Chapter 13 for additional cooling techniques.
3. You start to sweat later in activity and vasodilate longer (meaning your body tries to get rid of heat by sending more blood to the skin, known as convective cooling, instead of relying solely on sweating to cool you off for a longer period of time).
   Solution: Focus on hydration—keep food in your pocket and hydration in your bottle. Using the prehydration technique mentioned on page 231 before racing will help.
4. There is greater sensitivity to carbohydrates (meaning more blood sugar swings and less need for carbohydrates overall).
   Solution: Aim for a lower carbohydrate intake—between 30 and 40 grams per hour—and increase your calorie intake with mixed macronutrient

foods that contain relatively balanced amounts of fat, protein, and carbohydrates.

5. Your body uses protein less effectively (meaning that the type and quality of protein you eat and when you eat it become very important for building lean mass and holding on to it).

   Solution: Take 15 grams of whey isolate or 7 grams of EAAs 30 minutes before training and 40 grams of whey isolate or pea protein isolate 30 minutes postexercise (~6-10g EAAs). For optimal recovery, plan to evenly distribute protein across your meals, aiming for 30 to 40 grams per meal and 10 to 15 grams per snack.

6. Less power production (meaning you have to train for power, not for endurance).

   Solution: Focus on power training. The speed and strength of muscle contractions tend to diminish with age, thus power and speed become essential aspects of postmenopausal training. See Chapter 7 for specific exercises to boost your performance.

HARNESS THE PERIMENOPAUSAL POWER WINDOW

As we mentioned earlier, for many women, weight gain is one of the side effects of menopause they struggle with most. Physical activity helps. Research has even pinpointed the exact number of minutes of activity a week you need to keep weight gain at bay. In a landmark study, scientists tracked the exercise habits and weight fluctuations of more than 34,000 women (average age 54) for 13 years. On average the women gained about 6 pounds. Not surprisingly, there was a direct relationship between how much the women exercised and how much weight they did or did not gain. The number that best appeared to minimize weight gain? An average of an hour a day.

Also, if you're still in the perimenopausal window, dedicating yourself to a training plan that includes vigorous activity can really make a difference, according to a 2022 study published in *Menopause*, which analyzed the exercise levels, fitness, body composition, and metabolic rates of 72 women ages 35 to 60 split evenly into three groups: premenopausal, perimenopausal, and postmenopausal.

They found that fat mass was 7.1 kilograms (nearly 16 pounds) greater in the perimenopausal women compared with their premenopausal peers. It was also 1.4 kilograms (3 pounds) higher than the postmenopausal women. The perimenopausal women also had an average of 6.1 kilograms (13.4 pounds) less fat-free mass than the premenopausal women. There was a much smaller difference—just 0.12 kilogram or ¼ pound—between the perimenopausal and postmenopausal women, which shows the significance of the metabolic changes during the menopause transition years.

During an exercise test of increasing intensity, they found that premenopausal women were able to switch between burning carbohydrates and fat relatively easily in moderate intensity, with an increase in carbohydrate use in the higher intensities; but in both the peri and post groups, there was a heavy reliance on carbohydrates as fuel, regardless of intensity. What does this mean? It means that there is less metabolic flexibility that starts in the menopausal transition; but we know from other studies that high-intensity interval exercise helps with improving metabolic flexibility and body composition.

Though the women were fairly active, they didn't do much resistance training. All the women across the groups lifted just about once a week on average, with the perimenopausal women lifting the least often.

The researchers concluded that perimenopausal women may be able to avoid the loss of fat-free mass and unfavorable metabolic changes by engaging in activities that help maintain muscle mass and fat-burning capacity such as resistance training and focusing on HIIT training.

I couldn't agree more. That's why I tell the perimenopausal women I work with that if they do nothing else, they should lift heavy sh*t. You need that strong stimulus to maintain muscle as your hormone levels fluctuate and decline. Muscle cell studies show that when researchers take estrogen away from animals, their ability to regenerate muscle stem cells can drop 30 to 60 percent. Muscle biopsies in women during the menopause transition show the same thing. Resistance training that includes heavy lifting stimulates those cells and helps you maintain that muscle. Ideally, you should be lifting 3 days a week. (If you're an endurance athlete, you can drop that to lift twice a week in season.)

I also recommend sprint interval training—super-short 10- to 30-second all-out efforts—for women in the menopause transition as a way to maintain fat-burning metabolism and body composition. Many of my clients do their heavy lifting and sprint sessions on the same day with plenty of recovery between these hard days!

On a nutritional note, the perimenopausal women in this study also ate the least amount of protein, 64 grams (which is about 20 grams per meal) a day, compared to 71 grams among the premenopausal and 67 grams among the postmenopausal women. I'd tell them all to eat more protein, but especially the women in and through the menopause transition, because they absolutely need it to maintain muscle. Active women should aim for at least 1.8 to 2 grams of protein per kilogram a day, which is about 30 grams at each meal and 15 to 20 grams with snacks.

Once again, it's never the wrong time of your life to incorporate heavy lifting and high-intensity exercise and to boost your protein intake. But if you want to have the biggest impact on your metabolism and body composition as you reach menopause and beyond, starting early in your transition may be the most effective strategy.

MAINTAIN YOUR MOMENTUM

It's not officially a "symptom" of menopause, but research suggests you may also find yourself with a growing sense of sedentary inertia without even being aware of it. Though scientists have yet to understand the underlying mechanism, estrogen makes you move more. In a fascinating 9-month study on rats housed with running wheels, the rodents that had had their ovaries removed spent significantly less time (by about seven times) on their wheels than their peers who had dummy surgery that left their ovaries (and estrogen) intact. Observational studies on humans mirror these findings. Voluntary physical activity drops by about 230 calories a day during the transition to menopause.

Most of the women I counsel are already highly active. But this insidious sedentary creep concerns me, because as you may have heard, the hours you spend completely sedentary, especially sitting, can undo even a good bit of exercise. A meta-analysis published in 2015 found that even among people who were otherwise physically active (i.e., met the recommended guidelines and/or said they were active in their leisure time), sitting for long periods of time was associated with worse health outcomes including diabetes, heart disease, and cancer. Prolonged sitting also increased the risk of dying prematurely. Sedentary time and deleterious health outcomes were generally more pronounced at lower levels of physical activity than at higher levels, but the metabolic consequences of too much sitting are concerning no matter how active you are.

Research finds that 2 minutes of movement an hour is all it takes to protect yourself. In a study of more than 3,200 people, the US National Health and Nutrition Examination Survey reported that trading 2 minutes of sitting for 2 minutes of light activity such as walking down the hall each hour can lower your risk of premature death by 33 percent. A 2022 study on "activity snacks" like 15 body weight squats or a 2-minute walking break every 30 minutes improved muscle protein synthesis, which is especially great for menopausal women.

If you have a desk job, set an alarm to prompt you to move for a few minutes every 30 to 60 minutes to counteract the natural inclination to stay sedentary.

ROAR ▶▶▶ SOUND BITES

▸ With the onset of menopause, estrogen and progesterone diminish.

▸ Dropping hormones lead to a slew of changes that can result in disruptive menopausal symptoms and can make exercise feel harder, including less-compliant blood vessels (blood pressure changes are slower); it also gets harder to handle the heat.

▸ Menopausal women are more sensitive to carbohydrates, so they have more blood sugar swings and need less carbohydrates overall.

▸ Your body uses protein less effectively at this time of life, so the type and quality of protein you eat and when you eat it become very important to build and maintain your muscles.

▸ High-intensity power and strength training is *really* important once you hit menopause to prevent muscle loss, bone loss, and weakness with age.

4

DO YOU NEED TO TAKE A PREGNANT PAUSE?

THINGS ARE A LITTLE DIFFERENT WHEN YOU'RE WORKING OUT FOR TWO

I remember it as if it were yesterday . . . the moment my life changed forever. I was out doing my last bike intervals prepping for XTerra Maui. I felt off. I couldn't get any power, my heart rate was all over the map, and my boobs really hurt. In my head I was going over all the scenarios: "Did I not taper right? Am I getting sick? Is my period coming? Wait, when was my last period? Ohhhhhh sh*t. No way. It can't be!"

I finished the workout, more stressed than anything, thinking about the very real possibility that I was pregnant. But along the thought process, I tried to reason that I wasn't. "I can't be. I'm too lean to get pregnant. My periods have been regularly irregular. I can't be fertile." (Note this is generally not a healthy mindset, but I had just finished my last hard block of training and knew I had trained myself to an unsustainable body composition.) I got home, went upstairs, peed on pregnancy sticks (three of them), and they all said the same thing: positive.

"Sh*t, sh*t! Not before Worlds!" I went into my husband's home office and said, "Honey, got some news . . . first, we've got to go buy some more pregnancy tests because these three sticks all say the same thing, that I'm preggers; and next, if I am, I am still going to race in Maui. I've worked too hard to get there, and if anyone can handle the heat and knows about the female body, it's your wifey." Needless to say, we rushed into the car to buy some more tests, and, yep, they all said the same thing. I was pregnant. And yes, I did go race Maui and finished top 10!

Few times in a woman's life are as rife with confusion, controversy, and frankly a whole lot of misinformation than when she's pregnant. Friends, family, experts, even total strangers will tell you what you should and shouldn't be eating and whether or not you should be doing whatever exercise you're doing. Heck, if you followed the American College of Obstetricians and Gynecologists (ACOG) official guidelines from 1985, which cautioned women to keep their heart rate under 140 and restrict daily exercise to 15 minutes or less, you'd barely get out the door before you had to sit down and take a rest!

For the record, ACOG has since tossed those restrictions, but many myths and fears from "shaking the baby loose" with too much running to "cooking the baby" if you get too hot stubbornly persist. Barring pregnancy complications, exercising during pregnancy doesn't have to be that complicated, and it's really good for you—and the baby.

The current guidelines call for women to engage in 30 minutes or more of moderate physical activity most, if not all, days a week. In fact, research papers in the journal *Obstetrics and Gynecology* clearly call for women to engage in more vigorous activity (85 percent max heart rate or a 7 on a scale of 1 to 10), such as riding a stationary bike for 4 to 5 hours a week, during pregnancy to avoid complications such as gestational diabetes, of which high levels of physical activity can reduce the risk by 24 percent.

Yet only half of physicians recommend this amount of exercise, and the majority of pregnant women don't even come close to this recommendation. A mere 15 percent of pregnant women hit those very modest exercise marks. To this day, too many women who weren't active before they got pregnant are afraid to start, and too many who did exercise are scared into stopping completely.

THEN AND NOW

Historically, pregnant women worked in fields, and before modern appliances, they performed the hard physical job of feeding, clothing, and cleaning up after multiple children; however, modern medical associations decided we were too fragile to exercise much during gestation and started treating pregnancy almost more like a disease than a natural phase of many women's lives. Not all this advice is bad, per se. But some of it is.

And it's easy to see how any pregnant woman receiving these instructions would be scared sedentary. Check out these former guidelines (and what we know today).

- Maternal heart rate should not exceed 140 beats per minute. (No longer true.)
- Vigorous exercise should not exceed 15 minutes in duration. (No longer true.)
- Exercise in supine (lying down on the back) position should be done with caution (or avoided) after the fourth month of gestation. (True. In the second and third trimesters, the weight from lying on your back may compress the vein that carries blood from the uterus and could limit oxygen supply to the baby. If you use a bench, set it to incline.)
- Rise from supine (lying down, which you should be avoiding) position slowly to avoid a drop in blood pressure/dizziness. (True.)
- Avoid exercises that employ the Valsalva maneuver. (True. This maneuver, where you forcibly exhale while keeping your mouth and nose shut—generally to lift something heavy—places too much pressure in the abdominal area and can cause unsafe changes in blood pressure.)
- Avoid exercise in the heat or at levels that increase core temperature greater than 102°F, because hyperthermia poses a serious risk to the fetus. (True. Heat risk is real. But without a core-temperature pill, there's no way to know this. Oral temperature should not exceed 100° to 101°F. But you're generally

not going to be carrying a thermometer and taking your temperature while you're out there. The best way to avoid heat risk is to exercise in the cool parts of the day. If in the gym, exercise near ventilation and hydrate with a cold beverage. Use your head. You can feel when you're getting uncomfortably warm.)

- Caloric intake should be adequate for both exercise and fetus. (True. You need about 300 extra calories, not counting exercise. Extra calories for training depend on duration. As in any sound training program, go out well fed, eat during exercise lasting longer than 90 minutes, and eat a recovery snack with a mix of carbs and protein within 30 to 60 minutes of finishing.)
- Regular exercise (three or more times per week) is preferable to intermittent activity. (True. Moving every day for 45 to 90 minutes is ideal, even when you feel like crap. Light exercise helps with blood circulation and hormone fluctuations.)
- Avoid ballistic (jerky, bouncy) movements. (True. You want to go easy on your joints, which are already stressed.)
- Vigorous exercise should be preceded by a warmup and followed by a period of gradually declining activity. (Still true, pregnant or not.)
- Minimize competitive activities. (Not necessarily true. Contact sports are out. But golf or tennis—if you already play—are completely safe. Taking up a new sport isn't advisable.)
- Avoid deep flexion or extension of joints because of connective tissue laxity. (Mainly true. But if you've been doing these movements, such as yoga, prior to pregnancy and have the range of motion, then it's okay.)
- Consume liquids liberally. (True. Hydration is very important. Consume high-water fruits and veggies, soups, teas, watered-down juice, bubbly water, whatever you like. Amniotic fluid and increased blood volume demand increased fluid intake, as does thermoregulation.)

So let's set the record straight. Unless you have serious complications (see "Take a Break from Exercise" on page 75), you should definitely exercise during pregnancy. If you are athletic—and if you're holding this book in your hands, chances are good that you are—you can continue to be so even after you get the positive sign on the pregnancy test.

Training during pregnancy is good for you and the baby on many levels. Expecting moms who are physically active during their pregnancies improve their physical fitness. In fact, you might even see a bigger boost. In one study of female runners, those who kept running during their pregnancy actually improved their max VO_2 (the benchmark of aerobic fitness) 8 to 10 percent more than their nonpregnant peers. Exercise also helps to prevent excessive weight gain (especially in already-overweight moms; see the weight gain chart) and gestational diabetes; boosts mood; and improves posture, muscular strength, balance, and endurance. It can also help moms to sleep better and preps the body for the hard work of labor!

Recommended Weight Gain During Pregnancy

Women are often confused as to how much weight they "should or should not" gain during pregnancy. Below is the standard table based on your starting BMI. You can use this table as a general guideline, but the rate of pregnancy weight gain is very individual, of course. You may be outside of these ranges and still be perfectly healthy—as always, work with your doctor to meet your needs.

PREGNANCY BMI	BMI	TOTAL WEIGHT GAIN (LB)	RATES OF WEIGHT GAIN 2ND AND 3RD TRIMESTER (LB/WEEK)
Underweight	<18.5	28–40	1 (1–1.3)
Normal weight	18.5–24.9	25–35	1 (0.8–1)
Overweight	25.0–29.9	15–25	0.6 (0.5–0.7)
Obese	≥30.0	11–20	0.5 (0.4–0.6)

Source: Institute of Medicine

If exercise is doing all those great things for your pregnant body, imagine what it's doing for the mini-you growing in your uterus. Just as exercise keeps your blood vessels healthy and supple, it helps improve the health of your baby's so they're more resistant to future cardiovascular disease. Likewise, it builds a strong, healthy endocrine system and improves metabolism—yep, even in utero—so your baby has a lower risk of childhood obesity related diabetes. They're not only likely to have a healthier birth weight, but also children of vigorous exercisers have healthier body compositions at 5 years of age without any differences in height, head circumference, cognition, and brain development than children of sedentary moms.

To sum it up, exercising early in your pregnancy has a profoundly positive effect on your developing baby, as it stimulates placenta growth and function as well as the organs and systems of your baby. Staying active through the later stages of your pregnancy keeps your baby's growth and development on track. All this good stuff happens with just 30 to 45 minutes of exercise a day.

The Old Guidelines Are Out of Step with Modern Women

Even though exercise guidelines have changed, doctors will sometimes still caution their athletic patients to "take it easy" (they may not grasp that for a woman who clocks 60 miles a week and bangs out blistering track intervals every Tuesday and Thursday, a Sunday morning jog is "taking it easy").

This is exactly what Lizzette Perez demonstrated during the 2019 Boston Marathon when she ran the event while eight months pregnant. A lifelong runner, Perez found out she was pregnant a week after she qualified for the prestigious event. She continued running, got regular checkups, and when race day came, she "took it easy," which as she told ABC News, meant plenty of water breaks, snack breaks, and porta-potty breaks along the way. She finished in 5:49:20, healthy and elated. She gave birth to a healthy baby girl just over a month later.

At the elite level, tennis legend Serena Williams shut out her rival and won the 2017 Australian Open (her 23rd Grand Slam title) when she was 8 weeks into her pregnancy at the age of 35. She would return to the WTA (Women's Tennis Association) Tour six months later and win another title at the ASB Classic in Auckland, New Zealand, at the age of 38.

In 2022, 33-year-old Chelsea Sodaro shocked the world by winning the Ironman World Championship in Kona, Hawaii, after crushing the competition on the

26.2-mile marathon, running a mind-blowing 2:51:45—just 18 months after giving birth. As she told the Professional Triathletes Organisation (PTO) in a postrace interview, "We shouldn't have to choose between being world-class athletes and being moms."

Research is finally starting to catch up with these modern moms. In the first study of its kind, a group of Canadian sports scientists recently collected data from 42 elite runners throughout pregnancy, postpartum, and post-pregnancy to quantify the volume, intensity, and type of training the women did as well as their competition performance outcomes.

As you might expect, their average pace slowed down and their running volume decreased throughout their pregnancy, declining from about nine to about six sessions a week. Though they ran less, their total accumulated weekly training volume was nearly maintained throughout their pregnancy (until near the end, when it dropped from about 430 minutes a week to about 340 minutes a week) as they did more cross-training as their pregnancies progressed.

Most of the women returned to exercise about 6 weeks after delivery (Note: not full training, but a return to training plan), and they were back to about 80 percent of prepregnancy training loads by about three months postdelivery.

About 64 percent of the women said they intended to return to at least the equivalent or better running form post-pregnancy, and they succeeded. Among these women, there was no statistical decrease in performance one to three years post-pregnancy compared to prepregnancy. In fact, 56 percent of them improved their performance postpartum. Among those who had no intent to perform the same or better after having their baby, 10 percent still improved.

The women's return to sport was not without complications. Half of the participants reported an injury postpartum that delayed their return to running and/or competition. Most of those were musculoskeletal injuries, including sprains, strains, and bone stress injuries. The study authors concluded that it was possible that those who experienced injuries returned to training too quickly. That's possible, but I think it underscores the need to help guide women back to activity postpartum and, importantly, to help them fuel appropriately. Many female athletes are underfueled as a matter of course, which can exacerbate their injury risk postpartum when their fuel needs rise exponentially.

In the end, the authors concluded that "for the first time, we can confirm that those athletes with an intent to return to prepregnancy performance levels, that are able to remain injury-free, have equivalent to improved performance outcomes while maintaining ~2.5 to 3 times the training volumes of evidence-based published recommendations with no significant adverse maternal-fetal outcomes."

In other words, pregnancy and motherhood do not have to be the end of the line. We can and should encourage active women to continue their training during pregnancy and develop guidelines that reflect their high levels of baseline fitness and activity. We also need to help them return injury-free.

TRAINING DURING PREGNANCY: AN INSIDE GUIDE

A *lot* happens during the 40 weeks you spend growing a human inside you. Your blood volume expands 50 percent, or about a gallon jug's worth. You gain weight, gradually at first, just a few pounds during the first trimester and overall about 25 to 35 pounds for an average-weight woman (your doctor can guide you on the most healthy amounts for your individual pregnancy). Your body also starts preparing you to give birth by pumping out a hormone aptly named relaxin that increases the laxity and mobility in your joints so you can open up your pelvis to let the baby come out.

So even if you continue your regular activities, how you train is going to change because you're changing. And that's where some of the legitimate concerns arise. For one, that weight you're gaining isn't where you'd typically carry it—all in the front (though yes, you'll gain a bit in the back, too). So your center of gravity, balance, and coordination will be affected. That in combination with the loosey-goosey joints can increase your risk of injury. Your cardiovascular system is going to be taxed to the max because of the massive demands of the fetal-placenta unit (the placenta receives blood from both you and the developing baby). At term, your blood flow to the placenta is approximately 600 to 700 milliliters (one big bike bottle's worth) per minute. Add in the demands of your exercising muscles, and it's easy to see how sudden shifts in circulation can make your blood pressure take a plunge and cause dizziness. Finally, your core body temperature shifts pretty dramatically. As your metabolism speeds up, you create more heat. Fortunately, however, pregnant women do seem particularly good at regulating their core body temperature and don't have as dramatic an increase in body temperature during exercise as those who are not pregnant.

What's the real risk of all this for the baby? Well, "excessive" exercise may put her or him at risk of hypoxemia (inadequate oxygen), hypoglycemia (low blood sugar), and hyperthermia (excess heat). Sounds scary! But let's look a little more closely at what's really happening. While it's true that when you exercise you do reduce blood flow to the placenta and use precious resources such as oxygen and glucose (blood sugar) to fuel your working muscles, the body is very wise and good at meeting its (and your growing baby's) needs.

Nestled inside the placenta, the baby has relatively little demand for oxygen, and the vessels of the placenta allow for more oxygen extraction from the red blood cells than the mother's body does.

Frankly, pregnant athletes are generally unable to maintain what would be considered dangerously vigorous levels of training. It takes a lot of energy to grow a human, and many women are simply too fatigued to train at prepregnancy levels even if they want to. My coauthor, Selene Yeager, a triathlete and semiprofessional mountain bike racer, trained all the way through her pregnancy, but there were still days—especially early on—where she opted to curl up in the corner of her office and take a nap rather than even try to lace up her running shoes, because she was bone tired.

Also, by the second trimester, your heart at rest is working about 40 percent harder as it pumps out more blood with every beat, causing your heart rate to increase by 15 percent. When you consider how much harder your cardiovascular system is working even when you're just sitting around, common sense tells you that your exercise ceiling is going to be lower.

Not surprisingly, you need more oxygen—about 10 to 20 percent more at rest—when you're pregnant. Yet the very act of breathing gets harder as the baby grows and takes up more space, restricting your diaphragm. You may feel short of breath even before you take a single step or pedal stroke.

And let's talk weight gain. You not only have ever-increasing baby weight, but you're also going to have some fluid retention (many women get swollen legs, feet, and hands). As you grow increasingly heavier, you're going to slow down. That's just physics.

As mentioned earlier, your core temperature is elevated and you're more sensitive to ambient temperatures. Overheating remains one of the most worried-about risks for exercising moms-to-be. Play it smart. Exercise in the cool parts of the day or in air-conditioning. Drink cool fluids before, during, and after exercise. Walk instead of run to reduce heat production, and pay attention to your body!

As an active woman, you're used to pushing through discomfort. Obviously, pregnancy isn't really the time to be pursuing personal records, but it's actually very difficult to become anaerobic during pregnancy even if you want to. Your body is too busy doing other work. When you do feel energetic enough to do some vigorous exercise, you may indeed divert some blood flow from the uterus to your muscles, but this hasn't been shown to have a long-term impact on the baby. In fact, women who exercise have better blood flow to the placenta when they're not exercising, so it's likely beneficial for the baby's development in the long run.

TAKE A BREAK FROM EXERCISE

Though exercise is safe and smart during pregnancy, there still can be risks. Since it's pretty difficult to do studies on pregnant women, there's not a huge body of research on the absolute limitations of how much exercise your body can take while pregnant. But now 40 years into Title IX and millions of active, athletic moms both professional and amateur to learn from later, we have a good handle on where the real risks lie. You absolutely cannot exercise during pregnancy and immediately after if you have any of these conditions:

- Ruptured membranes
- Preeclampsia
- Stitch in the cervix
- Pregnancies of twins

Or are at a higher risk for the following:

- Premature labor
- Placenta previa
- Bleeding in the second or third trimester
- Significant heart and/or lung disease
- Previous miscarriage or premature birth
- Mild to moderate cardiovascular and/or respiratory disorder
- Poorly controlled systemic disease (such as hypertension)
- Twin pregnancy (after 28th week)
- Extreme morbid obesity
- Heavy smoker (*please stop*)
- Small for dates in current pregnancy

MOM-TO-BE EXERCISE RX

The best exercise prescription for pregnant women isn't dramatically different from that of a nonpregnant woman: Do cardio exercise, such as running, cycling, elliptical training, walking, and swimming, for 30 to 60 minutes most days a week. Add in some resistance training 2 to 4 times a week. Adjust according to how you feel as your body changes. The only activities that are off-limits are those that carry high risk of injury and/or put an inordinate amount of strain on you and the baby, such as scuba diving, downhill skiing, contact sports, and high-altitude training. The goal of strength training should be to increase strength and endurance in your upper and lower body for postpartum lifting, not for competition or to improve your physique. That means lower weight and higher reps. For instance, if you usually do leg presses with 50 pounds for 8 to 12 reps, try 30 pounds for 15 to 20 reps. Here are some trimester-by-trimester exercise guidelines:

First Trimester

For some women these first 3 months are the worst: Fatigue, morning sickness, and shifts in your blood circulation can leave you wiped out.

Cardio: Weight, balance, and stability aren't really a challenge yet. Do your favorite activities, eliminating those that carry excessive risk of crashing or hurting yourself like technical mountain biking. As always, listen to your body.

Resistance training: Focus on strength, stamina, and building muscle memory, which will serve you well once the baby is born. Core strength is a must. Perform exercises that strengthen your entire core (abs, back, waist, and pelvis) so it can support you like an internal corset, giving your body strength and resilience as your belly grows.

Second Trimester

This is often referred to as the golden period as energy levels return and you start to show and feel the baby moving. At this point your growing belly will start to alter your posture, stability, and balance. This is the phase in which you might experience round ligament pain, which is a sharp, jabbing feeling in the lower belly or groin on one or both sides. Round ligaments are the thick ligaments that connect the front part of your uterus to your groin where your legs attach to your pelvis. They can become strained during this trimester.

Cardio: Impact may become less comfortable as your belly gets bigger and your body feels heavier. Spinning, swimming, and low-impact fitness classes might be the ticket.

Resistance training: Focus on posture, core stability, and balance. Perform exercises to keep your spine in a proper neutral upright position, since this is when your back and neck will start to feel the strain of all the weight you are carrying in front. Core stretching and strengthening will help stave off round ligament pain.

Third Trimester

The homestretch can be the hardest for physical activity simply because weight gain and belly size have reduced your lung capacity. You may also feel general discomfort (aches, pains, urge to pee, swelling, and so on).

Cardio: Running might now become shuffling, and you may need to raise the bars on your bike (indoor or outdoor) to make room for your belly.

Resistance training: Focus on flexibility, joint mobility, and labor prep. Perform exercises to strengthen the pelvic-floor muscles. These will also keep the pelvis, spine, and hips mobile while relieving discomfort and preparing you for labor.

MYTH BUSTING: WHAT TO SAY TO THE NAYSAYERS

No matter what you do, there will be folks who wag their fingers and chastise your decision to keep your regular slot at SoulCycle rather than take to the couch during your pregnancy. Here are some of the most common myths my clients hear from the doomsayers in their lives and the reality check I give them to stand their ground.

MYTH: If you weren't exercising before you got pregnant, now isn't the time to start.

REALITY: Pregnancy is the ideal time to start moving. If you are just starting out, walking is the perfect place to start, and walking is not deemed unsafe. The real hazard is inactivity, which contributes to excess weight gain, high blood pressure, and aches and pains, as well as a higher risk of C-section and gestational diabetes.

MYTH: Exercise causes an increase in early pregnancy loss, stillbirth, or neonatal death.

REALITY: There is no evidence of any increase in miscarriage risk, stillbirth, or neonatal death with exercise. Quite the contrary, exercise improves placenta growth and fetal development.

MYTH: Resistance training during pregnancy can cause joint injury because relaxin makes ligaments feel looser, so you're at a higher risk of hurting yourself.

REALITY: The relaxin risk is mostly a theory. There is a lack of reputable studies showing increased risk of injury, though it makes common sense that there might be. Now isn't the time for breaking power lifting records, but you can and should still lift weights. Keep in mind that you're going to need to be strong once the baby comes, and strength training is the best way to prepare. In a 12-week study of 32 pregnant women who'd never done any weight training, the researchers found that they improved their strength (as measured on the leg press) by 36 percent by lifting just twice a week. They suffered no injuries, and their blood pressure didn't rise during or after the workouts. As soon as the women learned and employed proper breathing techniques, any minor side effects such as dizziness, headache, and pelvic pain subsided.

MYTH: If you are very athletic, you need to greatly dial down your exercise intensity. Otherwise, you'll go too hard, overheat, and deprive the baby of oxygen.

REALITY: You will naturally need to taper down your intensity. You are not going to be setting any personal bests or winning races in the next 9 months, so you shouldn't be doing high-intensity interval training right now. But maintaining your training is fully appropriate with your doctor's approval. Your body is accustomed to the stress of exercise, so your typical state of being and your existing metabolism are based on a level that includes exercise. There's a greater risk of weight gain, decreased fitness, and less-than-optimum fetal development if you suddenly stop exercising.

MYTH: Running is unsafe during pregnancy. You might shake the baby loose.

REALITY: As long as you have no pain or change in joints, it is fine. The baby is cushioned by amniotic fluid and cannot be shaken loose. Round ligament pain can inhibit pace, stride, and ability to maintain current speed and distance. So listen to your body; slowing down will happen, and that's okay.

MYTH: You shouldn't work your abs. Lying flat on your back can compress the vena cava and cut off oxygen to the placenta.

REALITY: You need a strong core, and doing Kegels isn't enough! True, you should ditch the crunches (honestly, they're not very functional anyway, since they only work the rectus abdominals and not much else). Instead try key core moves such as side planks (see page 115). Most of all, get in touch with a pelvic floor specialist early on to learn how to train and/or relax your pelvic floor muscles; then ensure you have sessions with them in the weeks post–vaginal birth.

REAL MOMS ON THE MOVE

The best evidence of the benefits of exercise comes from the real women I've worked with over the years. Here's a snapshot of four first-time moms, their exercise decisions, and their outcomes.

THE RECREATIONAL EXERCISER

A 35-year-old woman who exercises most days a week for general fitness and enjoyment, including yoga once a week, cardio two times a week, and resistance training one time per week. Prepregnancy her BMI is 22 and her body fat is 26 percent.

During her pregnancy, she increased her aerobic exercise to 3 or 4 days per week at 70 to

85 percent of her maximum heart rate in accordance with the current guidelines. She strength-trained 3 days per week with two gym circuits and a prenatal Pilates class. She also practiced prenatal yoga.

She carried the baby for 39 weeks and gained 22 pounds overall. The baby was born weighing 7 pounds, 11 ounces. She did not experience any complications such as gestational diabetes, preeclampsia, or morning sickness.

THE COMPETITIVE TRIATHLETE

A 28-year-old competitive triathlete who trains 15 to 18 hours per week doing a combination of swimming, biking, running, TRX training, and yoga. Prepregnancy her BMI is 19 and her body fat is 14 percent.

Since there were no specific pregnancy guidelines for athletes, she dialed back her physical activity to the current guidelines. She lowered her aerobic exercise to walking and swimming three times per week. She did a low-weight strength-training routine three times a week consisting of two gym circuits and a prenatal Pilates class. She also practiced prenatal yoga.

She carried the baby for 41 weeks and gained 41 pounds overall. She was unsuccessfully induced, which resulted in an emergency C-section. The baby was born weighing 8 pounds, 6 ounces. The mom developed gestational diabetes, severe morning sickness, and edema and had a slow return to sport (greater than 18 months).

THE ELITE RUNNER

A 32-year-old competitive runner who logs 77 to 80 miles per week with two hard workouts and a 100-minute-long run every week. Prepregnancy her BMI is 18.2 and her body fat is 14 percent.

During her pregnancy, she continued training at the same prepregnancy level with a few modifications. She reduced her intensity and distance on the track and added strength training for posture and core strength. She defined her runs by time rather than distance.

She carried the baby for 38 weeks and gained 15 pounds overall. The baby was born at 7 pounds, 6 ounces. She did not experience any complications such as gestational diabetes, preeclampsia, or morning sickness. She was able to continue running until she gave birth and resumed running 6 weeks postdelivery.

THE ELITE CYCLIST

A 38-year-old competitive cyclist who logs 18 to 20 hours per week training during the race season from February to October. She also strength-trains and practices Bikram yoga. Prepregnancy her BMI is 18.2 and her body fat is 14 percent.

She suffered from severe nausea and vomiting throughout her entire pregnancy (hyperemesis gravidarum), which put her at risk of low birth weight and other complications. She felt relief only when she was physically active. During the first trimester, she continued to cycle outdoors but reduced her intensity and distance.

She didn't vary the terrain from normal, but she did stop group riding for fear of group crashes. She continued to strength-train for posture and core strength and kept up Bikram yoga. In her second trimester, she still cycled outdoors but on flatter roads, limited hills, and on non-technical mountain bike trails. She added swimming to her routine and replaced Bikram yoga with vinyasa. In her third trimester, she still cycled outdoors on flat roads with a modified road bike; she also went hiking and swimming and continued strength training. She actually rode her road bike on the day she went into labor.

She carried the baby for 39 weeks and gained only 6 pounds total. Because of the lack of weight gain, induction was scheduled, but she went into labor naturally the night before. The baby was born at 7 pounds, 3 ounces without complications or health issues. She did not experience any additional complications and was able to return to cycling 3 weeks postdelivery.

EATING FOR TWO OR JUST YOU

Let's be perfectly clear. Even though you are in fact nourishing yourself to sustain two lives, you are not literally eating for two when you're pregnant, because one of you is really pretty small! That's not to say you don't need to take in more fuel for both of you. You do, but generally only about 100 to 300 more calories a day, with the higher end as you progress through your pregnancy.

In fact, fascinating research shows that your intestines change during pregnancy to allow you to absorb more energy and nutrients from the same amount of food while you're pregnant, so you don't need to be a nonstop eating machine for 9 months. Pretty cool, when you think about it.

Of course, it is always important to eat a balanced, whole food–based diet—and it's even more important when you're pregnant, because what you eat is the main source of nutrients for your baby. If there is any time to make the switch to avoiding ultraprocessed foods, it is now.

By eating a healthy, balanced diet, you're more likely to get the nutrients you and your baby need. But you will need more of the essential nutrients (especially calcium, iron, and folate) than you did before you became pregnant. Most women can meet their increased needs with a healthy diet that includes plenty of fruits, vegetables, whole grains, and proteins. According to ACOG, you should try to eat a variety of foods from these basic food groups. If you do, you are likely to get all the nutrients you need for a healthy pregnancy.

Key Nutrients You Need

According to ACOG, you and your baby need these key nutrients and dietary components for a healthy pregnancy:

Calcium: Helps to build strong bones and teeth. Main sources include milk, cheese, yogurt, and sardines. During pregnancy, you need 1,000 milligrams (mg) daily.

Iron: Helps red blood cells deliver oxygen to your baby. Sources include lean red meat, dried beans, peas, and iron-fortified cereals. During pregnancy, you need 27 milligrams daily.

Vitamin A: You need this vitamin for healthy skin, eyesight, and bone growth. Carrots; dark, leafy greens; and sweet potatoes are good sources. During pregnancy, you need 770 micrograms daily.

Vitamin C: Promotes healthy gums, teeth, and bones and helps your body absorb iron. Good sources include citrus fruit, broccoli, tomatoes, and strawberries. During pregnancy, you need 85 milligrams daily.

Vitamin D: Aids your body in the absorption of calcium to help build your baby's bones and teeth. Sources include exposure to sunlight, fortified milk, and fatty fish, such as salmon. During pregnancy, you need 600 International Units (IU) daily.

Vitamin B_6: Helps form red blood cells and helps your body use protein, fat, and carbohydrates. You can find vitamin B_6 in beef, liver, pork, whole grain cereals, and bananas. During pregnancy, you need 1.9 milligrams daily.

Vitamin B_{12}: Helps form red blood cells and maintains your nervous system. You can find this vitamin only in animal products. Good sources include liver, meat, fish, poultry, and milk. During pregnancy, you need 2.6 micrograms daily.

Folate (folic acid): A B vitamin important in the production of blood and protein, it also reduces the risk of neural tube defects (a birth defect of the brain and spinal cord). You can find folate in green, leafy vegetables; liver; orange juice; legumes (beans, peas, lentils); and nuts.

You must get at least 400 micrograms of folate daily before pregnancy and during the first 12 weeks of pregnancy to reduce the risk of neural tube defects. During pregnancy, doctors recommend you get 600 micrograms daily.

Protein: You need additional protein to support the growth of your baby but also your own lean mass (you are getting stronger by having to support more total body weight). In general, aim for 75 to 100 grams of protein per day. Lean meat, poultry, fish, and eggs are great sources of protein. Other options include dried beans and peas, dairy products, and nut butters.

Water: Dehydration is a huge issue during pregnancy, and ironically I ended up in the emergency room with an IV a few times from morning sickness during my own pregnancy. Trying to stay hydrated with a queasy stomach isn't easy. The best way to maintain hydration is to eat watery fruits and vegetables; have soups, teas, and sparkling waters; and add a dash of salt to plain water. You can also use a low-carbohydrate electrolyte drink but not sugar-free; you do not want the sugar substitutes. Boosting fluid absorption is essential, and it can help to drink this during labor as well.

BEWARE PREGOREXIA

At any given time, one-third of American women are trying to lose weight, according to the most recent Gallup Health and Healthcare poll. Worse, a recent survey by *Self* magazine in partnership with the University of North Carolina at Chapel Hill reveals that 75 percent—three-quarters—of women have disordered eating behaviors that include serious illnesses such as anorexia and bulimia. What does this have to do with pregnancy? Well, those same women often get pregnant, and those body issues and food obsessions don't necessarily go away. In fact, sometimes they worsen. Though pregorexia, the fear of gaining weight during pregnancy, isn't yet a formally recognized medical condition, it is very much a real concern.

Experts estimate that about 30 percent of pregnant women actually don't gain enough weight. Though not all of them are pregorexic, it's a growing concern as celebrity culture celebrates women who have the perfectly sized baby bumps and get back into prepregnancy shape quickly. Eating disorders—including those that come about during pregnancy—aren't something you can handle alone. If you are restricting calories, skipping meals, deliberately exercising to excess, and/or obsessing about food and weight gain, tell your doctor and ask to be referred to a specialist. You can beat this and be healthy for you and your baby. But you can't do it alone . . . and you aren't alone.

• • • • •

Finally, during pregnancy, some foods can cause harm to a developing baby. Be sure that all meats are thoroughly cooked to avoid exposure to toxoplasmosis, salmonella, and other harmful organisms. Eliminate alcohol and reduce or eliminate caffeinated beverages (soda, coffee) from your daily intake.

ROAR ▶▶▶ SOUND BITES

- Exercise during pregnancy is encouraged (unless there is a serious medical condition) for both your and your developing baby's health.

- Your body is smart; it will tell you what you can and cannot do (e.g., you won't be able to go anaerobic).

- Weight gain is a normal, healthy part of pregnancy; expect to gain about 15 to 35 pounds, depending on your starting weight.

- The best exercise prescription for pregnant women isn't dramatically different from that of a nonpregnant woman. Do cardio exercise, such as running, cycling, elliptical training, walking, and swimming, for 30 to 60 minutes most days a week. Add in some resistance training 2 to 4 times a week. Adjust according to how you feel as your body changes.

- It takes fewer calories to "eat for two" than traditionally thought: generally only about 100 to 300 more calories a day, increasing to the higher end during the second and third trimester.

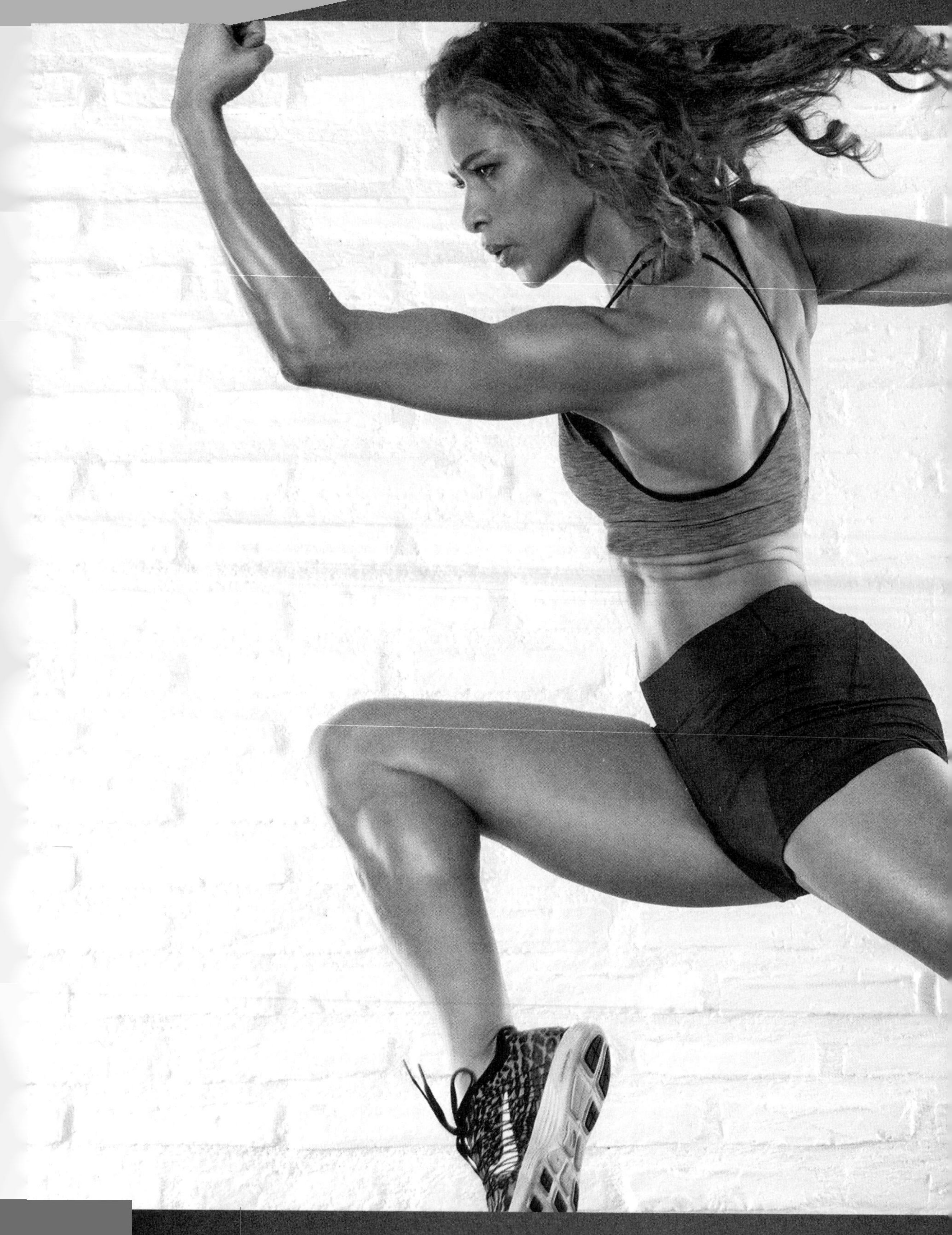

PART II

YOUR FEMALE FITNESS FOUNDATION

5

WEIGHTY MATTERS

STRONG, HEALTHY BODIES COME IN MANY SHAPES AND SIZES. HERE'S HOW TO MAKE THE MOST OF YOURS.

What is it about body weight and women? We are constantly bombarded with messages about weight, leanness, optimal body weight for performance, health, and of course appearance. I have yet to meet a woman who has always had a healthy relationship with her weight. In fact, most women I've worked with, competed against, or just generally have gotten to know have had at least one period of disordered eating, if not a full-blown eating disorder, in their lives. Frankly, most women battle with their bodies most of their lives—myself included.

The core of the problem, I believe, is the very notion that there is one magic weight we should be. It simply doesn't exist. Across my competitive life, my race weight has varied by nearly 20 pounds. I raced an Ironman at 147 pounds, my bike race weight was 132 pounds, my XTerra weight was 136 pounds, and now I sit at 128 pounds doing mostly heavy lifting and gravel riding. Yet despite the fact that I was competitive at all those weights, I was always striving to be thinner, since that was the message that coaches had drilled into my head from an early age. I've seen it across the board from all ages of female athletes. At some point their coaches have said, “If you would only lose X amount of weight, you’d be so much faster,” and the idea stayed with them. But remember my core philosophy: You have to work *with* your physiology, not against it.

One of the best recent examples of this is world champion cross country mountain bike racer Evie Richards, who shared her story with the BBC. When she was just 16 and in the British Cycling Academy, Evie’s periods stopped. Over a span of five years, she had only three menstrual cycles—which her doctors called “normal” for a professional female athlete.

She knows now she suffered from REDs (see page 32), but the message she got as a teen was that elite athletes should eat as little as possible and try to be as light as possible to go fast. She obsessed about her weight until her mother told her she looked like “a bag of bones.” And she still didn’t think it was a bad thing. She had been told that she wasn’t built to be a climber—and you need to climb hills fast to win at the elite level—so getting rail thin was the goal. Except it wasn’t working.

As she shared with the BBC, she worked on her mindset and fueling and said, “When I became world champion, I showed everyone that I don’t need to be thin to be fast up the hills.” She also has her menstrual cycle back and is a happier athlete.

YOU ARE MORE THAN A NUMBER

It’s tempting to end the chapter right there, really. Eat healthy (see Chapter 10 for specific how-tos), find your set point, and be happy. But I realize that you’re looking for a bit more guidance than that. My first bit of advice is to step off the scale for at least a month. Too many women allow themselves to be defined by a number, and it’s generally one that is grounded in nothing more than a notion of what they think they should weigh.

Though I understand wanting to track progress if you’re trying to achieve a certain body composition, the scale isn’t the best measurement of success. How good you feel and how your clothes fit are better indications of progress. I would also encourage you to identify your somatotype, which is your natural shape and size. Most of us can slot our overall build into one of three general categories, recognizing that you can be a mix of two and that there are a wide variety of shapes and sizes even within these categories.

- **Ectomorph:** You tend to be long limbed and not particularly muscular. You can be thin without necessarily having a lean body composition.
- **Mesomorph:** It is relatively easy for you to build muscle mass. You are medium-boned and proportionally built.
- **Endomorph:** You tend to have a curvier build. You may have a larger bone structure and store fat relatively easily.

Once you identify your somatotype, start following the specific eating and training advice in this chapter and see what happens. Give yourself at least a month to let your body adjust before you step back on the scale. Or, even better, skip the weigh-in altogether and get your body composition tested with dual-energy x-ray absorptiometry (DXA), so you know how much of your mass is lean tissue and how much is fat. When I did this, I could see that during peak racing periods, my body fat ranged from 11 to 15 percent across various weights (which put me squarely in an endurance athletic range regardless of the number on the scale). Importantly, even with this low body fat percentage, I was still menstruating on a regular basis.

It's also important to recognize that there is no magical body composition percentage for every athlete. Yes, if you're a competitive body builder, you'll need to be on the very lean end of the scale, but it matters far less if you're a power lifter. Endurance athletes are successful in a wide range—always take your somatotype into consideration, so you're not working against your body type.

Women naturally have more fat than men because we have a greater amount of essential fat (fat needed for bodily functions, from forming reproductive tissue to aiding the absorption of vitamins consumed in different foods). The body fat ranges for optimal health are 14 percent to 30 percent for women and 6 percent to 25 percent for men. Aiming for as low as you can go is not going to automatically help you gain performance benefits, and lower is not always better. As I noted above, I naturally sit on a low end when training hard and peaking for a race, but I maintained my endocrine health and my body fat percentage changed across the years and seasons.

The issue is when people try to achieve a certain number that is unrealistic for their body—which can backfire and actually make you unhealthy.

Here are the ranges according to fitness levels. Note: Research shows that at the higher end of this chart, your risk of metabolic disease increases, BUT you can absolutely be fit at any weight and body composition, and fitness is protective of health. Also, no matter where you fall on this chart, your goal should be to increase your muscle mass regardless of fat mass, since research is showing that skeletal muscle mass is a better predictor of mortality than BMI and fat mass.

BODY FAT RANGES ACROSS HEALTH AND FITNESS LEVELS

	WOMEN (%)	MEN (%)
Essential fat	10–12	2–5
Athletes	12–22	5–13
General fitness	16–25	12–18
Good health	18–30	10–25
At risk	≥31	≥25

Eating as an Ectomorph

Ectomorphs are the body type that is the most resistant to weight gain because of a fast metabolism. People with this body type generally have little observable body fat, are only lightly muscled, and have a small frame (and joints). Basically, your genetic makeup limits your ability to put on muscle mass. When training, focus on power and resistance training to build strength.

To optimize body composition as an ectomorph, eat good-quality fats with moderate protein intake of about 30 to 35 grams per meal (four meals per day if you have a pretraining mini-meal) along with good-quality carbohydrates.

SAMPLE MEAL PLAN TO KEEP YOUR METABOLISM ON POINT AS AN ECTOMORPH

TIME	FOOD OR WORKOUT
WAKE UP: 6:00 A.M. PRETRAINING: MINI-MEAL	Coffee 6 oz (180 ml) vanilla almond milk with 15 g protein powder OR 1 piece sprouted whole grain toast with 1 Tbsp almond or another nut butter
6:30–7:45 A.M. POWER TRAINING	Running hill repeats, followed by plyometrics
8:00 A.M. POSTTRAINING: BREAKFAST (Try to eat within the 30-minute recovery window.)	Coffee or green tea Quinoa Bowl (see recipe on page 329) OR 2 pieces sprouted whole grain toast with 2 Tbsp almond or other nut butter Green Goddess Smoothie (see recipe on page 329)
10:30 A.M. SNACK	1 piece fresh fruit with ¼ cup mixed nuts and 4 oz (120 ml) low-fat Greek yogurt
12:30 P.M. LUNCH	Sandwich with 2 slices sprouted whole grain bread with 2 Tbsp hummus, sliced tomato, avocado, and carrots ½ cup quinoa or barley with 1 hard-cooked organic egg or 4 oz lean protein 1 piece fresh fruit: apple, orange, kiwifruit, or banana OR Mixed green salad with 4 oz cold-water fish or grilled chicken over spinach with chopped apple, walnuts, flaxseeds, peppers, cucumbers, artichokes, or other veggies ½ cup quinoa or sprouted brown rice

TIME	FOOD OR WORKOUT
3:30 P.M. SNACK	Green tea, kombucha, or coffee with one of the following: 15 veggie sticks (carrots, celery, snow peas) and 2–3 Tbsp hummus OR ½ cup (120 ml) plain 2% Greek yogurt with ½ cup fresh berries and 1 Tbsp sliced roasted almonds OR 2 slices sprouted whole grain bread with 2 Tbsp almond or other nut butter
5:30 P.M. PREDINNER SNACK	15 veggie sticks (carrots, celery, snow peas) and 2–3 Tbsp hummus
7:30 P.M. DINNER	Seafood red curry with eggplant and broccoli over 1 cup brown rice or quinoa OR 6 oz salmon or lean bison (170 g) with a side of 1 cup steamed veggies 2 cups mixed green salad with ¼ cup berries, ½ apple, ½ grapefruit, 10 cherry tomatoes, and ¼ cup black beans or chickpeas, topped with 2 scrambled egg whites, sea salt, and pepper OR 2 cups stir-fry veggies of your choice with 4–6 oz lean protein (palm size) over 1–1½ cups cooked purple or red rice or quinoa Mixed green salad with spinach, apple, berries, grapefruit, tomato, light balsamic vinaigrette, and 2 Tbsp pumpkin or sunflower seeds
8:30 P.M. EVENING SNACK	20 g casein protein with 4 oz tart cherry juice

Eating as a Mesomorph

Mesomorphs can generally lose and gain weight easily and are able to build muscle quickly. This body type tends to have a long torso and short limbs. Women with a mesomorph body type are often strong and athletic. Mesomorphs excel in explosive sports—that is, sports calling for power and speed. The reason for this talent lies in the type of muscle mesomorphs possess. Mesomorphs have a higher percentage of fast-twitch fibers and will gain muscle mass more quickly than any other body type.

Basically, your genetic makeup suits power and strength. For training, focus on moderate endurance training, high-intensity interval training (HIIT), and plyometrics. You can add in Pilates or yoga to assist with mobility and fluidity.

To optimize body composition as a mesomorph, eat good-quality fats with moderate carbohydrates and time your protein intake, aiming to have 30 to 40 grams of protein at every meal, and 10 to 15 grams of protein in your snacks.

SAMPLE MEAL PLAN TO KEEP YOUR METABOLISM ON POINT AS A MESOMORPH

TIME	FOOD OR WORKOUT
WAKE UP: 6:00 A.M. PRETRAINING	Coffee 6 oz (180 ml) unsweetened vanilla almond milk with 15 g protein
6:30–7:45 A.M.	Hydration during workout CrossFit or endurance tempo
8:00 A.M. POSTTRAINING: BREAKFAST (Try to eat within the 30-minute recovery window.)	Coffee 3 egg whites with 1 yolk (cooked however you prefer), ¼ avocado, 2 corn tortillas, 1–2 oz Cheddar cheese, ¼ cup low-fat cottage cheese, with 2–3 Tbsp salsa OR Sauté of purple potatoes, spinach, and beets with 4 oz lean protein topped with sliced orange or grapefruit
10:30 A.M. SNACK	2 hard-cooked eggs with 1 piece fresh fruit ¼ cup mixed nuts
12:30 P.M. LUNCH	Mixed green salad with 4 oz cold-water fish or lean protein over spinach or kale with chopped apple, walnuts, flaxseeds, peppers, cucumbers, artichokes, or other veggies OR 6–8 sushi rolls with avocado and 1 cup miso soup OR 1 6-inch quinoa tortilla filled with ⅓ cup hummus, 4 oz fish or chicken, and unlimited veggies (lettuce, cucumbers, tomatoes, etc.) 1 piece fresh fruit: apple, orange, kiwifruit, or banana OR 4 oz (120 g) grilled chicken with 1 small sweet potato, 2 cups mixed green salad, and ½ avocado

TIME	FOOD OR WORKOUT
3:30 P.M. SNACK	Green tea or coffee with one of the following: Mix ½ Tbsp nut butter with ½ oz vanilla protein powder and a splash of water to make a spread. Serve with ½ medium banana.
OR 5:30 P.M. PREDINNER SNACK	1–2 Vegan Nut Butter Balls (see recipe on page 333)
7:30 P.M. DINNER	2 cups stir-fry veggies of your choice over 1 cup cooked sprouted brown rice or quinoa Small side salad of mixed greens with palm-size serving of protein (e.g. tempeh) and olive oil vinaigrette OR Quinoa, Broccoli, Apple, and Pomegranate Salad with Lime Vinaigrette (see recipe on page 330). Save some for lunch with 2 slices sprouted whole grain bread and 1–2 tsp salted butter OR Warm Potato Salad with Broccoli and Cranberries and Orange Vinaigrette (see recipe on page 333) over arugula with 4 oz lean protein of choice
8:30 P.M. EVENING SNACK (~2 HOURS BEFORE BED)	20 g casein protein with 4 oz tart cherry juice

Eating as an Endomorph

Endomorphs naturally tend to have curvy, fuller figures and may have the tendency to gain weight easily.

As an endomorph, maintaining muscle is important. Aim to eat a higher amount of protein spread evenly across the day. Training-wise, emphasize strength training and include some high-intensity interval days. As an endomorph, focusing on eating a wide variety of veggies, grains, and fruit to have a very diverse gut microbiome is essential, as is hitting the upper range for protein intake to maximize body composition and to control insulin and blood sugar.

SAMPLE MEAL PLAN TO KEEP YOUR METABOLISM ON POINT AS AN ENDOMORPH

TIME	FOOD OR WORKOUT
WAKE UP: 6:00 A.M. PRETRAINING	Coffee ½ banana or apple with ½ cup (120 ml) Greek yogurt OR 6 oz (180 ml) unsweetened vanilla almond milk with 1 scoop protein powder
6:30 A.M. HIIT SESSION	Running: 10- to 15-minute warmup, then 4 rounds of: 200-meter sprint, 30 jumping squats, 200-meter sprint, 20 pushups, 200-meter sprint, 10 burpees, 20 Tabata V-ups (or situps), and cooldown
POSTTRAINING (Try to eat within the 30-minute recovery window.)	½ cup Greek yogurt with 10 almonds and ½ apple OR 1 slice sprouted whole grain toast with 3 oz Cheddar or Colby cheese with sliced tomato and avocado OR Breakfast (as below, within 30–45 min posttraining)
BREAKFAST	Coffee 2 poached eggs with spinach sauté (use butter or grapeseed oil) on 2 slices of sprouted whole grain toast OR ½ cup steel-cut oats soaked overnight in almond milk, topped with 1 Tbsp walnuts, ¼ cup blueberries, and ¼ cup 2% Greek yogurt OR Green Goddess Smoothie (see recipe on page 329) OR 2 protein pancakes (use flapjack mix or a protein powder–based recipe) with fresh blueberries or strawberries
11:30 A.M. SNACK	2 hard-cooked eggs with 1 piece fresh fruit

TIME	FOOD OR WORKOUT
1:30 P.M. LUNCH	1 6-inch whole wheat pita filled with ⅓ cup hummus, unlimited veggies (lettuce, cucumbers, tomatoes, etc.), and 1 cup fat-free cottage cheese or ½ cup tuna in water 1 orange or 2 tangerines OR Large mixed salad with 4–6 oz (115–170 g) grilled chicken over spinach with almonds or walnuts, berries, tomato, cucumber, and chopped apple. Sprinkle with hemp oil and sea salt. OR 1 medium white corn tortilla spread with 2 Tbsp almond or other nut butter, topped with ½ cup low-fat Greek yogurt or ricotta cheese and 4 crushed strawberries
4:30 P.M. SNACK	Green tea or coffee with one of the following: 1 apple with 2 oz low-fat cheese OR 2 slices lean turkey lunchmeat with 4 strawberries OR 1 cup steamed edamame with 1 oz Brazil nuts
6:30 P.M. DINNER	4–6 oz (115–170 g) lean beef, chicken, or cold-water fish, with 1 cup steamed veggies 2 cups mixed green salad with ¼ cup berries, ½ chopped apple, ½ grapefruit, 10 cherry tomatoes, and ¼ cup black beans or chickpeas, topped with 2 scrambled egg whites, sea salt, and pepper OR 2 cups stir-fry veggies of your choice with 4–6 oz lean protein (palm size) over 1–1½ cups cooked purple or red rice or quinoa Mixed green salad with spinach, apple, berries, grapefruit, tomato, light balsamic vinaigrette, and 2 Tbsp cashews or almonds
8:30 P.M. EVENING SNACK	20 g casein protein with 4 oz (120 ml) tart cherry juice

EATING ADVICE FOR EVERY BODY TYPE

Many people come to me for advice for optimizing their body composition, and in many of those cases they would like to lose some body fat. I always stress that they should focus on making muscle first and foremost, and then they can make some adjustments to lose some body fat if they desire. There are a number of ways to do that, but counting calories isn't one I recommend. That's because the quality of your food is far more important for optimizing body composition than the number of calories it contains. The entire low-fat debacle was based on the idea that fat is more calorie-dense than carbs or protein, so if we don't eat it, we'll eat fewer calories and get lean. But it didn't work out that way. We ate empty calories that didn't satisfy us, and our metabolic health suffered.

What's more, the whole notion that 3,500 calories equals 1 pound (hence, shave 500 calories a day to lose a pound a week) is completely false. (Moreover, recent research has shown that this number is actually closer to 4,200 calories because of the effects different foods have on our hormones.) Higher-calorie foods such as nuts, avocado, olive oil, and so forth are exactly what you need to be healthy. Besides, research shows that the mental effort of counting calories causes stress, fatigue, and burnout and leads to bingeing because you feel miserable and deprived.

And if all that wasn't enough, a recent study of men and women who created a 3,500-calorie deficit by either dieting or exercising showed that when the women exercised, their appetite remained stable, but when they slashed calories by eating less, the hormones that affect appetite spiked and they got hungrier and ate more. If you are looking to lose some body fat, I stress that dieting isn't natural and doesn't work. Don't do it. Do this instead:

Eat low on the food chain. Eat food that you recognize as food from the earth, choosing local and/or organic when possible, as pesticides can cause inflammation and interfere with normal metabolism.

Time your intake. Don't go into an exercise session totally fasted, especially in the morning, when cortisol levels are at their highest; just a small snack with protein and carbs (about 150 calories total) before you head out will counter some of the cortisol.

The most important thing, though, is postexercise recovery. Get that protein (30 grams) within 30 minutes of finishing your session. It doesn't have to be a special supplement; it can be a split meal. For instance, you have the protein component of your breakfast within 30 minutes of your workout, then have the rest of your meal within 90 minutes of finishing your session. This will still work to knock down cortisol.

Don't fast. Please, please, don't do intermittent fasting. Fasting drives cortisol up, creating an elevated baseline of cortisol, which promotes fat storage. If you do decide that you want to follow the trend of fasting, just stop eating after dinner, then have breakfast when you wake up, so you have a longer overnight fast than if you snacked in the evening (technically called *Time-Restricted Eating;* time-restricted eating aligns the eating and fasting cycles to the body's innate 24-hour circadian system and is associated with better metabolic health and reduced risks of obesity). When training or exercising first thing in the morning (yes, even super early), women do better in a fed state (see timing your intake!). Not only does this help improve the training session by giving your body the fuel it needs to hit intensities and create an adaptive stress, but it also signals to the hypothalamus that nutrition is available, so you don't go into the repercussions of low energy availability (see the section on REDs, page 32).

Maintain a base. Aim for about 180 to 200 grams of good-quality carbohydrate intake a day through grains, fruit, veggies, and low-sugar/fermented (hello sourdough!) bread.

Focus on body composition, not weight on the scale. It is less stressful, and we aren't in the superskinny "Kate Moss is cool" era any longer, no matter what marketers want to bring it back. Strong is the new skinny!

DOES EXERCISE TIMING MATTER?

Women will sometimes ask if there's a "best time" of day to exercise for fat loss. Obviously, exercise whenever you do it is better than no exercise at all. That said, recent research indicates that when it comes to reducing abdominal fat (which is the type that generally has the most negative metabolic consequences), morning exercise might be preferable for women.

A study of 27 trained women and 20 trained men reported that among the women, morning (6 to 8 a.m.) exercise reduced abdominal fat (-10 percent versus -3 percent) and blood pressure compared to evening exercise, and evening (6:30 to 8:30 p.m.) exercise enhanced upper body strength (15 percent versus 9 percent) and power (37 percent versus 8 percent). Among the men, evening exercise increased fat burning and reduced systolic blood pressure and fatigue. The precise mechanism behind these outcomes needs further study but is likely linked to the physiological response to our circadian rhythms.

HEAR HER ROAR

EATING 1,000+ MORE CALORIES EACH DAY AND FINALLY AT GOAL BODY COMPOSITION

Cammie Urban, 48, came to me specifically to "up her game." She was a mountain bike racer in her early twenties, but she took a break when she had kids. When her high school–age daughter started racing, Cammie was eager to jump back into competition. But she wasn't producing the power she wanted to be successful. Unsurprisingly, she simply wasn't eating enough—not even close.

"My daughter and I were both cutting calories to lose weight. But it turns out we were actually doing more harm than good because we weren't fueling properly. My muscle was really breaking down because I wasn't giving it the glucose it needed for fuel or the protein it needed to rebuild. We were also avoiding fat at all costs—another big mistake," says Cammie.

As a result, they were hungry all the time and weren't getting lean, but instead they were actually losing muscle and power along with it. The first thing I had them do was eat a big breakfast—a bowl of steel-cut oats with blueberries and protein powder—especially on training days. Next, they eat on the bike (see Chapter 11 for specific exercise-fueling guidelines) and have a recovery drink the moment they get off their bikes. They are now eating more nutrient-dense foods, including healthy fats, quinoa, and other grains, along with plenty of protein, and of course veggies and fruit.

"I've just about doubled my food intake," says Cammie. "Before I was limiting myself to 1,300 calories a day. Now I'm closer to 2,500 to 2,700, I'm leaner than ever, and my power has gone up. I'm never hungry on the bike, and I have great confidence that I'm fueling myself optimally."

That confidence resulted in a masters world championship title. Amazing what the right fuel can do!

KEY ACTIONS

1. Get quality sleep; at least 7 to 8 hours. Less than 7 hours is associated with greater cardiovascular and metabolic disease risks and reduces the amount of time your body has to repair.
2. Increase vitamin D, calcium, and magnesium as well as protein and fat intake, and eat more throughout the day. Limit dried fruit and instead eat more fresh citrus fruits.

3. Eat a wide variety of fruits, veggies, and grains to improve the diversity of your gut microbiome.
4. Increase B_{12}-rich foods such as eggs and fish.

A NOTE ABOUT THIS FOOD PLAN

As we approach menopause, our bodies become more sensitive to carbohydrates and have a harder time repairing (which is why we need more frequent doses of amino acids). The concept behind this plan is to encourage the selection of nutritious foods that enhance liver and muscle glycogen storage and to improve body fat loss as well as lean-mass preservation and gain. Expanding overall food choices will allow for greater micronutrient (vitamin and mineral) intake.

Body-composition changes are also affected by the types of carbohydrates you consume and when you eat them. The body is primed for a carbohydrate load first thing in the morning and toward early afternoon (trying to boost blood glucose levels for the brain, heart, lungs, kidneys, and other organ systems). As the day wanes, the body becomes more adept for protein, especially in the midafternoon and toward bedtime. Protein is key for many cellular processes and muscular repair, which occur while you sleep. The key to general eating is to plan several small meals throughout the day, with even doses of protein for each meal and greater emphasis on complex carbohydrates in the morning and around training.

CAMMIE'S DAILY FUEL PLAN TO OPTIMIZE BODY COMPOSITION AND RECOVERY

The emphasis here is not on weight change but on improving overall body composition. Based on Cammie's body composition, height, and current weight (around 125 pounds), focus was placed on eating at regular intervals throughout the day and implementing some high-intensity interval training. By fueling her body when she needed it, she recovered faster and became leaner and stronger. With a focus on health and performance, this was the best power-to-weight ratio for Cammie.

Grams of carbohydrate per day: 195–210
Calories: 780–840

Grams of protein per day: 115–125
Calories: 460–500

Grams of fat per day: 80–95
Calories: 720–855

Baseline calories per day: 1,960–2,195
(40% carbohydrate, 25% protein, 35% fat)

Keep in mind that this caloric intake is a recommended baseline, and it is specific to Cammie's plan. The lower end of the spectrum is for rest and recovery days; the upper end of the spectrum is for long training days and does not include calories from training food. When the volume and intensity of exercise increase, the body's caloric and nutrient needs will change.

MEAL PLAN

This meal plan includes a morning strength-training session and an afternoon ride. Carbohydrate choices are essential—choose nutrient-dense, complex carbs. Try to eat more veggies and fruit for your carbohydrate choices outside of training. (See Chapter 10 for daily nutrition recommendations.) Incorporate 80 to 95 grams of fat in your diet each day. The main focus is on protein with a bit of fat and carbohydrates. The recommended carb choices are mainly fruit and veggies along with some healthy bread.

SAMPLE MEAL PLAN FOR MORNING STRENGTH SESSION AND AN AFTERNOON RIDE

TIME	FOOD
WAKE UP: 6:30 A.M. **7:00 A.M. BREAKFAST**	Latte with low-fat milk or milk alternative 2 poached eggs with spinach sauté (use butter or grapeseed oil) on 2 slices sprouted whole grain toast OR ½ cup steel-cut oats soaked overnight in almond milk, topped with 1 Tbsp walnuts, ¼ cup blueberries, and ¼ cup 2% Greek yogurt OR Green Goddess Smoothie (see recipe on page 329)
8:30–10:00 A.M. STRENGTH TRAINING	Hydration only: 16 oz fluid with 5 g branched-chain amino acids (BCAAs) added
10:30 A.M. POSTSTRENGTH RECOVERY	10 almonds in ½ cup cottage cheese, sprinkled with cinnamon OR 1 apple with 1 oz cheese
12:30 P.M. LUNCH	6–8 sushi rolls with avocado and 1 cup miso soup OR 1 6-inch quinoa tortilla filled with ⅓ cup hummus, unlimited veggies (lettuce, cucumbers, tomatoes, etc.), and 4 oz (115 g) fish or chicken 1 piece fresh fruit: apple, orange, kiwifruit, or banana OR 1 gluten-free bagel with lox, cream cheese, tomato, avocado, salt, and pepper, with ½ cup Greek yogurt or kefir or cottage cheese, 20 almonds, and ½ apple OR 4 oz (115 g) grilled chicken with 1 small sweet potato, 2 cups mixed green salad, and ½ avocado

TIME	FOOD
4:30–6:00 P.M. TRAINING RIDE	Hydration: 0.10–0.12 oz per lb (6 to 6.5 ml per kg) per hour hydration beverage. Drink this beverage with food about 60 minutes into your ride (assuming you ate breakfast). Calorie intake on the bike should be 1.3–1.6 food calories per lb (3 to 3.5 food calories per kg) per hour. 1 nut butter sandwich (2 slices low-fiber bread with 1 Tbsp almond or other nut butter and 1 tsp jam), Date Brownie (see recipe on page 332), 5 small new potatoes (cooked and salted), 3–4 Salty Balls (see page 212 for recipe) If you have eaten within 2 hours, you can afford to be low on intake the first hour, then use potatoes or sandwich bites for fuel.
6:30 P.M. RECOVERY SNACK (Try to eat within the 30-minute recovery window.)	16-oz smoothie made with 1 frozen banana, ½ cup milk/milk alternative, 1 scoop protein powder (20–25 g), and ½ cup low-fat (unsweetened) yogurt
8:00 P.M. DINNER	Seafood red curry with eggplant and broccoli over 1 cup brown rice or quinoa OR 1 cup steamed veggies 6 oz (170 g) salmon or lean bison or Quorn over 2 cups mixed green salad with ¼ cup berries, ½ chopped apple, ½ grapefruit, 10 cherry tomatoes, and ¼ cup black beans or chickpeas, topped with 2 scrambled egg whites, sea salt, and pepper OR 1 cup broth-based soup (miso, vegetable) 6–8 oz (170–220 g) lean protein (salmon, chicken, lamb, or try sautéing mushrooms and chickpeas with tamari and sweet chili sauce) with 1 heaping cup broccoli cooked with 1 tsp olive oil Mixed spinach salad: 1½ cups spinach, ½ chopped apple, ½ grapefruit, 1 Tbsp seeds, crumble of feta cheese, and 4 avocado slices (equivalent to ⅓ avocado)

STRENGTH PROFILE: OLYMPIC LIFTING AND STRENGTH COACH

Kasey Warrenton, 32, came to me as she was migrating out of strict Olympic lifting into her first strongman competition. She was concerned because she had inconsistent energy levels, reducing her ability to train and progress. "One morning I'll wake up and be jumping out of bed, then the next I am so tired I can't face the alarm, but there is no pattern to it!" She ate a healthy, mostly whole-foods diet and tried to hit her macros every day—but she wasn't getting stronger and was noticing an increase in belly fat.

"I was adding in way too much, from an activity level. I was still trying to coach Olympic lifting three times a week, as well as do my own training (which was adding up!). Plus, my boys were running around and I had to constantly keep after them. I can see now that I was not planning my food needs, and I was skipping optimal windows for recovery, not to mention not eating nearly enough to build strength and muscle. Stacy keeps reminding me that it takes abundance to create muscle; and since I was barely eating what my body needed on a recovery day, it is no wonder I was tanking!" says Kasey.

As a result, she was tired all the time and was unable to hit the loads she wanted to progress for her new sport. The first thing I had her do was fuel for each session, including time on her feet coaching. Next we made sure she was hitting at least 1.1 grams of protein per pound of body weight on most days, bumping that up to 1.4 grams on heavy, hard training days in the luteal phase (protein needs go up about 12 percent in this phase). Just because she was strength-focused did not mean she could neglect the carbs! We made sure to hit at least 4 grams of carbs per pound (9 grams per kilogram) per day in her heavy training blocks, dropping it to 2.7 grams of carbs per pound (6 grams per kilogram) in her recovery weeks (see Chapter 11 for specific exercise-fueling guidelines). Although Kasey was eating "clean," she was not eating a wide variety of foods, so we upped the intake of healthy fats, quinoa, and other grains; plenty of protein; sourdough bread (yes, bread!); and, of course, veggies and fruit.

"I am now super conscious to eat in and around my training; specifically getting good protein and carbs in within the hour; not waiting until I get home and then chasing my boys," says Kasey. "Before, I was just focused on getting my macros in but, looking back, that only added up to about 1,800 calories a day. Now I'm closer to 2,500; I am stronger, leaner, and my energy is consistent, which really helps with the training loads! I am now pressing my old squat weight, and I laugh that my warmup deadlift sets used to be my 3-rep max!"

ROAR ▶▶▶ SOUND BITES

▶ Your weight and body composition depend on your somatotype: ectomorph, mesomorph, or endomorph. Eat and exercise for your physiology.

▶ Don't get caught up in the numbers on the scale. Body composition is what counts, especially how much muscle you have.

▶ One pound does not equal 3,500 calories. Stop counting calories.

▶ Don't train fasted. As a woman, especially, it can promote fat gain and reduce positive fitness adaptations.

▶ Fuel your body in and around training, specific for what you have planned; it is especially important to eat postworkout to stop the catabolic (breakdown) state and reduce the chances of falling into low energy availability (LEA).

6

CORE STRENGTH, STABILITY, AND MOBILITY

INJURY PREVENTION FROM THE INSIDE OUT

Core strength has been a hot term in the fitness industry for decades. Unfortunately, in far too many instances, it's become synonymous with six-pack abs. That does the rest of your core, which includes your back, obliques (sides), and glutes, a disservice. Neglecting those important supporting players can also set you up for injury, especially as a woman.

As a woman, you generate the lion's share of your strength and stability from your lower body, as that is where you have a higher proportion of your muscle mass. And though women do have powerful legs, we often have relatively poor core strength by comparison, which can set us up for a world of hurt in places such as the soccer field or basketball court.

In the wake of Title IX in the United States and more opportunities for girls to play sports globally over the past 50 years, there has been a tidal wave of ligament blowouts. Statistics show that the relative risk of ACL injury in female athletes is three to eight times greater than in males (depending on the sport). That not only hurts your playing ability (not to mention long-term mobility) but also rattles your confidence and robs you of the stress relief and joy you receive from playing your sport.

A few of the factors that make us more susceptible to these types of injuries are out of our control. Our undulating hormones may make our connective tissues more lax at certain times of our cycle. We have wider hips than men. In fact, research finds that until puberty, male and female pelvic structures are similar. With the onset of puberty, the female pelvis becomes wider, reaching its full width around 25 to 30 years. From 40 onward, it actually begins to narrow again. That wider structure makes us more likely to be a bit knock-kneed and therefore at risk to cave in and tear the ACL when we jump and land (it also can lead to excessive foot pronation and ankle issues). We're also generally smaller than men. That means the ACL itself is smaller, as is the notch through which the ligament connects to the femur. It's not just your knees. Women's shoulders are vulnerable as well. Weaker shoulder muscles and looser supporting tissues mean our shoulder joint is less stable than men's. Before you go cursing your genetic makeup, however, know this: Injuries to both areas are easy to avoid. It just takes some attention to your core—*your full core*, which I define as everything but your head and arms and legs.

STRENGTHEN YOUR STEERING WHEEL

I once heard a very wise physical therapist (PT) describe the butt—an essential and overlooked part of your core—as the steering wheel and stabilizer for the legs. If you don't have a solid command of the steering wheel, the legs will go every which way. Brilliant analogy! I've actually seen it in action. The same PT showed me early video clips of what became one of the most powerful and dominant tennis players in the world jumping off a box. As she landed, you could clearly see her knees collapsing inward—an ACL risk—because she was using her quads—her dominant muscles—to do all the work. That's a very common imbalance in women, and your quads can't stabilize you, which sets the stage for not only ACL risk but also any number of lower-body strains and sprains as some muscles pull double duty while others fail to pull their weight.

When your glutes (butt muscles) are strong, they snap into action first to keep your pelvis rock steady and allow your quads to go where they're supposed to go rather than collapsing inward. Moving upward from the waist, strong abs, obliques, and back muscles help keep everything in line, so you move as one solid unit.

Note, nowhere in this process do I recommend doing crunches. You want your core exercises to make you look like a tall, straight bamboo stalk, not a bendy straw. Too many of us already resemble bendy straws from all the hunching we do. Crunches perpetuate that bendy straw posture because they do absolutely nothing for your glutes and back, which hold you upright, while putting you in the same forward flexed position you're in all day long. Honestly, crunches aren't even that great at strengthening your abs. In a head-to-head face-off published in *Medicine and Science in Sports and Exercise*, researchers found that the plank position made the abdominals work twice as hard as traditional crunches. As a bonus, planks strengthen your shoulders, back, and glutes, which improves your posture and helps you stand straighter.

While we're talking planks and posture, I want to call attention to the inner unit of your core, which is the deepest abdominal muscles that act like a weight belt to hold your whole midsection—front and back—firm and tight. That inner unit needs to be strengthened before you even think about forming a six-pack.

When your entire torso—collarbone to hip bones—is strong and solid, so are you. You'll stand straighter, move better, and be far less likely to get hurt. Case in point, take dancers, who, unlike many traditional sport athletes, concentrate on developing core strength as the foundation of their every move. One very telling study compared the biomechanics of 40 elite modern and ballet dancers (20 men and 20 women) and 40 team sport athletes (20 men and 20 women) as they performed single-legged drop landings from a 12-inch platform.

Dancers of both sexes and the male team athletes all landed with their knees straight and steady. The female athletes? Not so much. Like so many women athletes, their knees caved inward. The dancers also had greater trunk stability than the team sport players. Not surprisingly, both male and female dancers have a far lower incidence of ACL injuries than team sport athletes.

Research has shown that when women perform preventive exercises to strengthen these key areas, they absolutely have fewer injuries, says Holly

Silvers-Granelli, MPT, PhD, owner of Velocity Physical Therapy in Santa Monica, California, who has developed an ACL injury prevention protocol called *prevent injury and enhance performance* (PEP). "We know that women have muscle imbalances and movement patterns that put them at a higher risk for these injuries," she says. "We also know that we can decrease the number of ACL injuries that are occurring, because we've done it."

Though sports clubs have been slow to implement ACL injury prevention programs, the ones that have, such as the Pepperdine University basketball program, have seen huge success. At Pepperdine, Silvers-Granelli's plan reduced ACL injuries by 100 percent by the next season—the players had zero blown ligaments, compared to their usual two per year. In a separate study of more than 2,100 female soccer players, there was an 88 percent reduction of ACL tears among those practicing PEP training for a year.

Despite this, in the seven years since the first edition of ROAR came out, Silvers-Granelli says ACL injury frequency remains a massive issue and that despite extensive scientific evidence to support injury mitigation, the adoption and adherence rates for these prevention programs remain low. Her group continues to expand their risk factor profile to now include anatomy, hormones, biomechanics, environment, genetics, and medical resources. But Silvers-Granelli notes that the root of the problem lies in continued inequity in sports: "Women and girls have been underfunded compared to males," she says. And equal access to coaching, strength and conditioning, and equipment play confounding roles in this problem. In other words, we still have a long way to go.

A PLAN TO STRENGTHEN YOUR CORE AND HELP PREVENT INJURY

These key moves from the PEP plan will help keep your core and steering wheel stable and strong. For optimal results, do 2 sets of each exercise 3 days a week.

WALKING LUNGE

(1 minute or 3 sets of 10 reps)

Strengthens the glutes and quad muscles and improves balance and stability

Take a giant step forward and lunge forward, leading with your right leg. Drop the back knee straight down, keeping your front knee over your ankle (you should be able to see your toes). Push off with your right leg and lunge forward with your left leg, repeating the move. Control the motion and try to prevent your front knee from caving inward.

MAKE IT HARDER:
Hold dumbbells.

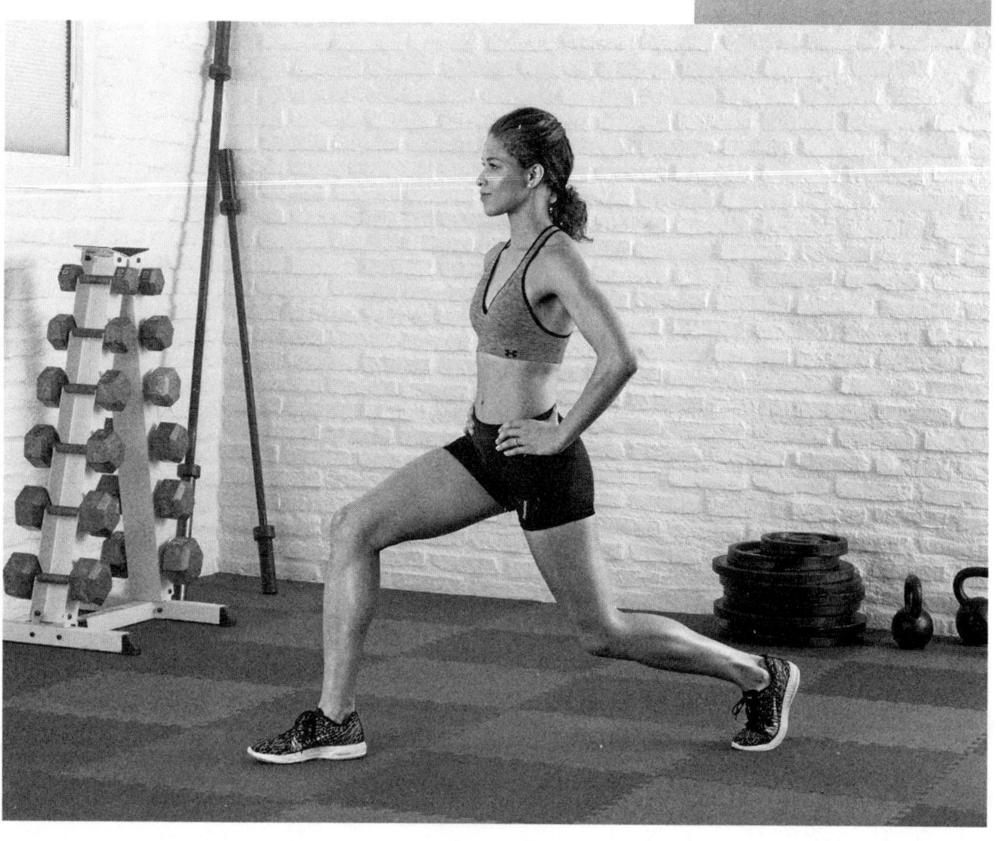

SINGLE TOE RAISE

(1 minute or 2 sets of 30 reps)

Strengthens the calf muscle, improves glute strength, and increases balance

Stand up with your hands on your hips. Bend the left knee up and contract your right glute and tighten your abs to maintain your balance. Slowly rise up on your right toes while keeping your balance. You may hold your arms out parallel to the floor to help stabilize. Slowly lower to the ground for a full set and switch to the other side.

MAKE IT HARDER:
Hold dumbbells.

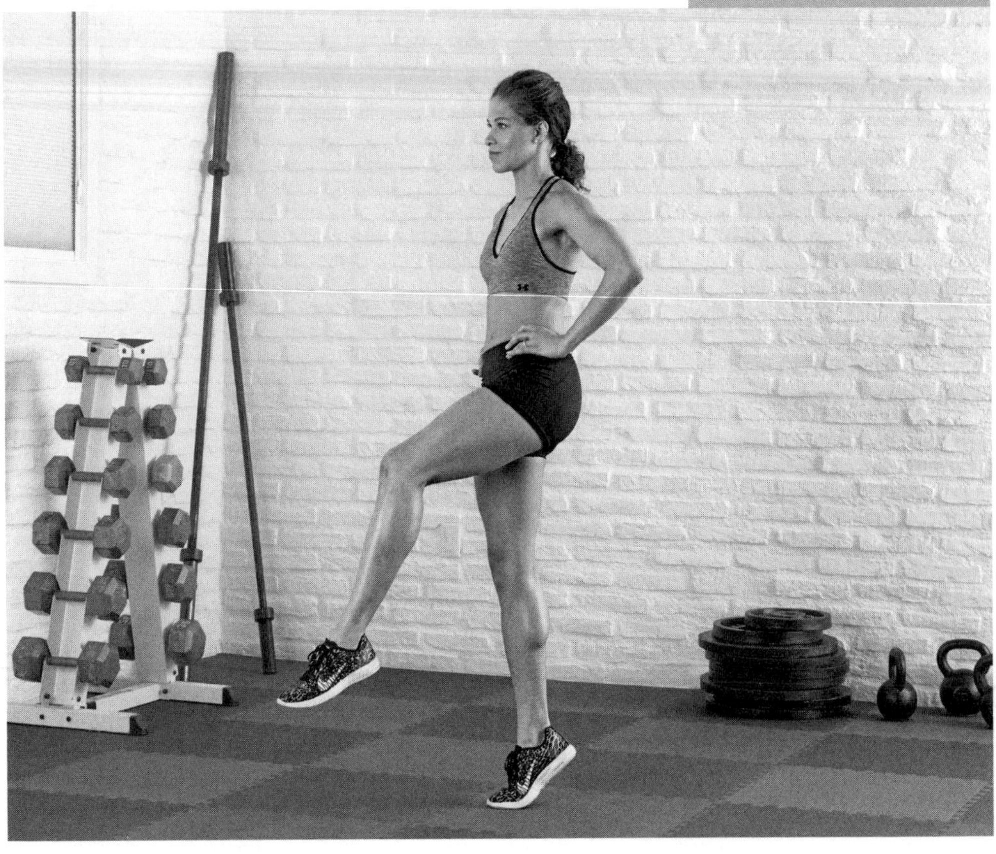

BRIDGE WITH ALTERNATING HIP FLEXION

(15 reps per side)

Strengthens the outer hip muscles and glutes

Lie on your back with your knees bent and feet on the ground. Raise your butt up off the ground and squeeze. Lift your right foot off the ground and make sure that your right hip does not dip down. Lower your right foot and repeat the move on the left side for a full set.

MAKE IT HARDER:
Perform a full set per side rather than alternating.

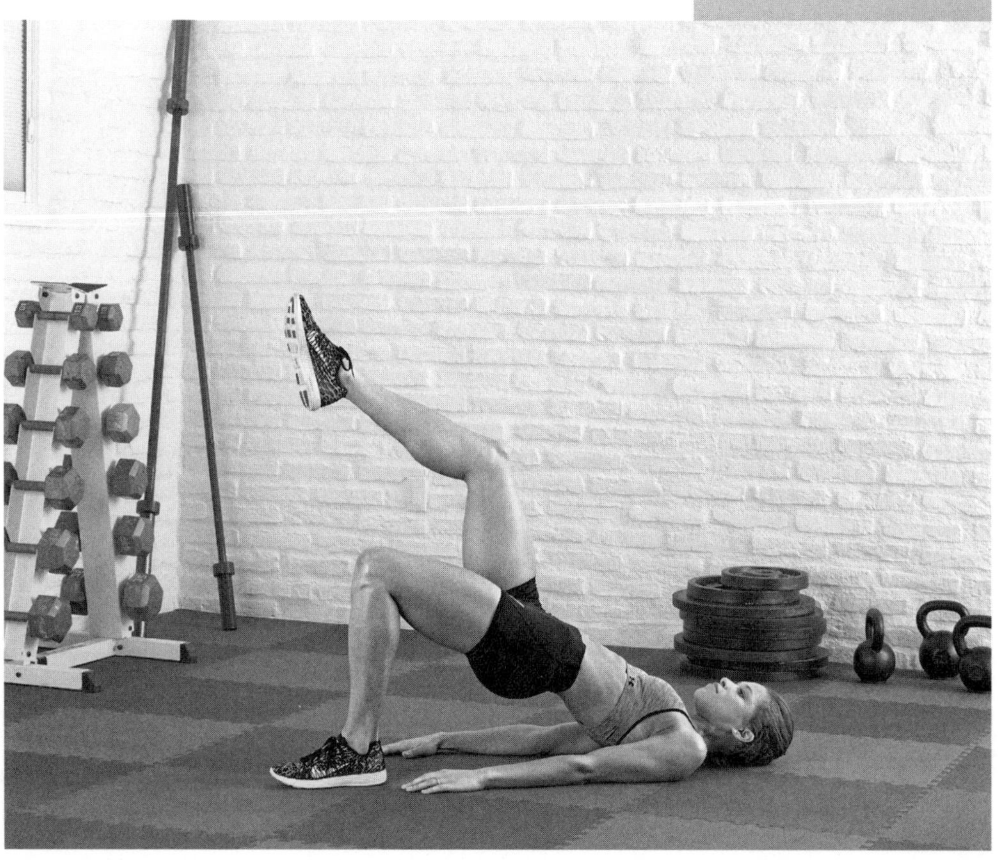

PLANK WITH KNEE DIPS

(10 dips per side)

Strengthens the abdominals, shoulders, hips, and glutes

Get into a pushup position, extending your arms so your hands are on the floor directly beneath your shoulders and your legs are straight with your weight on the balls of your feet. Keep your abs taut and your body in a straight line. Pull your abs in and slowly drop and tap the floor with your left knee. Straighten your left leg and repeat the move with the right knee. Return to a straight plank position for a full set.

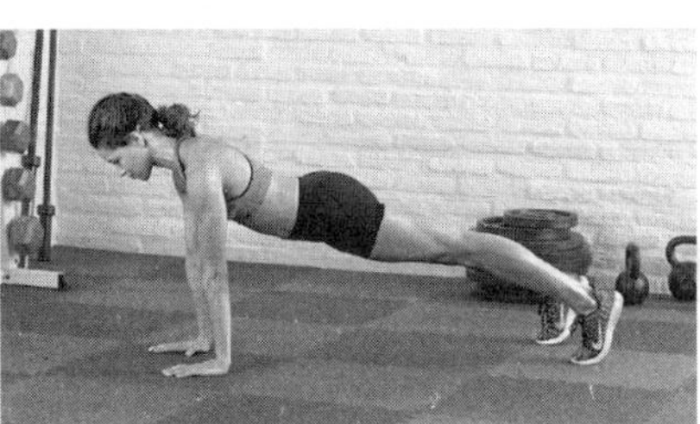

MAKE IT HARDER:
Perform the same move with your elbows bent.

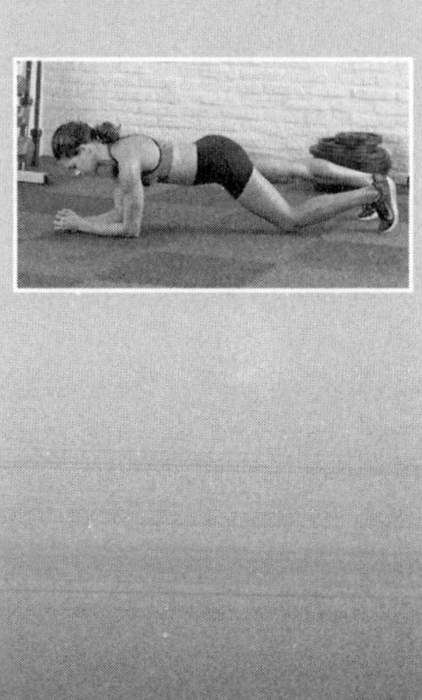

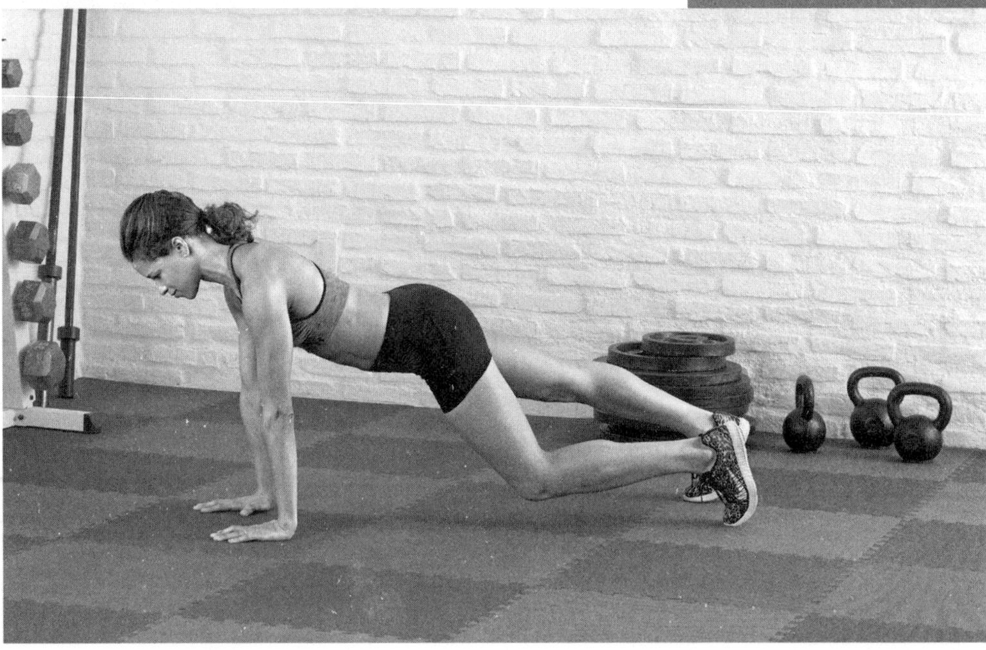

SIDE PLANK

(Hold for 20 to 30 seconds per side.)

Strengthens the abdominals, obliques, and shoulders

Lie on your right side with your legs extended and feet and hips stacked. Prop your upper body up on your right elbow and forearm. Raise your hips until your body forms a straight line from your ankles to your shoulders. Hold this position. Flip around so that you're lying on your left side and repeat. For a beginner modification, bend your knees and keep your lower legs on the ground.

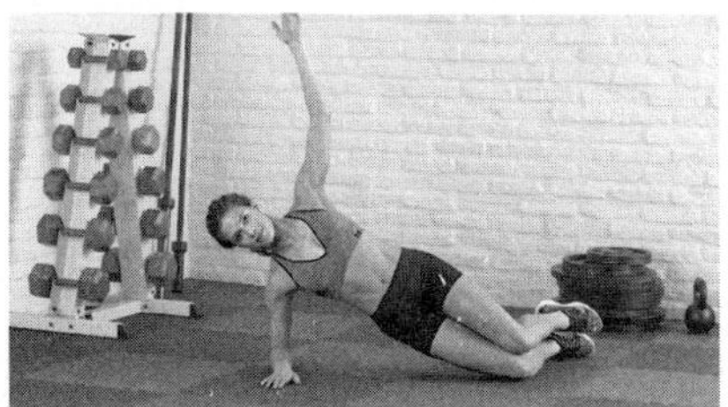

MAKE IT HARDER:
Add a twist. Bend your top (nonsupporting) arm and put that hand behind your head, elbow pointed toward the ceiling. Keeping hips stacked, slowly rotate your torso, bringing your elbow toward the floor. Rotate to start. Repeat for a set of 6 to 8 reps. Then switch sides.

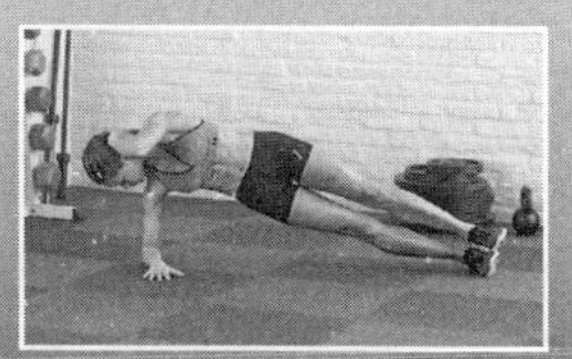

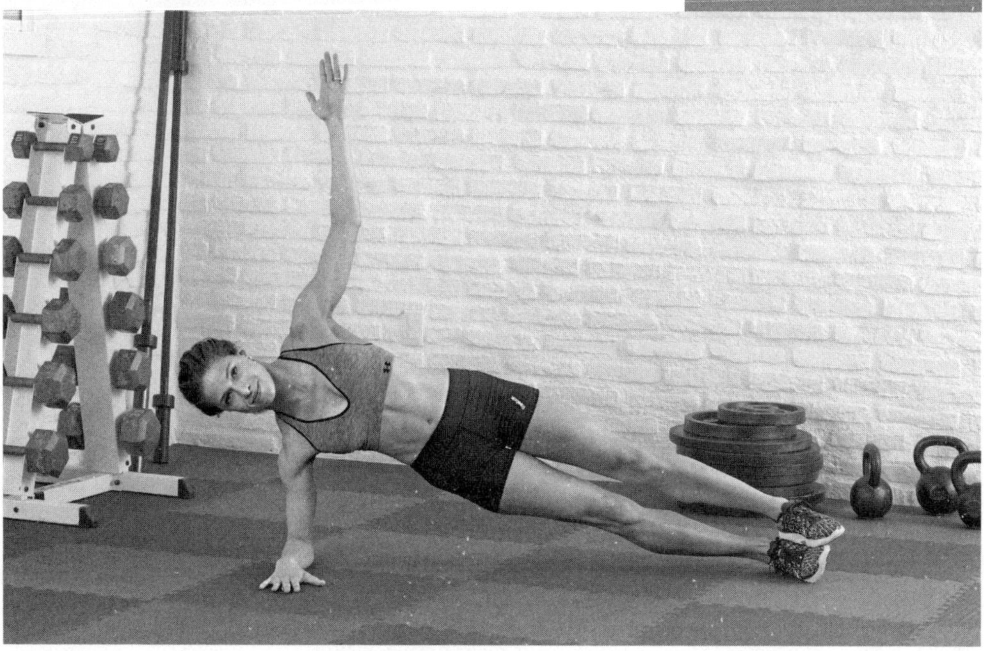

WHAT'S YOUR ACL RISK?

Are you at high risk for ACL injury? Medical director for the WNBA Las Vegas Aces Laura Ramus, PT, ATC, who is the residency director at DMC Sports Physical Therapy and has run programs devoted to ACL tear prevention, says you can answer that question with a few simple screens. "We examined almost 1,000 athletes and came up with an eight-point screening program to predict an athlete's risk," she says. Her goal is to make this screening preseason protocol for girls entering sports, but you can use it, too. Here's what to look for:

FOOT TYPE: Check your feet. Do you have either flat feet or high arches? Both increase ACL injury risk. Flat feet predispose you to pronation (a foot that collapses inward), so your knees are more likely to cave in when you land. High-arched feet are rigid, so your ankles may not flex enough when you jump, putting more stress on your knees.

FLEXIBILITY: Bend your wrist and try to touch your thumb to your arm. If you reach, you're excessively flexible, which increases your risk because your muscles have to work extra hard to keep your body in proper alignment when you stop suddenly and/or change directions on the run.

QUAD DOMINANCE: Hop up and down. What muscles do you feel working most? If you feel your quads springing into action first, you, like many women, are quad dominant. You need to practice engaging your glutes and using them as your prime mover to protect your knees.

LANDING STABILITY: Stand on a step or box and jump down. Your knees should bend straight out in front of you when you land. Caving in is a big red flag for ACL injury risk.

GLUTE STRENGTH: Glute strength and pelvic stability are paramount for healthy knees. Stand on the edge of a step so your foot runs parallel with the step and let one leg dangle off the edge. Does your pelvis stay square or droop? Any dipping means weak glutes and puts you at risk.

CORE STRENGTH: Lie on your back and bend your hips and knees 90 degrees. Contract your abs and try to pull your knees to your chest. Can't make it? You're far from alone. Most of the athletes Ramus screens can't. It means you have a tight back, weak core, and poor trunk stability, which are directly related to a higher risk of ACL injury.

LEG DOMINANCE: Draw a square on the floor and hop forward and back and side-to-side as many times as you can on your right leg for 30 seconds. Then repeat with your left. The results should be within 10 percent of each other. If not, you have too much leg dominance on one side.

SQUAT FORM: Hold a broomstick overhead and squat down so your hips fall below knee level. Your heels should stay firmly planted on the floor and the stick directly overhead. If your heels come up or the stick falls forward, you're a candidate for an ACL injury.

THINK MOBILITY OVER FLEXIBILITY

You can't address core stability without talking about flexibility, and more importantly, mobility, which is what women should really concentrate on. Simply being flexible, as many women are, is not necessarily advantageous when it comes to having optimum mobility—the ability to move your body the way you want without being restricted by stiffness or imbalances, or, of course, injury.

To explain it, I've called in the assistance of mobility expert Kelly Starrett, DPT, of the Ready State, whose book *Becoming a Supple Leopard* is one of the best books on the subject I've ever seen.

"Flexibility describes the properties of a rubber hose," says Dr. Starrett. When most people talk about flexibility, they're talking about their range of motion around a joint, which has more to do with connective tissues such as ligaments than it does muscles. We know that women have higher levels of a hormone aptly named relaxin that softens and relaxes ligaments in the joints, creating elasticity of the connective tissues. This may weaken the ability of your lumbar spine (lower back) to withstand impact and twisting forces, which increases your risk of knee injuries and lower-back injuries, which are even more common during PMS and menstruation.

There are also women who are hypermobile, such as longtime yogis and gymnasts. "When your tissues are more lax, your joints don't have the integrity they should because they're stretched out," says Dr. Starrett. This impairs your proprioception, the sense of where your limbs are oriented in space and in relation to one another, which is a huge factor in mobility and stability. When you're not getting that proprioceptive feedback, your movement patterns are thrown off. That's why it's actually advantageous to have a little healthy stiffness in the joints as opposed to being very lax.

Dr. Starrett says, "A stiff athlete leans into the stiffness for support as they move. When you're hypermobile, you have to actually know the end of your range of motion in a conscious way."

Everyone's lumbar spine has some wedge-shaped vertebrae—similar to wedge-shaped bricks or stones that architects use to create arches—that create the natural curvature of the spine. Women have three of these wedge-shaped vertebrae as opposed to just two in men. This again is one of Mother Nature's pregnancy-preparation designs. As a pregnant woman's belly grows, she can lean back farther (up to 28 degrees) through the spine to balance her center of gravity over her hips and maintain her balance. The downside of this adaptive feature is that some women become permanently stretched into a position of exaggerated lumbar curvature, which in turn tips your pelvis forward and starts inhibiting muscles in the trunk and pelvic floor, which can lead to incontinence problems.

BRACE YOURSELF

A properly braced neutral spine is the bedrock from which all safe, dynamic, and high-volume athletic movement is generated, says Dr. Kelly Starrett, who teaches a bracing sequence I highly recommend all women practice until it becomes automatic. The beauty of this sequence from Dr. Starrett's book *Becoming a Supple Leopard* is that it starts with your feet and works systematically up to your head to ensure that you address any improper postures that you might have adopted over time. Practice this on its own a few times a day and employ it before strength training.

STEP 1: SCREW YOUR FEET INTO THE GROUND

Position your feet directly under your hips and parallel to each other. Now screw your feet into the ground by exerting force in an outward direction from your hips. Externally rotate your right hip and press your right foot into the ground in a clockwise direction and externally rotate your left hip and press your left foot into the ground in a counterclockwise position.

STEP 2: SQUEEZE YOUR BUTT

Set your pelvis in the proper, neutral position by squeezing your glutes. Activate your glutes and then reduce the tension to maintain a neutral pelvic position.

STEP 3: INHALE AND LOCK IT IN

Your glutes set your pelvis in position, and your abs lock it in. Lock your pelvis and rib cage in place by taking a big breath in through your diaphragm with your glutes squeezed.

STEP 4: EXHALE AND BALANCE YOUR RIB CAGE

Exhale, and as you do, balance your rib cage over your pelvis and tighten your belly. You're not sucking in or drawing in your belly. You're stiffening it into place as you exhale. This creates intra-abdominal pressure around your spine.

STEP 5: NEUTRALIZE YOUR HEAD AND SHOULDERS

Rotate your shoulders back, widen your collarbones, and turn your palms up toward the sky. As you do, center your head over your shoulders, focusing your eyes forward. The goal is to set your head and shoulders in a neutral position and to align your ears over your shoulders, hips, and ankles.

STEP 6: FULLY BRACED

Let your arms fall to your sides so your thumbs point forward and your shoulders remain externally rotated. You should be standing with your ears over your shoulders, your rib cage over your pelvis, and your hips over your knees and ankles, fully braced and ready to go.

Even if you never get pregnant, your spine can become similarly compromised if you spend a lot of your time in high-heeled shoes, because they put you in a similar position where your body is being tipped forward—this time by the high heels—and you compensate by leaning back. "I see a lot of professional women who have their lumbar spine in a terrible position all the time, and the body adapts around that position," says Dr. Starrett.

Your spine isn't the only joint structure that is affected by spending inordinate amounts of time walking around in heels. With your feet in plantar flexion, your ankles are also affected. "Women who wear high heels most of the time end up with shorter heel cords, which in turn prevents the ankle from rotating and moving through its full range of motion when you're not in high heels," says Dr. Starrett. "You start to walk and strike the ground with your feet turned out to accommodate the shortened heel cord." In a 2010 study, researchers found that women who wore heels 2 inches or higher 5 or more days a week had calf muscles that were an average of 13 percent shorter and Achilles tendons that were significantly thicker than their flat-shoe-wearing counterparts.

Put it all together—the naturally curved lumbar spine, possibly shortened heel cords, and the wider pelvis that creates a bit of knock-kneed stance—and you can see why proper mobility absolutely trumps flexibility. Wearing heels as little as possible can help, as can the strengthening moves in the simple plan for injury prevention beginning on page 110. The exercises not only help to build injury-preventing strength but can also improve your stability and mobility.

ROAR ▶▶▶ SOUND BITES

▶ Your "core" is more than your abs: It's everything but your limbs. Women especially need to strengthen theirs to protect their joints.

▶ Kick the crunches to the curb. You spend enough time bending forward. Switch to planks instead.

▶ Flexibility is overrated and sometimes detrimental. Aim for optimum mobility instead.

▶ Too much time in high heels can harm your calves and back.

▶ Your glutes and hips are your body's steering wheel. Keep them strong for better balance and stability.

7

POWER UP

BEING STRONG IS ESSENTIAL

As a woman, you have few precious natural resources as important as your muscles. They're what keep you strong, able, and independent. They're also frighteningly easy to lose. Around age 30, women begin to lose muscle density. Lean muscle mass slips away to the tune of about 3 percent per decade between the ages of 30 and 80, while strength declines 30 percent between the ages of 50 and 70 and takes a major nosedive after that.

The researchers of the landmark Framingham Disability Study drove this home when they reported that 40 percent of women between the ages of 55 and 64, 45 percent of women between 65 and 74, and 65 percent of women between 75 and 84 reported they could not lift 10 pounds! Ten pounds! That's a bag of cat food.

As women, we start out with less muscle than our male peers, and we lose more with age because our hormones aren't conducive to muscle making. Although estrogen (specifically estradiol/E2) is anabolic in nature, progesterone counters it with a significant catabolic influence when it is elevated. So yeah, it can be harder for us to build muscle, especially as we age. But it's not impossible!

It just means you need to train hard. All the cardio in the world won't cut it. Research on women, especially past age 40, shows that even high levels of aerobic activity don't translate into any meaningful changes in lean body mass. The only solution is strength training, strength training, strength training. And I don't mean doing "toning" exercises with 5-pound dumbbells. I mean high-intensity power training—heavy lifting for pure strength. This kind of training stimulates your neuromuscular system, activating the maximum amount of muscle fibers. It also keeps those high-energy, powerful type II muscle fibers engaged, which is essential because those are needed for speed, and they're the first to go.

Research shows that when endurance athletes slow down with age, a major reason why is that their muscles simply aren't contracting as quickly and as powerfully as they used to. This slowdown is preventable—and fixable—with strength training.

Strong legs lead to a more powerful foot strike and rebound off the ground when you're running. They punch pedals with more force when you're sprinting out of the saddle on your bike. And they propel you against gravity when you're climbing hills. As if all that weren't enough reason to grab some weights, resistance training also strengthens your connective tissues and can help you avoid injury.

The best part is that the benefits of strength training are nearly immediate. Even before your muscles get bigger and stronger, you wake up sleeping muscle fibers and develop neuromuscular connections that result in strength gains after just a few sessions.

THE ROAR RULES FOR MAKING MUSCLE

Here's what you need to know to optimize your strength-training results.

Lift heavy. While there are certainly exceptions, far too many women still simply will not lift weight that is heavy enough to optimally increase strength and stimulate hypertrophy (muscle growth). For this to happen, you need to challenge and stimulate your muscles so they break down and repair bigger and stronger.

How heavy is heavy enough? Pick up a weight and lift it 8 times. How hard are those last 2 reps? You have chosen the right weight if you are barely able to eke out that final rep while maintaining good form. If you could easily do two or three more, you need to go heavier. That being said, there is an endless stream of videos online of poorly coached weight lifters using far too heavy weight while contorting themselves in awful ways that are bound to lead to injury. Don't do that either. Heavy weight plus good form equals great results. Too little weight is a waste of time. More than you can lift with good form is counterproductive. You can also opt for body-weight exercises, which can be extremely effective as long as you reach the same point of fatigue, which is quite easy to do with pushups and single-leg squats. When lifting, always remember to brace yourself, keep a strong neutral spine, and engage your core for maximum efficiency and results.

As a general rule, aim to perform two or three sets of about 6 to 8 repetitions (or less) in the suggested time frame. Perimenopausal and postmenopausal women should prioritize lifting heavy, aiming for three to five sets of 3 to 5 reps with 3 to 5 minutes of recovery between sets at 80 percent of their 1 rep max. Lifting heavy helps stimulate muscle maintenance and development as hormones shift and decline.

Lift often. Try to fit strength training into your schedule 2 to 3 days a week. Three is preferable, but you'll still see benefits from two. Twenty minutes of focused work is all it takes!

Mix it up. There are countless exercises to choose from, and variety is your friend when it comes to making muscle. Remember, your body adapts to the challenges you present it with. When you keep doing the same exercises over and over, your body gets bored and you stop making gains, or worse, you backslide! No one wants to do hard work for nothing. So mix up your routine at least every 2 to 3 weeks.

BODY-WEIGHT MOVES

I find one way to keep it fresh is to drop the dumbbells, get out of the gym, and do some total-body power moves, and for the more advanced, do these with a weighted backpack or weight vest. Medicine balls and kettlebells are great for this (more on that later), but you can get a killer workout without any equipment. The following are my go-to moves for strengthening with body weight, no equipment required.

SQUAT

(60 seconds)

Strengthens the glutes, hamstrings, quads, and core

Stand with your feet hip-width apart and toes pointed forward. Push your butt and hips back as if you're sitting in a chair and lower down as far as possible while keeping your weight on your heels and extending your arms overhead. Return to the starting position and repeat.

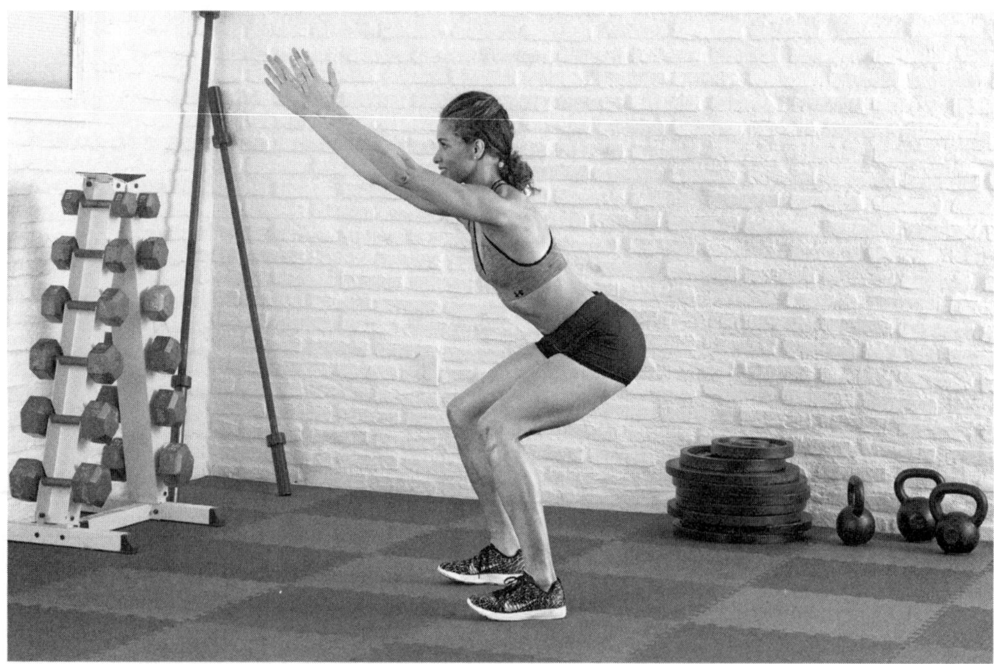

PISTOL SQUAT

(however many you can!)

Strengthens the glutes, hamstrings, quads, calves, and core

Stand on your right foot with the left foot off the floor and leg extended in front of you. Bend your right leg and press your hips back, lowering yourself down as if you're sitting in a chair. Drop as low as possible while keeping good form, trying to get the back of your thigh and your calf to touch (this might take a while!). For more support, hold on to a stable surface with one hand. Return to the starting position and repeat on the left leg.

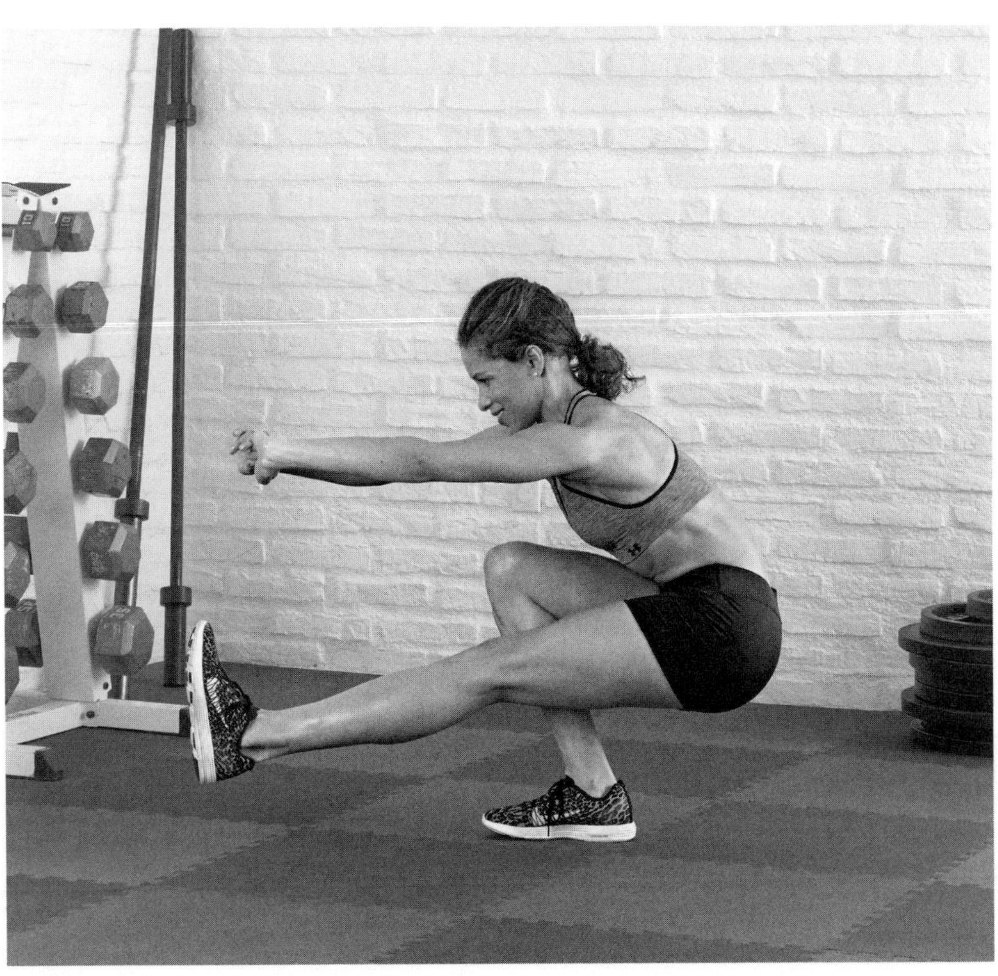

X LUNGE

(60 seconds)

Strengthens the glutes, hamstrings, quads, and core

Stand with your feet shoulder-width apart, toes pointed forward, and hands on hips. Take a giant step diagonally forward with your right leg, crossing in front of the left. Keeping your back straight, bend your knees and lower your hips toward the floor until your right leg is bent 90 degrees. Push back to start. Repeat with the other leg.

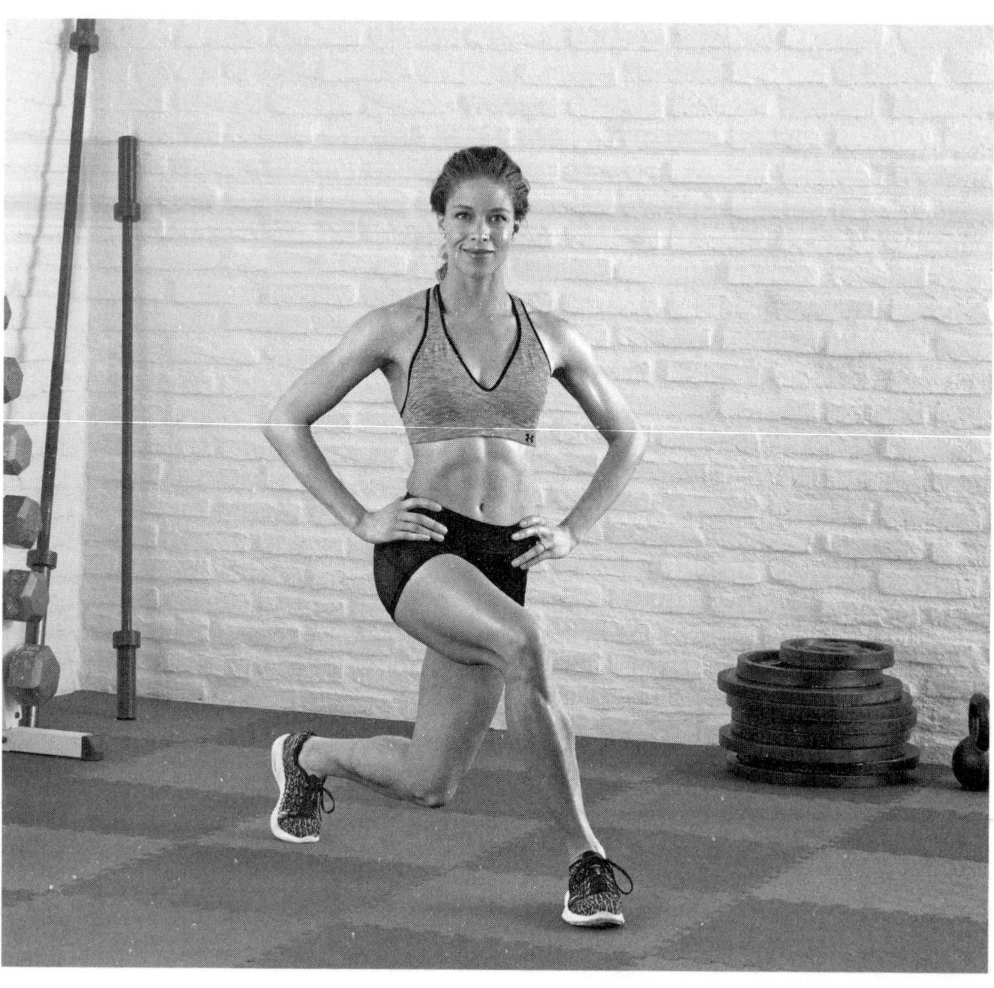

PUSHUP PLANK JUMP

(60 seconds)

Strengthens the chest, shoulders, triceps, core, glutes, hamstrings, quads, and calves

Start in a pushup position, engage your core, and lower down into a full pushup. Press back to the starting position and immediately jump your feet toward your hands, stopping in a crouched position with your arms extended parallel to the floor. Jump back into the starting pushup position. Repeat.

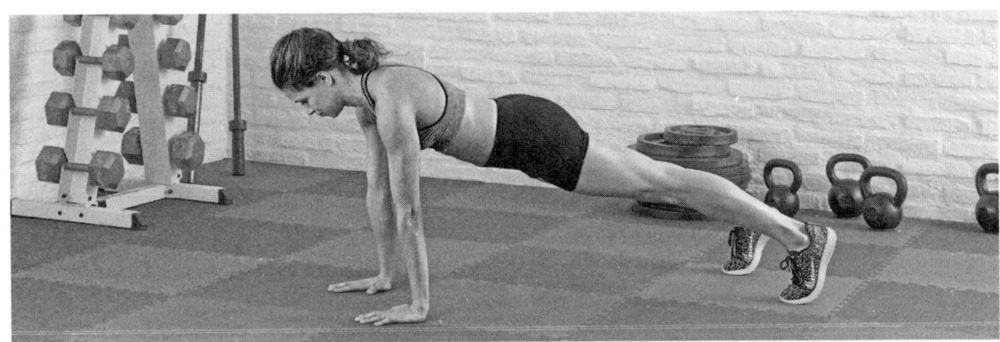

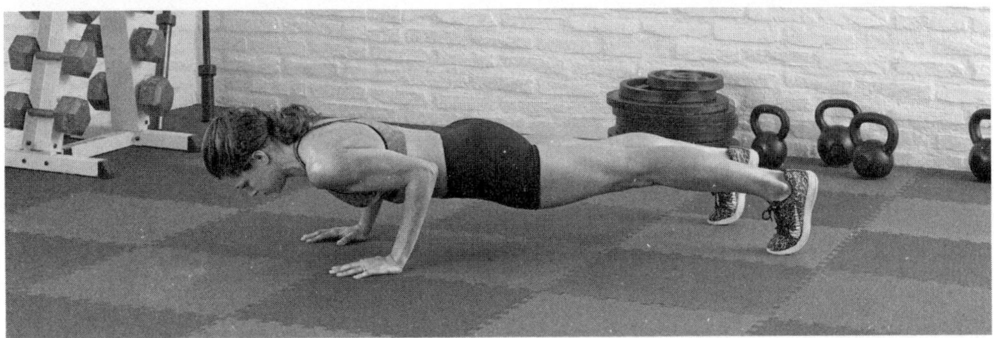

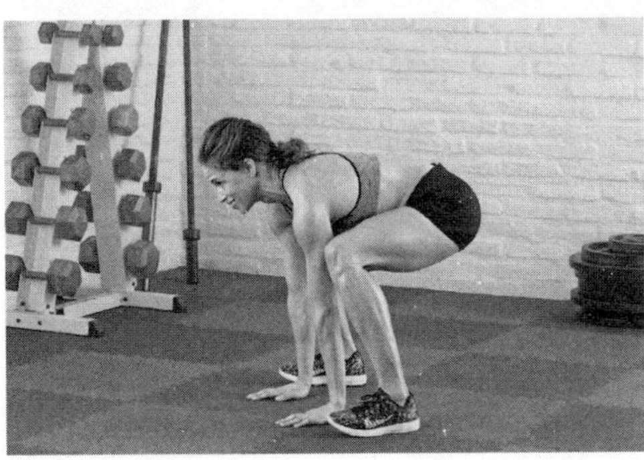

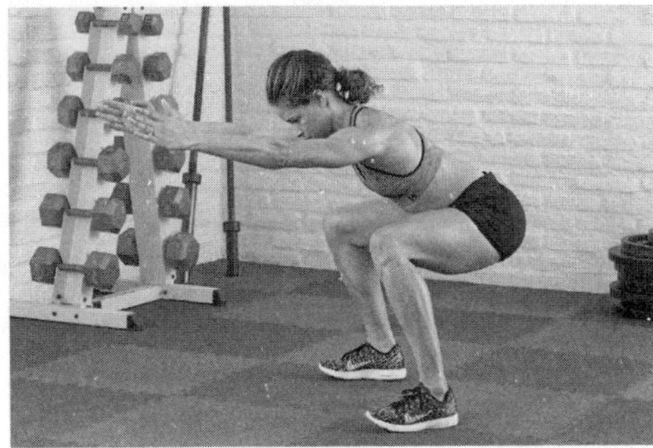

BURPEE

(60 seconds)

Strengthens the chest, shoulders, triceps, core, glutes, hamstrings, quads, and calves

Begin in a squat position with your hands on the floor in front of you. Kick your feet back into a pushup position. Immediately return your feet to the squat position. Leap up as high as possible from the squat position. Land softly, keeping your feet, knees, and hips in alignment and pointed straight ahead. Repeat.

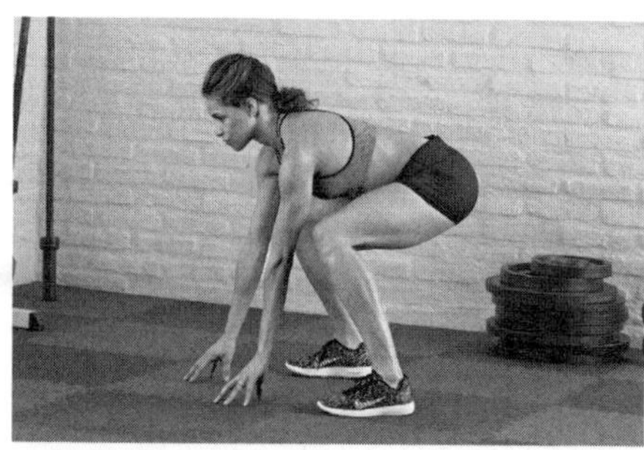

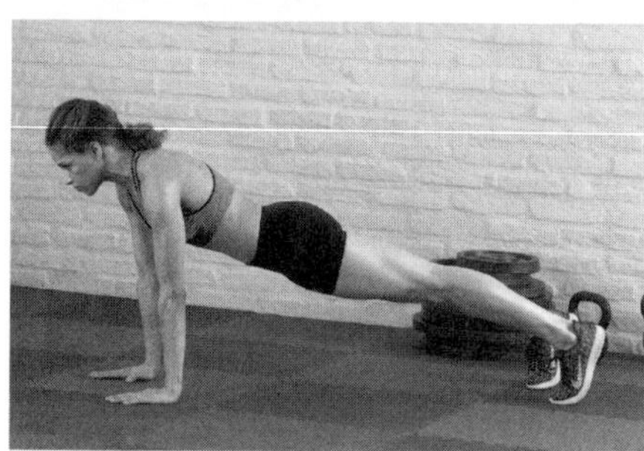

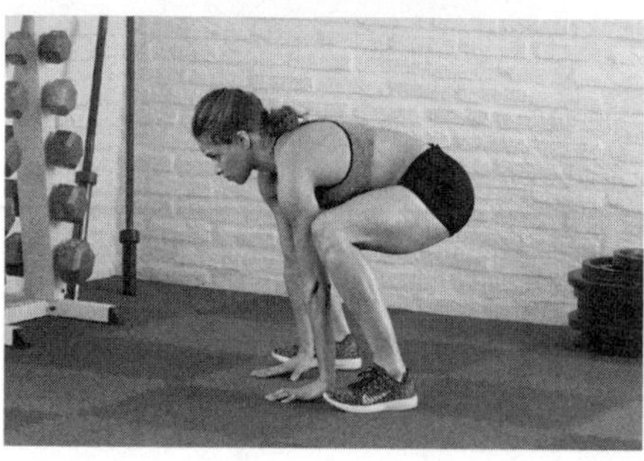

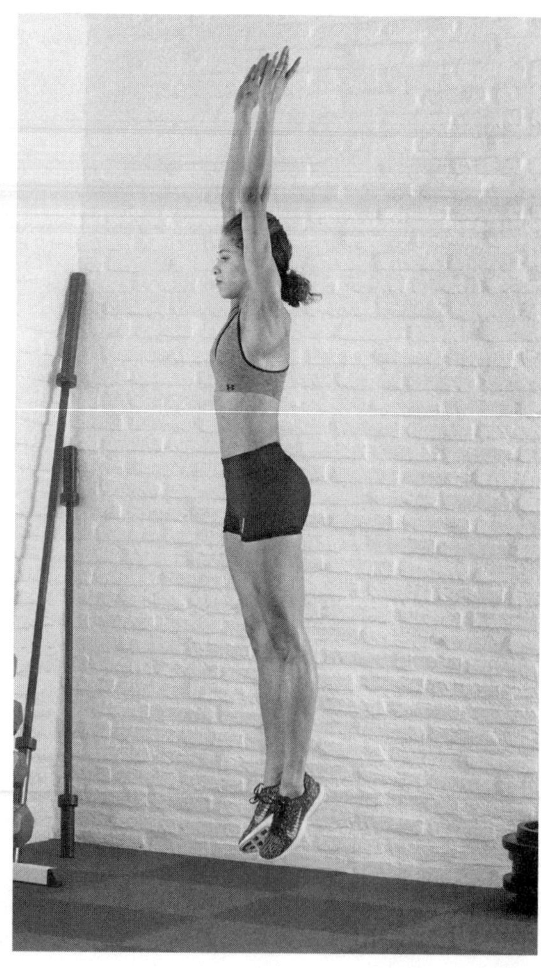

PLYOMETRIC JUMPS

Jumping builds explosive strength and bone strength. Just do it!

SINGLE-LEG JUMPING LUNGE

(30 to 60 seconds)

Strengthens the glutes, hamstrings, quads, calves, and core

Stand with your right leg forward and your left leg extended behind you. Bend your right knee and dip your left knee toward the floor so you're in a lunge position. Place your arms straight out in front of you or out to the sides. Swiftly jump up and switch legs in the air, landing in the opposite position. When the back knee grazes the ground, jump again. Keep jumping continuously without resting for a full set to each side.

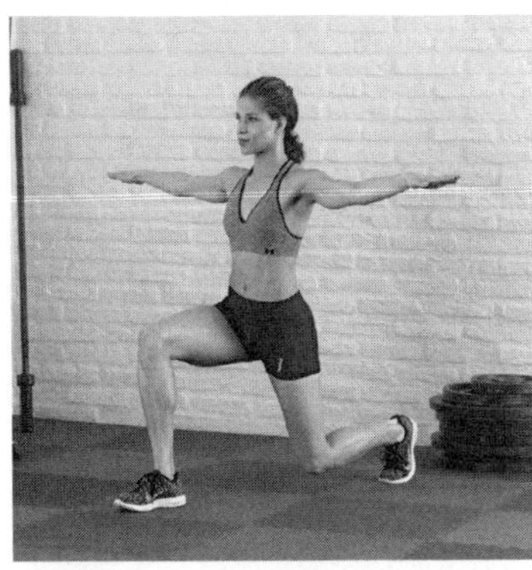

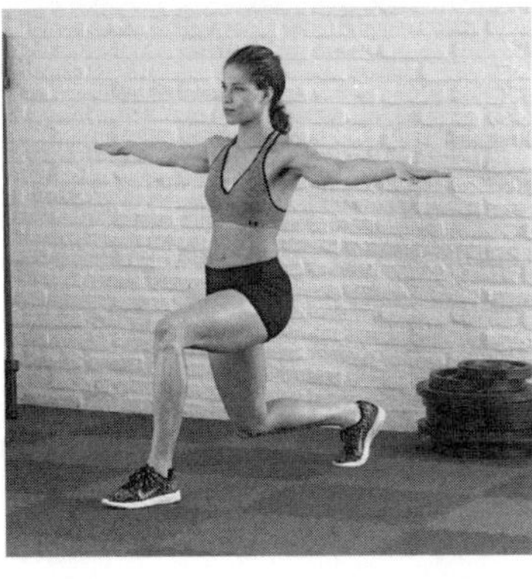

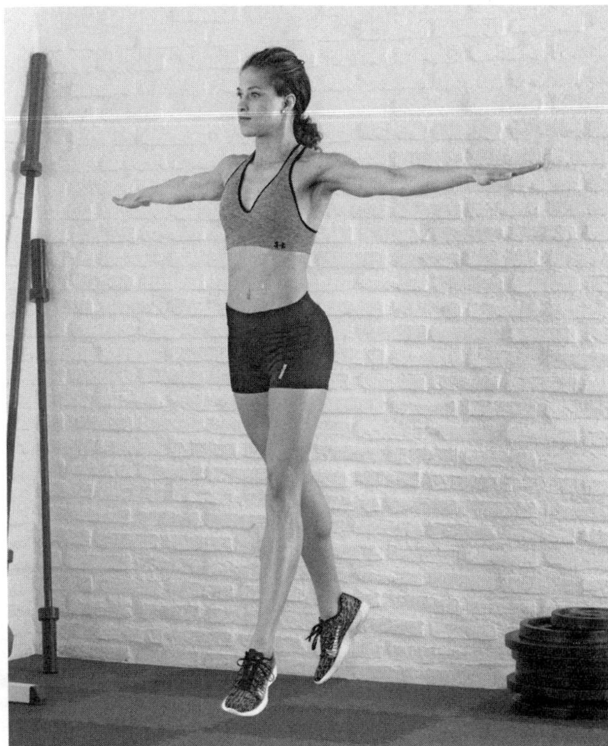

HIGH-KNEES POWER SKIP

(60 seconds)

Strengthens the glutes, hip flexors, hamstrings, quads, calves, and core

This looks like exaggerated skipping. Bound off your right foot, springing off your toes while thrusting your left knee forward and up. Land softly on the ball of your left foot, bending the left leg and immediately bounding forward again. Complete a full set to each side.

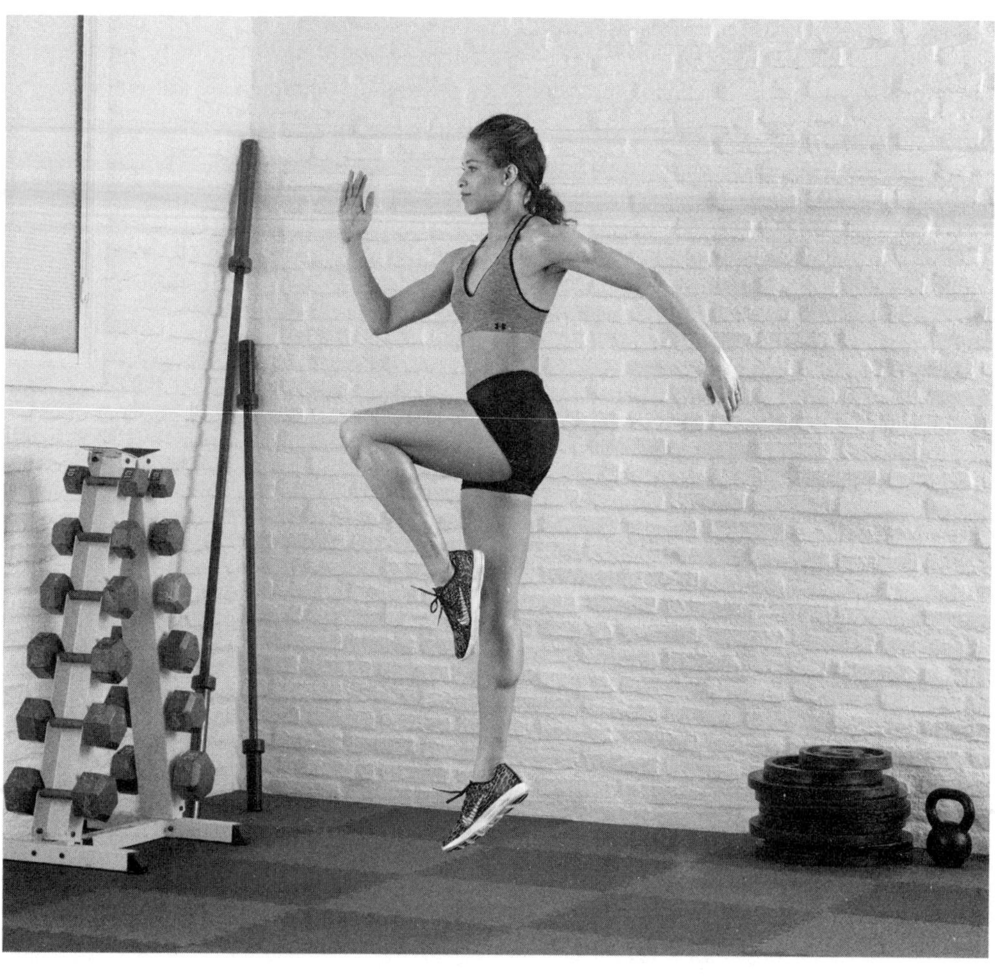

TUCK JUMP

(30 to 60 seconds)

Strengthens the glutes, hip flexors, hamstrings, quads, calves, and core

Stand with your feet shoulder-width apart and toes pointed straight ahead. Squat slightly as if sitting in a chair. Jump up, bringing both knees toward your chest. Try to bring your thighs parallel to the floor. Land softly, keeping your feet, knees, and hips in alignment and toes pointed straight ahead. Repeat.

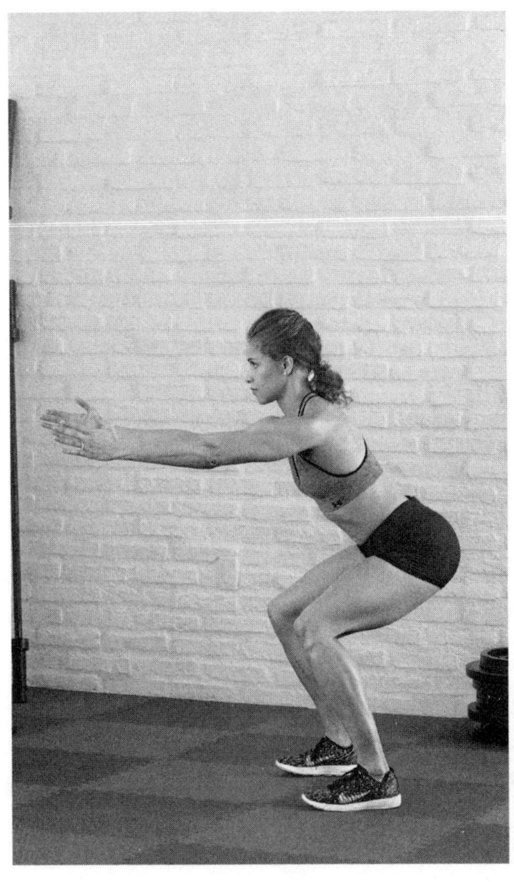

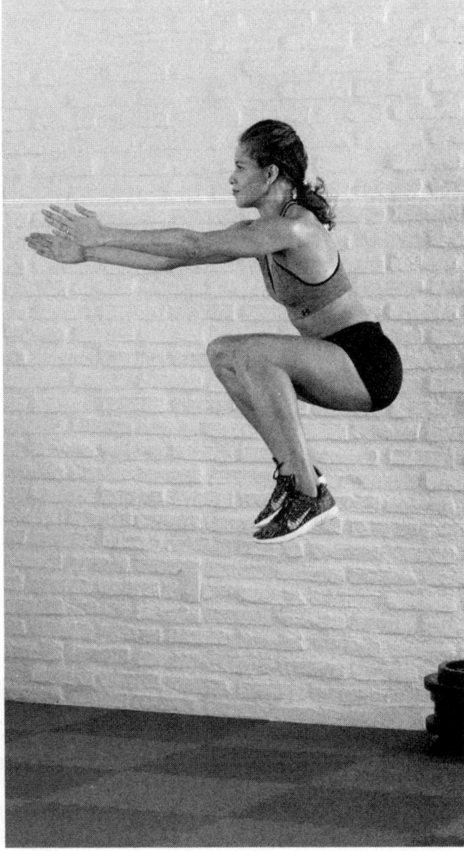

JUMP SQUAT

(30 to 60 seconds)

Strengthens the glutes, hamstrings, quads, calves, and core

Stand with your feet shoulder-width apart and toes pointed straight ahead. Squat as if sitting in a chair, extending your arms behind you. Swing your arms forward and jump up, extending arms overhead. Land softly, keeping your feet, knees, and hips in alignment and toes pointed straight ahead. Repeat.

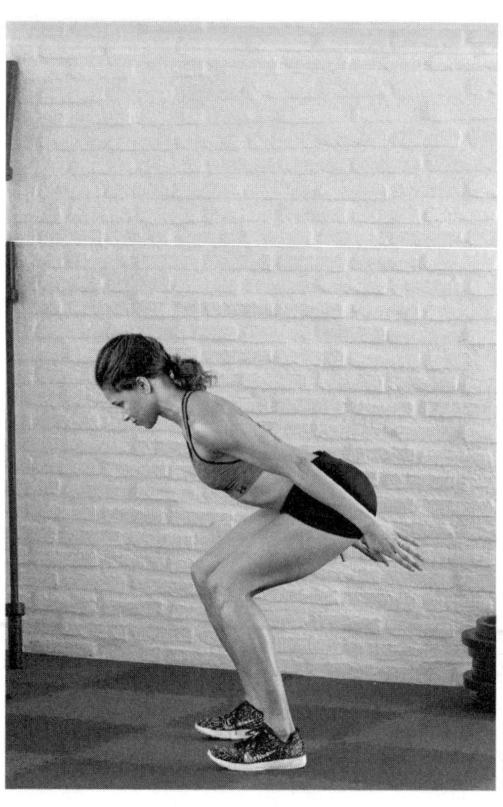

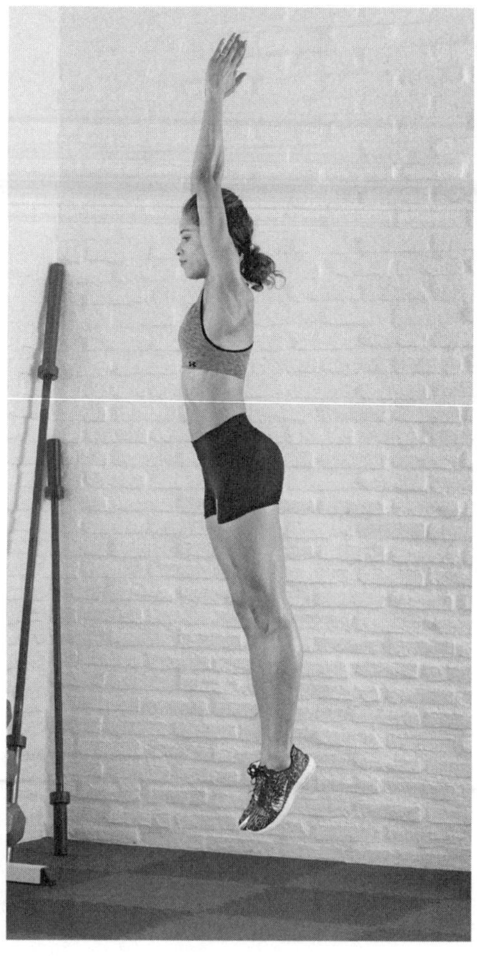

BOX JUMP

(30 to 60 seconds)

Strengthens the glutes, hip flexors, hamstrings, quads, calves, and core

Stand in front of a stable platform about 12 to 18 inches high. Squat down, swinging your arms back behind you. In one explosive move, swing your arms forward, spring up, and land on the box with soft knees, keeping your feet, knees, and hips in alignment and pointed straight ahead. Step down and repeat.

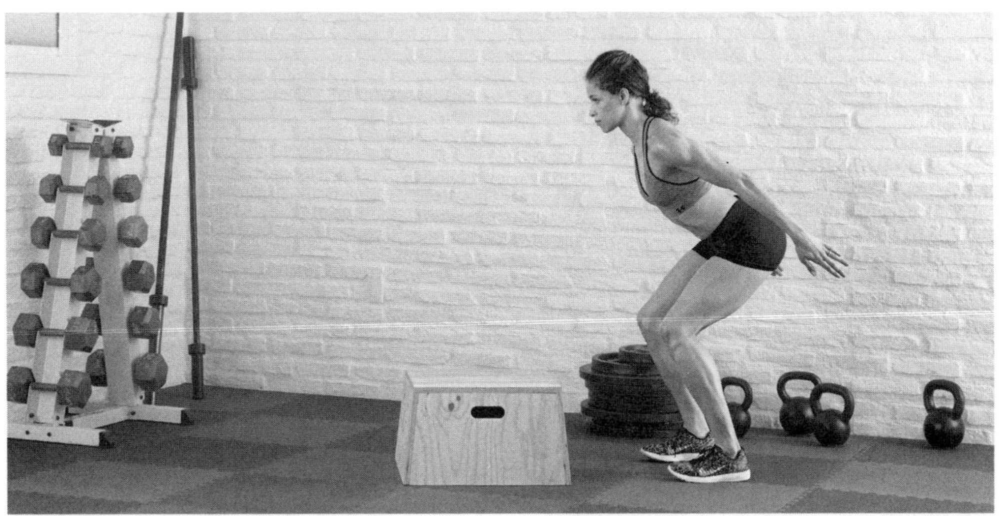

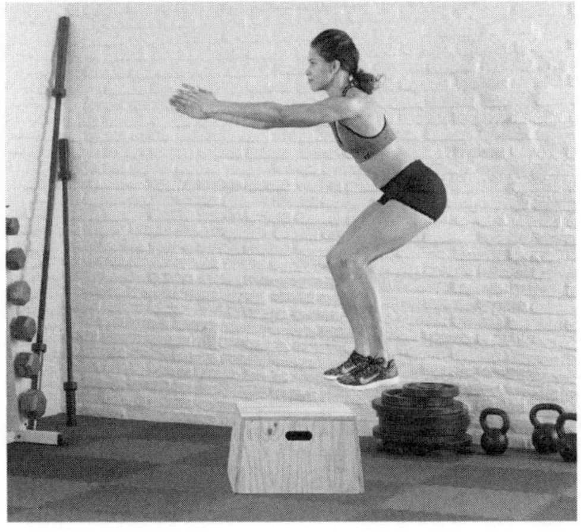

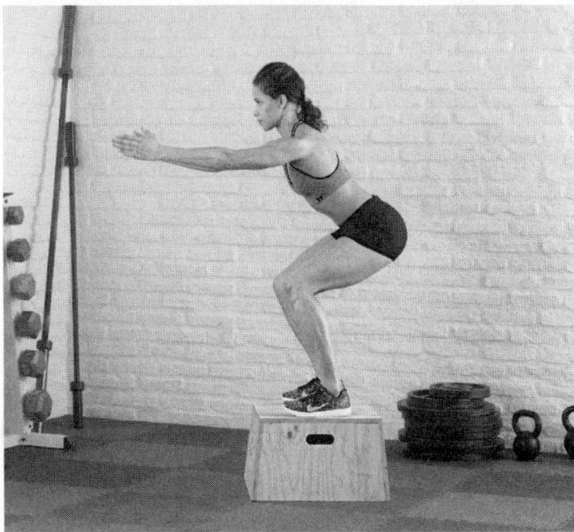

MEDICINE BALL MOVES

I love medicine balls because they're fun. There's a reason so many sports use balls, right? They make everything, even exercise, feel like a game. They're also really functional and effective. Most medicine ball moves work multiple muscles and are great for your core. Start with a ball that weighs 10 to 12 pounds.

MEDICINE BALL TWIST

(30 to 60 seconds)

Strengthens the abs and obliques

Sit on the floor while holding a medicine ball in both hands with shoulders relaxed, elbows bent, and arms pulled close to the sides of your body. Place your knees and feet about hip-width apart, heels on the floor, knees bent, and back straight. Pull your abs in tight, and with a straight back, lean back from the hips until you feel your abs engage. Keeping heels on the floor, abs engaged, and arms close to your body, twist from the waist to the left side. Twist back to the center starting position. Twist to the opposite (right) side. Return to the starting position to complete 1 rep. Continue alternating sides.

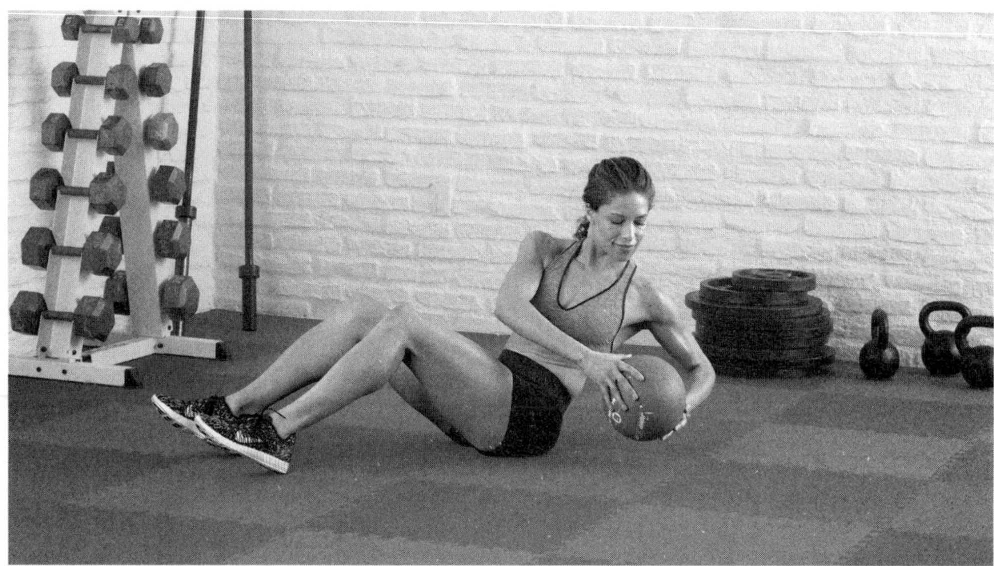

WALL BALL

(30 to 60 seconds)

Strengthens the glutes, hamstrings, quads, calves, shoulders, arms, and chest

Stand a couple of feet away from a wall, facing the wall, and holding a medicine ball at chest level, just below your chin. Perform a squat. Quickly and explosively stand back up, lift up onto your toes, and extend your arms forcefully to "pass" the ball to the wall so it bounces back to you. Catch the ball and bring it back to your body as you drop into another squat. Repeat.

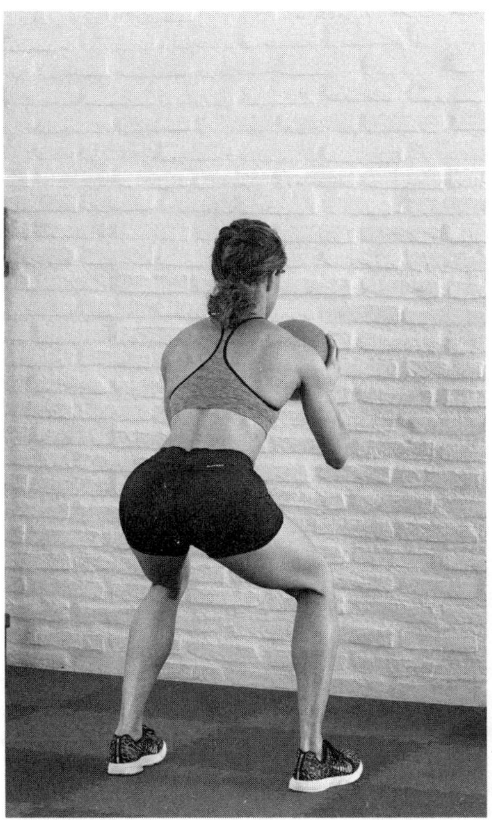

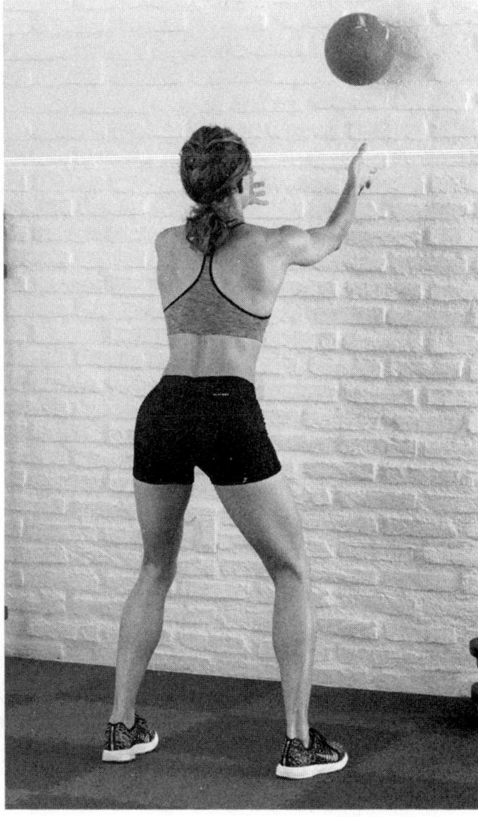

BALL SLAM

(30 to 60 seconds)

Strengthens the shoulders, lats, arms, and abs

Stand with your feet shoulder-width apart, knees slightly bent, and hold a medicine ball overhead. Contract your abs and throw the ball down to the ground in front of your feet with as much force as possible. Catch the ball as it bounces from the floor. Lift the medicine ball back to the starting position. Repeat.

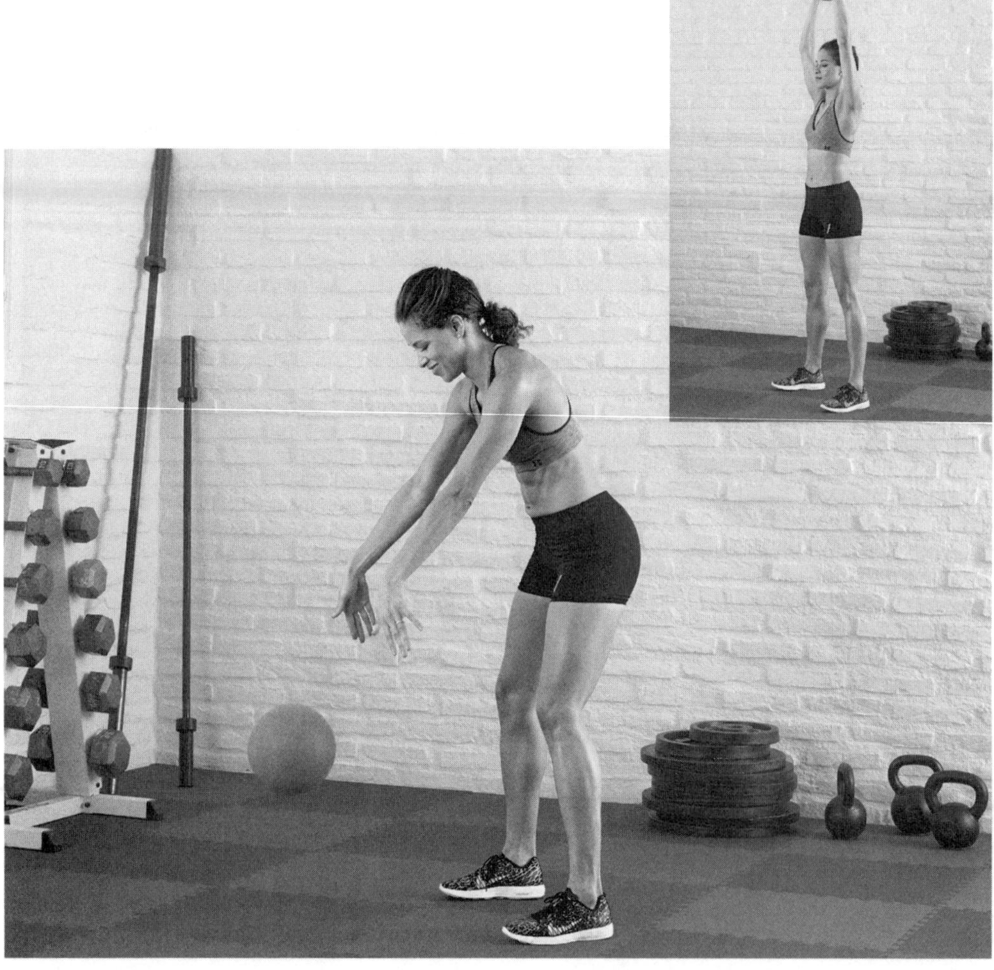

MEDICINE BALL CLEAN

(30 to 60 seconds)

Strengthens the glutes, hamstrings, quads, core, arms, and shoulders

Stand with feet slightly wider than shoulder-width apart. Place a medicine ball on the ground between your feet. Squat down with your hands outside of the ball and arms perpendicular to the ground. Grasping the ball, stand back up and push your hips forward as you simultaneously shrug your shoulders, drop into a squat, and bring your hands under the ball, so the ball is level with your head. Return to the standing position. Return the ball to the floor and repeat.

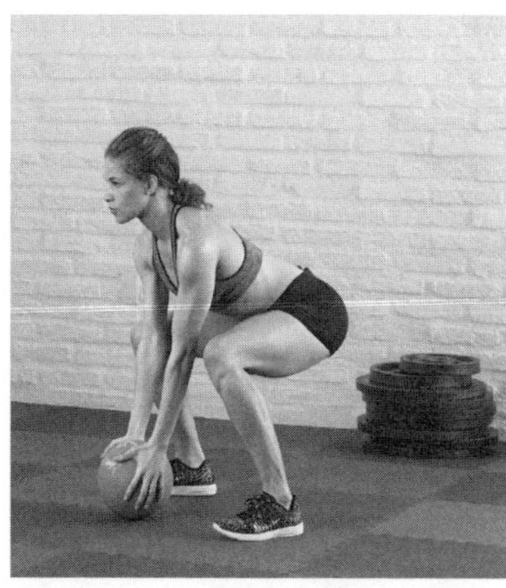

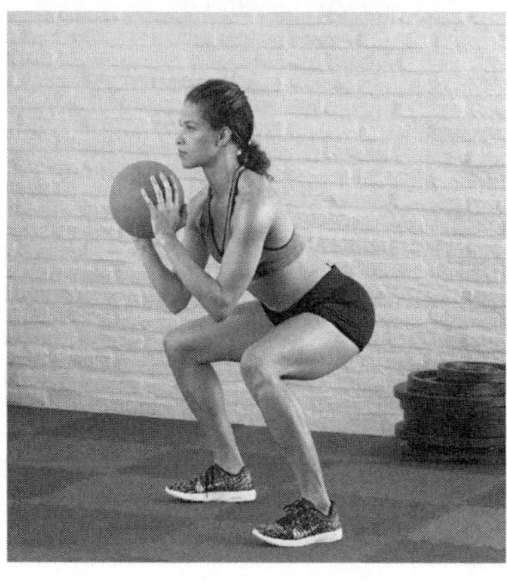

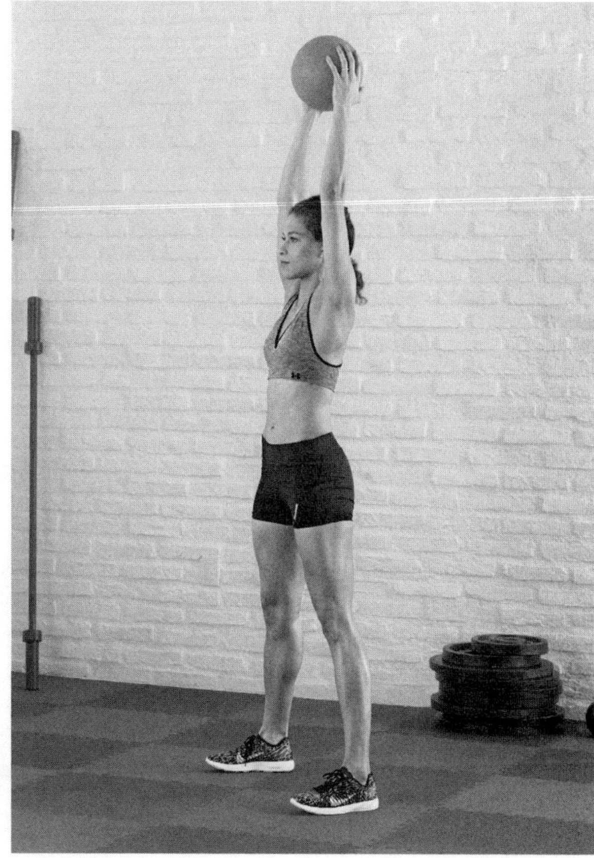

MEDICINE BALL THRUSTER

(30 to 60 seconds)

Strengthens the glutes, hamstrings, quads, core, arms, and shoulders

Stand with feet hip- to shoulder-width apart, feet facing forward, and hold a medicine ball close to your chest. Bend your hips and knees and squat back as if sitting in a chair until your thighs are parallel to the floor. Stand up, pushing your heels into the ground and extending your arms to press the medicine ball straight overhead. Return to the starting position. Repeat.

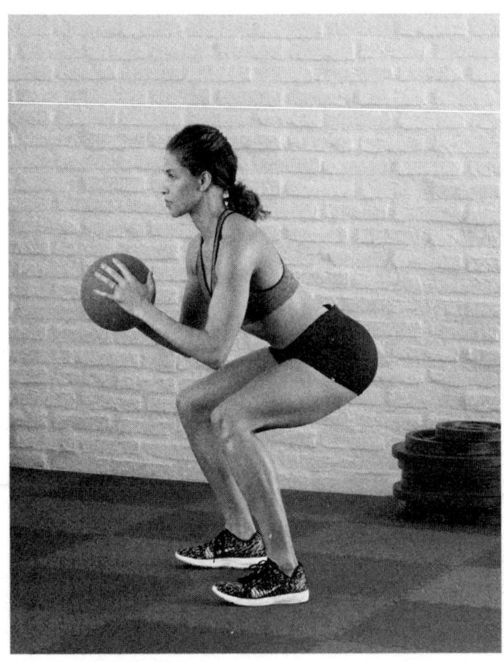

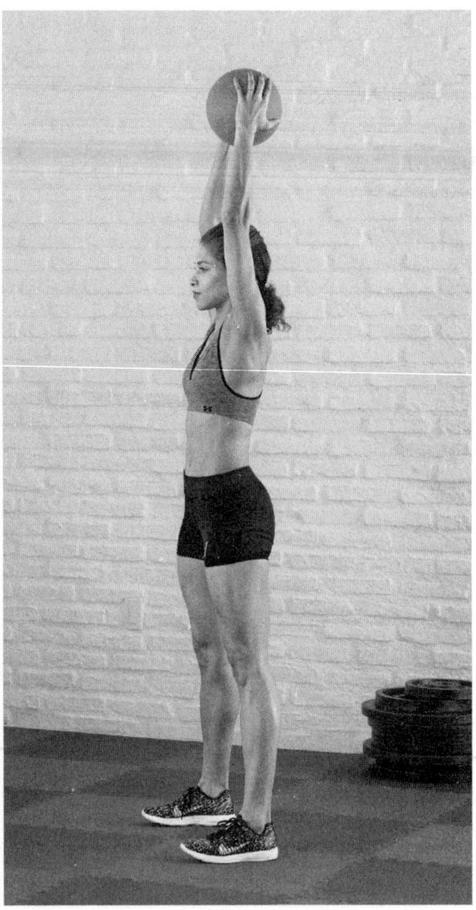

KETTLEBELL MOVES

Because the weight hangs below your hand, kettlebells provide an unstable form of resistance that puts your whole body on alert for every move. A 2010 study led by the American Council of Exercise reported that a 20-minute workout with kettlebells provided a perfect one-two cardio-strength punch to keep you aerobically fit while strengthening your hips, core, legs, and arms. The study also found that high-intensity kettlebell workouts burned about 272 calories in 20 minutes (about 14 calories a minute—the equivalent of running a 6-minute mile).

SINGLE-LEG DEADLIFT

(8 to 10 reps)

Strengthens the glutes, hamstrings, quads, and core

Hold a kettlebell by the handle in your right hand and stand on your right leg. With that knee slightly bent, bend at the hip, extending your left leg behind you for balance. Continue lowering the kettlebell until your torso is parallel to the ground. Return to the starting position. Repeat for a full set and switch sides.

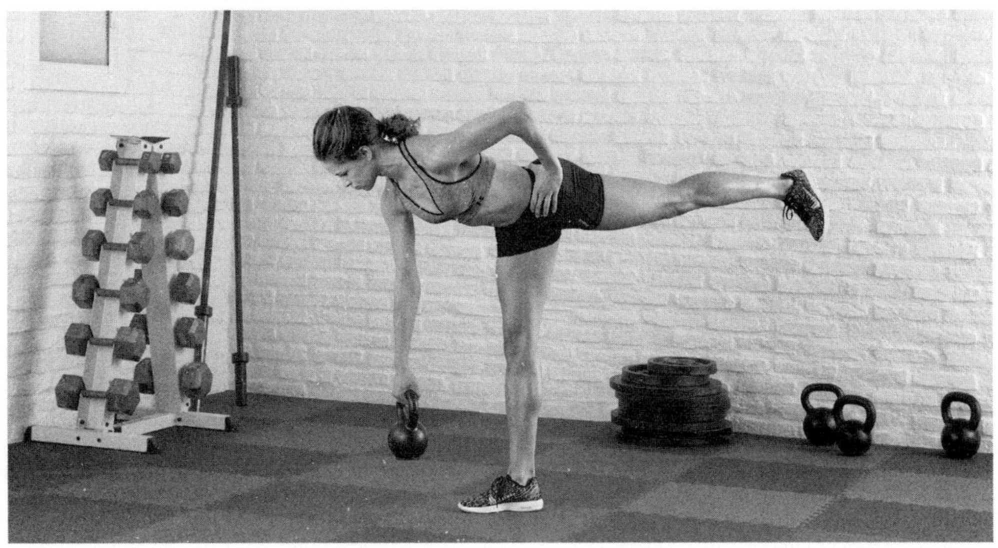

HANG HIGH PULL

(8 to 10 reps)

Strengthens the glutes, hamstrings, quads, core, arms, shoulders, and upper back

Stand with your legs in a straddle stance, toes pointed out 45 degrees, and hold a kettlebell in both hands, allowing the weight to hang down in front of your body. Perform a squat, lowering your hips down and back, lowering the weight until your thighs are parallel to the floor. Forcefully extend back to a standing position, bending your elbows out and up and pulling the kettlebell to chin height. Lower the weight back to the starting position. Repeat.

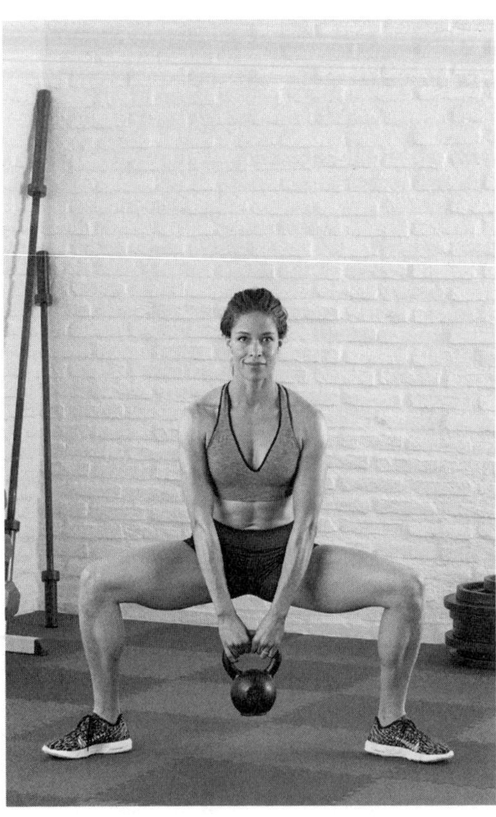

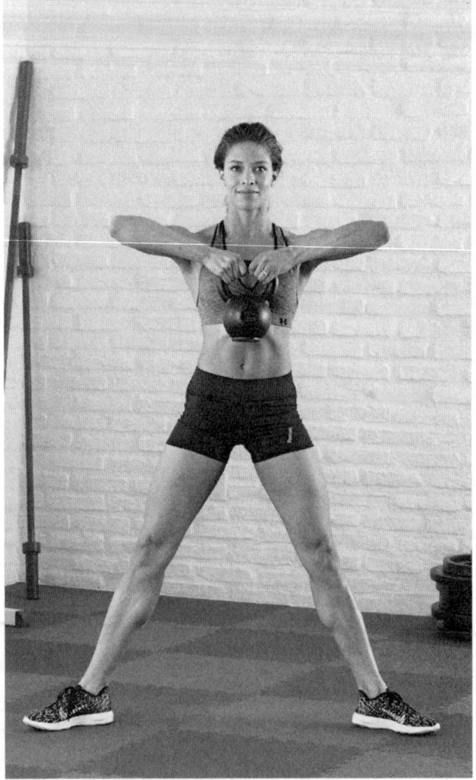

SNATCH, PULL, AND PUSH PRESS

(8 to 10 reps)

Strengthens the glutes, hamstrings, quads, core, arms, shoulders, and upper back

Stand with your feet shoulder-width apart, toes turned out about 45 degrees, holding a kettlebell with both hands. Squat down and place the kettlebell on the floor between your feet. Stand up and lift the weight to chest height. Grab the sides of the handle and push the kettlebell straight overhead. Lower it to your chest and assume the original grip before placing the kettlebell on the ground and returning to the starting position. That's 1 rep.

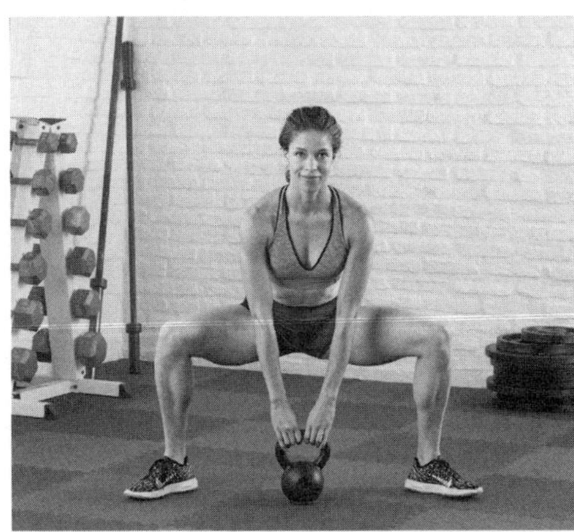

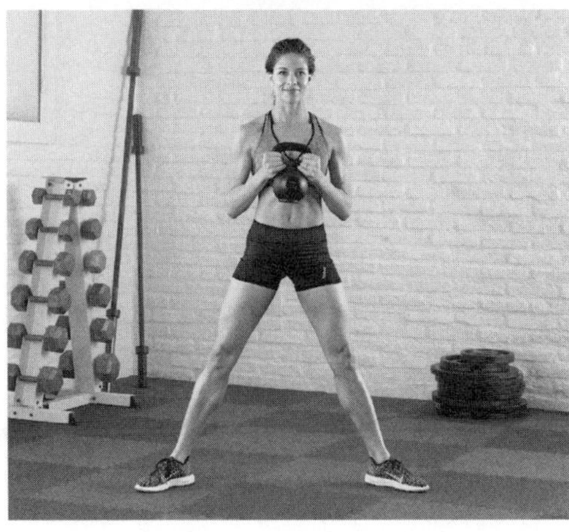

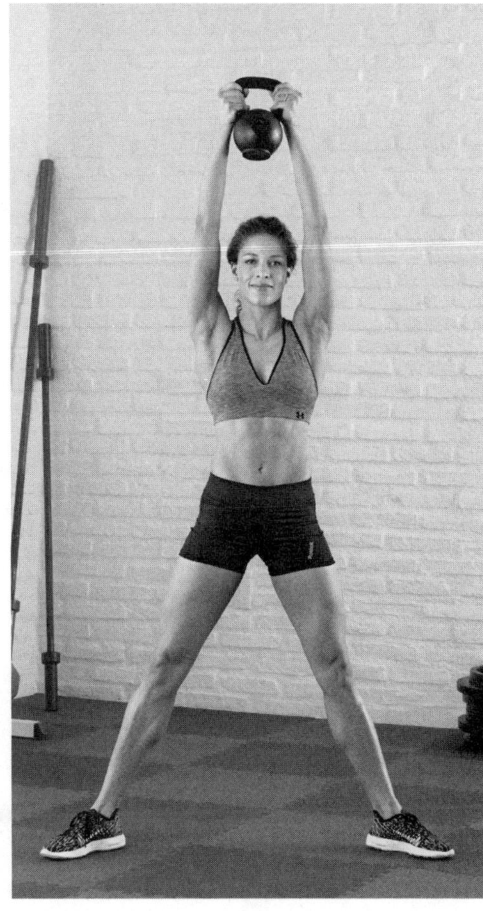

HALF GET UP

(5 reps on each side)

Strengthens the abs, shoulders, and hip flexors

Lie faceup on the floor, legs straight, holding the kettlebell in your right hand straight above your shoulder. Bend your left knee, place your foot on the floor, and prop yourself up on your left arm. Keep the weight directly in line with your shoulder and sit up until your back is straight. Reverse the movement to return to the starting position. That's 1 rep.

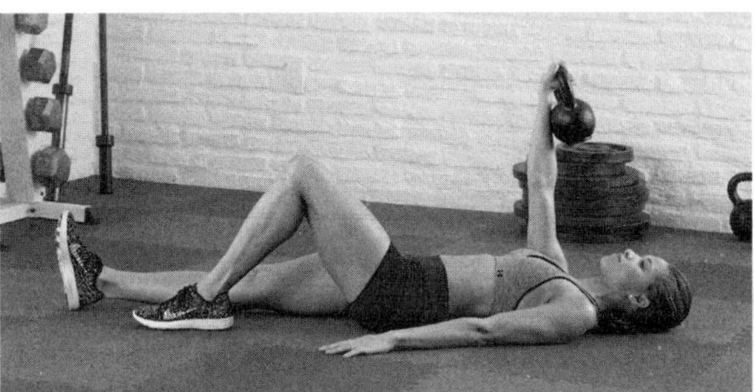

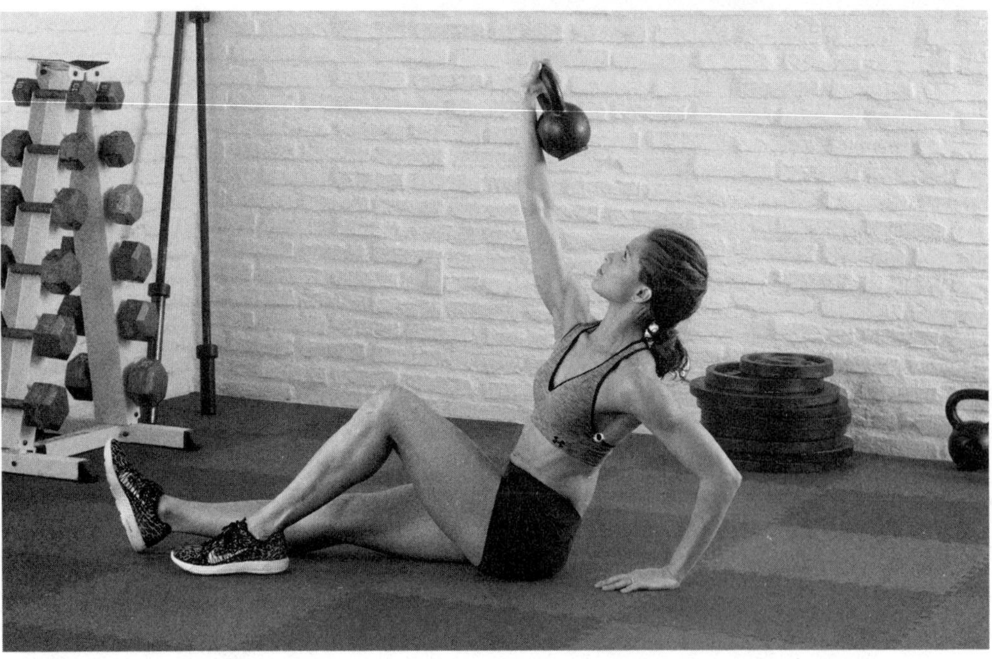

SWING

(10 reps)

Strengthens the glutes, hamstrings, quads, core, arms, shoulders, and upper back

Stand with feet shoulder-width apart, toes pointed out, and knees slightly bent. Hold a kettlebell using a two-handed, overhand grip, arms extended straight down in front of you. Keeping a neutral back, bend your hips back until the kettlebell is between and behind your legs. Squeeze your glutes to extend your hips and swing the weight up. Allow the weight to swing back between your legs, bending hips and allowing knees to bend slightly. Extend hips and knees to swing weight back up to chest level. And repeat.

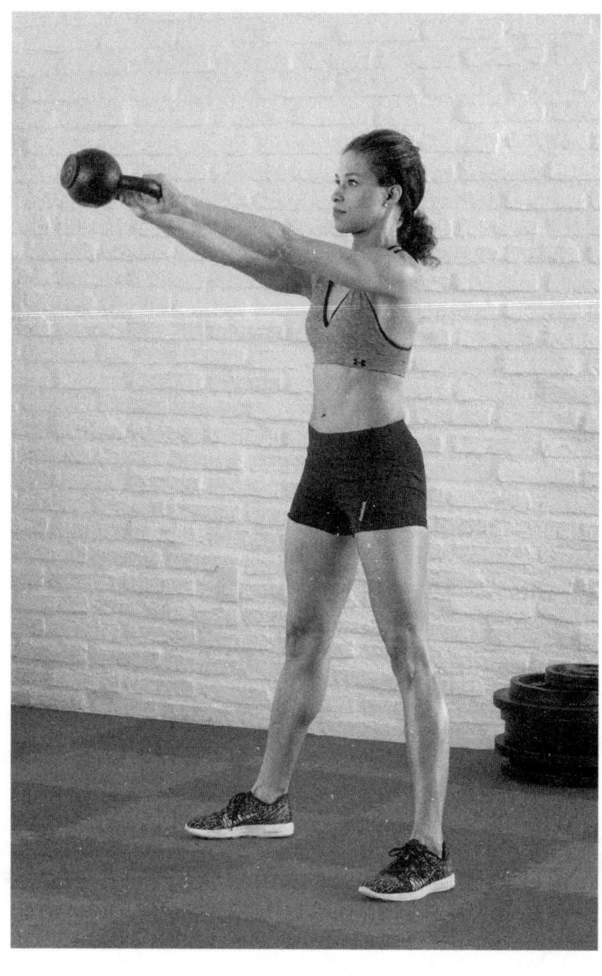

SPLIT SQUAT KETTLEBELL PASS

(8 to 10 reps)

Strengthens the glutes, hamstrings, quads, core, arms, and shoulders

Hold a kettlebell by the handle in your left hand, arms at sides, palms facing in. Stand with your left foot 2 to 3 feet in front of your right, toes pointing forward, back heel off the floor. Bend your knees, lowering your hips toward the floor, as you pass the bell under your front leg to your right hand. Then pass it over your front leg to your left hand as you straighten your legs. Continue for 8 circles, then reverse arm directions. Switch legs and repeat.

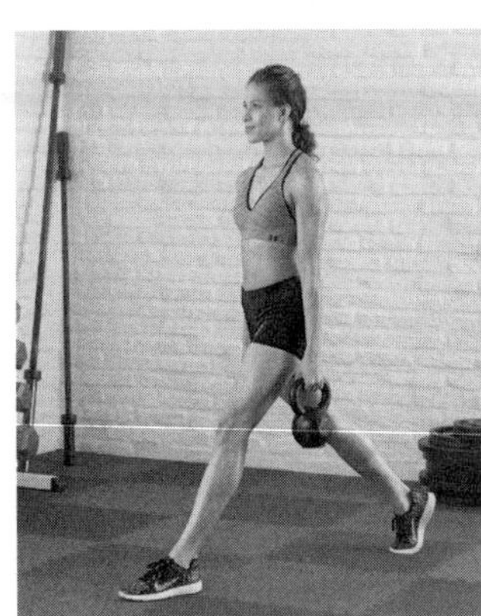

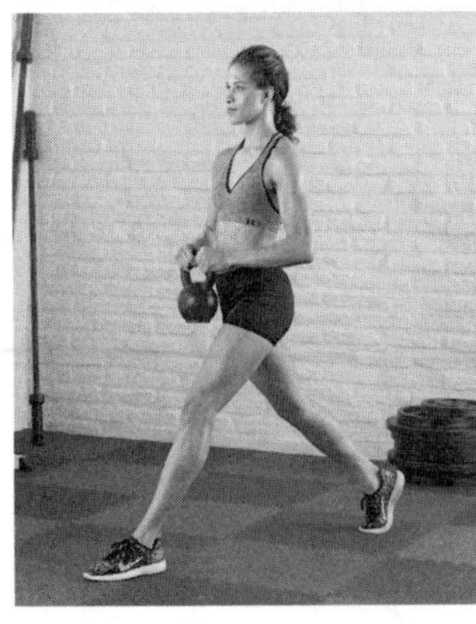

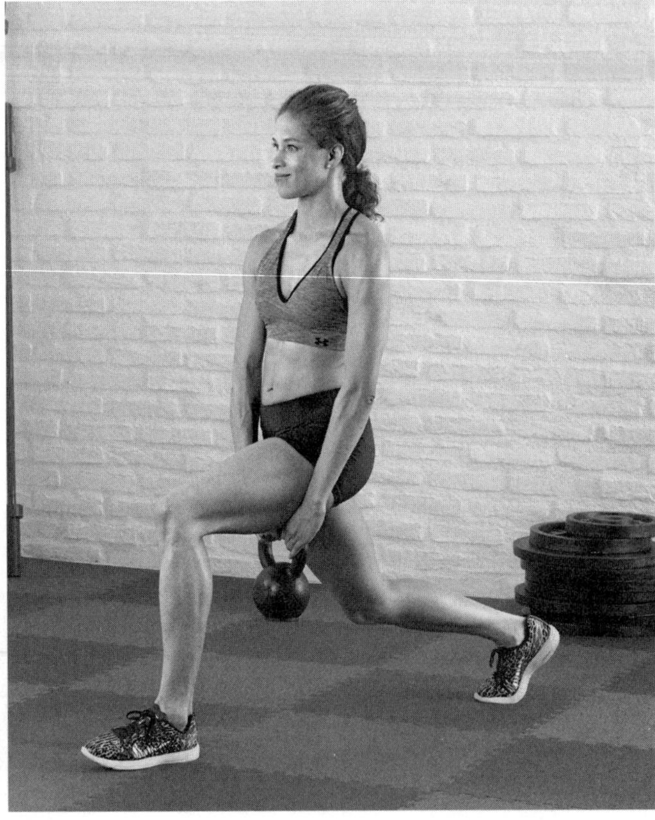

YOUR CYCLE OF STRENGTH

Your period can definitely impact how strong you feel when you strength train. Research shows it *may* also impact your strength gains.

In a study published in the *International Journal of Sports Medicine*, researchers followed two groups of women for a month. One group lifted weights every third day throughout their cycle. The other lifted just once a week during their high-hormone phase and every other day when their hormone levels were low. The women who synced their strength training to their low-hormone weeks and rested more when hormones were high saw a 32 percent increase in strength—more than twice the 13 percent gain of those who lifted the same way regardless of where they were in their cycle.

That said, despite early evidence showing some promise of phase differences, the research is equivocal and every woman's cycle (or hormonal contraceptive phase) is different. The best way to match your strength training to your cycle is to simply go with how you feel. Rather than push through a lousy bout with PMS, give yourself a break and do some yoga, take a little spin on your bike, or just take the day off. Research shows you are better off taking a break than following a rigid schedule despite your cycle.

POWER MOVE MATRIX

Keep your results coming by keeping your workouts interesting. Here's a simple monthly schedule that will keep every muscle challenged. When you reach the end, just start again from the top. Aim to do some strength training an average of 2 or 3 days a week (keeping in mind that you can adjust for your menstrual cycle if you're feeling particularly lousy).

WEEK 1: 3 body-weight moves; 2 jumps; 2 medicine ball moves; 2 kettlebell moves

WEEK 2: 3 jumps; 2 body-weight moves; 2 medicine ball moves; 2 kettlebell moves

WEEK 3: 3 medicine ball moves; 2 body-weight moves; 2 jumps; 2 kettlebell moves

WEEK 4: 3 kettlebell moves; 2 medicine ball moves; 2 body-weight moves; 2 jumps

POWERFUL CARDIO

As a former Ironman triathlete and bike racer, I understand the love of aerobic exercise and endurance training. Endurance training can improve cardiorespiratory fitness, lipid profiles, and insulin sensitivity. It can lower blood pressure and boost mood and brain health. Plus, women are built for endurance, as we're seeing women outright win ultra-running races like the 2021 Ultra-Trail World Tour and 2021 Race Across America (RAAM). That's why I don't devote much space in this book to straight-up cardio training. If you like it, by all means keep doing it—just make sure you also make time for strength training. I also recommend that women include interval training in their cardio routine.

High-intensity training is powerful medicine. It fires up your fast-twitch muscle fibers, which are those quick-burst, high-energy fibers that generally sit on the sidelines during endurance exercise. (They're the first to go with disuse and age.) It strengthens and increases the amount of your energy-producing mitochondria, improves insulin sensitivity, and significantly reduces abdominal visceral fat as well as training your body to burn more fat for energy when you're not exercising. Research shows it also helps increase lean muscle mass, as well as improve power and cardiovascular fitness. And you don't need a ton of it to reap the benefits. Just a couple of sessions a week will do!

You can do high-intensity interval training (HIIT) as part of an exercise class or online training program. Or you can do them on your own. HIIT intervals are done at 80 to 95 percent max effort (the shorter the interval, the higher the effort). They last 45 seconds to 4 minutes with variable recovery (also known as rest between intervals or RBI) in between, but usually a 1:1 work:rest ratio because the intervals are not supramaximal. The usual goal of HIIT is to tap into max VO_2/sustainable anaerobic efforts for metabolic conditioning.

I am also a huge proponent of a subset of HIIT training known as sprint interval training (SIT), which are efforts done at 110 percent supramaximal intensity. SIT intervals are 30 seconds or less with variable recovery; it can be as little as 30 seconds or as much as 3 to 4 minutes of complete recovery. Because these are so hard, it may be only 2 or 3 efforts are achievable at the beginning of this kind of training. Working up to 8 to 10 efforts is the ideal.

The following are examples of HIIT and SIT workouts.

HIIT Training

- Warm up with 10 minutes of mobilization and muscle activation.
- Then 2 minutes ON, 2 minutes OFF, 5 times.
  (The 2 minutes ON interval is at 85 to 90 percent max, running, cycling, rowing, elliptical, kettlebell swings, your favorite barbell movement, etc. The 2 minutes OFF is at 50 percent or less effort, so you have FULL recovery.)
- Repeat 5 times. (As you become fitter, you can rest 10 minutes and do another round.)
- Cool down 5 to 10 minutes to bring heart rate down, and then finish with mobility work.

Total: 30 to 40 minutes with 10 to 20 minutes of active work.

SIT Training

- Warm up with 10 minutes of mobilization and muscle activation.
- Then 30 seconds ON, 2 minutes OFF, 5 times.
  (The 30 seconds ON can be running, cycling, rowing, elliptical, kettlebell swings, your favorite barbell movement, etc. The efforts should be hard and FAST. The 2 minutes OFF is active recovery at 50 percent or less effort to rapidly bring your heart rate down, gain control of breathing, and have some metabolic and central nervous system recovery.)
- Repeat 5 times.
  Cool down 5 to 10 minutes to bring heart rate down, and then finish with mobility work.

Total: 27:30 minutes with 2:30 minutes of active work.

ARE FEMALES MORE FATIGUE RESISTANT?

As women close the sex-difference gap in endurance sports such as marathon running, a debate about whether women will eventually catch the men has caught on. A few immutable factors work against us. Though we're not just small men, we are generally smaller, especially in the heart and lungs, which has a large impact on our exercise capabilities. We do, however, have some unique advantages that account for our ability to get pretty close to the men even if we don't completely pass them across the board. One is our fatigue resistance. In a study of 20 ultraendurance runners—half male and half female—researchers found that after a 110-K (68.3 miles) trail-running race, the men's calf muscles were nearly three times as fatigued as the females', and their quad strength was considerably more diminished. This muscular resilience could partly explain why women tend to close the gender gap the longer the race gets and why women like Courtney Dauwalter have beaten men and won the overall in ultraendurance running events in recent years.

ROAR ▶▶▶ SOUND BITES

- You must strength train to maintain your muscle mass and strength. Women who don't can expect to lose at least 3 percent of their muscle mass per decade after age 30.
- Strength training improves your endurance performance, too.
- Lift heavy weight. Be scared of muscle loss; don't be scared of "bulk." (It is incredibly hard for women to develop very large muscles; it takes a LOT of training and food!)
- Variety is key to keeping your muscles stimulated and strong.
- You may be able to make greater strength gains during your low-hormone phase, so if you're not feeling like pushing hard during PMS, that's okay. Save it for the following week.

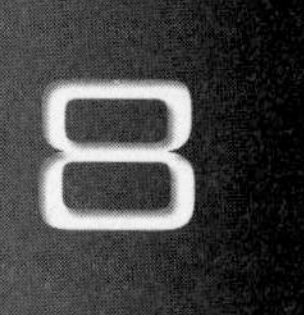

GO WITH YOUR GUT

YOU MAY HAVE MORE CONTROL OVER CHOCOLATE CRAVINGS, SICK DAYS, AND YOUR MOODS THAN YOU THINK

There's no question that what you eat is essential for health and performance. But what you put in your mouth is only part of the equation. What is happening in your gut is just as if not sometimes more important. In fact, the specific bacteria that live in your gut, or your digestive tract, particularly in your stomach and intestine, influence pretty much everything in your body, including your moods, cravings, metabolism, immunity, fat storage, and so much more that we probably don't even know about yet. The gut microbiome refers to all of the microbes in your intestines, which act as another organ that's crucial for your health. So, it is absolutely crucial to take good care of your gut and to foster a healthy gut, along with developing good eating and fueling habits.

Before we dig in here, it's essential to note that the modern science of understanding gut colonies and their influence on health is still in its infancy. New studies are coming out by the day, and as with all science, different reports can sometimes show conflicting information. This chapter reflects our best understanding of this topic at this moment in time. But stay tuned. Much, much more information will be coming out in the months and years to come.

THE ARMY INSIDE

Let's start with the basic function of the gut—digestion. As you know, your gut takes the food you eat and breaks it down so it can be absorbed into your bloodstream and sent out to your organs and muscles. The process is a bit like composting. A rich array of active bacteria and healthy flora is needed to fully break it all down and create fertile ground. Otherwise, it all just sits there in a heap. Active bacteria in your gut are essential to good digestion, and as you will see in this chapter, good digestion is the foundation for good health. It means you're getting the most nutrition out of every morsel you eat. The by-products of some digestive processes, especially the fermentation of indigestible fibers, also creates the production of short-chain fatty acids (SCFA) that help protect against inflammation, help retain your skeletal muscle mass, and perform other vital metabolic functions like reducing insulin resistance.

A healthy, diverse gut microbiome is also essential for immunity, as healthy intestinal microorganisms can help keep inflammation in check and keep the immune system in balance. It also helps us synthesize various vitamins, like the B vitamins and vitamin K, as well as some amino acids.

As healthy as they can be for us, it's important to realize that these bacteria are also serving themselves. Digestion is not a one-way street where we can simply dump in food for the bacteria to break down and send on its way. Though we benefit from them, the microorganisms hosted by a human body aren't really working for us. They are interested in their own survival and reproduction; however, they can't survive on their own, so by design they have a symbiotic relationship with the human host. In other words, the relationship can be beneficial to both parties, but this is not always the case. For example, there are microorganisms in your gut that ferment polysaccharides (chains of sugar) into energy for you to use, which is a positive by-product of their activity. Others, however, expend their energy fighting one another, suppressing the growth of other microorganisms to optimize their own living conditions.

Sometimes this is to your benefit, as in the case of a genus called *Bifidobacterium*, which tends to alter the gut environment in positive ways at the expense of not-so-beneficial bacteria. But other microbial turf wars can be detrimental to human health. Ever experience stomach upset when taking antibiotics? This is because antibiotics kill both good and bad bacteria, allowing less-beneficial organisms the chance to overgrow and produce toxins.

Like any good army, gut bacteria are solely focused on care of their own, which is no small job, as there are a lot of them. Your intestines contain more than 100 trillion microorganisms. That is 10 times more than any other cell in your body. If you have too many of one type and not enough of another, things can easily get out of whack. In our fast-moving lives when we are often overtired, overstressed, undernourished (although overfed), and grinding our immune system down to tatters, it is very easy for our gut flora to go a little haywire, which in turn affects our total-body health.

Let's take a closer look. With trillions of microorganisms, there's no way you can get to know them all, but we can identify a few general varieties as examples. A typical adult's intestines contain approximately six or seven different bacterial phyla (divisions of the main bacteria) that we know affect your overall health.

The two most dominant phyla are:

Firmicutes: These play a major role in fat storage; the stronger the Firmicutes population in your gut, the greater the conversion of your food into energy. This energy can be stored or used immediately by your body.

Bacteroidetes: Unlike Firmicutes, these bacteria use a lot of the sugar they consume for themselves, reducing the energy storage load on the host—you!

These phyla are less abundant, but still important, because they all act to keep each other in check, preventing any one type from taking over and creating a healthy, balanced gut.

Actinobacteria: Found in potatoes, wheat, and rice.

Verrucomicrobia: Found in cultivated soil.

Euryarchaeota: Methane forming and salt loving.

Proteobacteria: This group contains nearly a third of all known bacteria, including *Escherichia coli* (*E. coli*), the most studied of all the bacteria. *E. coli* comes in many strains, some of which can be pathogenic, causing diarrhea in children and urinary infections in older adults. However, *E. coli* may also be nutritionally beneficial to its hosts, as it releases vitamins such as vitamin K.

It is essential (and fascinating) to understand that these battles are not limited to your intestines. They influence your entire being. These microbes can actually alter the neurotransmitters in your brain, which in turn manipulate your food cravings and influence your food choices.

When it's 10:30 at night and you're struggling with inexplicable anxiety and battling to resist the call of a chunk of dark chocolate, it is not a lack of self-control or a freak-out. It's your gut flora sending some seriously strong messages to your brain. Yes, your gut talks to your brain. In fact, it has your brain on speed dial via the vagus nerve, which connects your digestive tract to the tenth cranial nerve in your brain.

You can see this at work in studies where researchers examine gut bacteria among people with common cravings. These studies show that your gut microbes manipulate your eating behavior by tinkering with the taste receptors in your gut (yes, you have taste receptors there, too) to make you want more of the types of food that feed them and help them grow. For instance, research has demonstrated that individuals who have strong chocolate cravings have different dominant colonies of bacteria in their intestines compared to those who are indifferent toward chocolate. It is possible that eating chocolate promotes the growth of the bacteria that flourish on chocolate, thus altering the gut microbiota composition and creating additional chocolate cravings. This might help explain why some people have a hard time giving up chocolate, but once they do, their cravings subside, as the chocolate-loving bacteria die off without the fuel to promote their growth.

As mentioned earlier, your gut bacteria also assist in numerous biological functions including the production of hormones, regulation of immunity, and even the manipulation of your moods, which is especially noticeable when you are lacking certain key microbes. For example, as levels of important gut flora, such as the *Lactobacilli* strain (part of the Firmicutes variety), decline, various symptoms of psychological distress such as anxiety, poor sleep, and high heart rate increase. On the flip side, research shows that mood significantly improves when healthy levels of these bacteria are restored. In a survey of 710 college students, those who ate the most food with live cultures, such as yogurt, pickles, kimchi, and sauerkraut, enjoyed lower levels of social anxiety, which commonly causes sweaty palms and a racing heart, than those who ate the least.

Starving any of your important flora through fasting limits the nutrients the bacteria need to grow and thrive. As a result, your pain perception increases as your gut sends the message that you're not in the condition to work very hard until you get the nourishment you need.

GUT MICROBIOME AT A GLANCE

The gut microbiome is a massive universe within us and can be challenging to wrap your head around. Here's a guide to how it breaks down.

Microbiome: the collective genetic material of microorganisms inside a particular environment (in this case, all the microscopic bugs and their genes in the gut).

Microbiota: the community of microorganisms themselves (so just all the bugs, including bacteria, fungi, viruses, etc.).

Microbiota diversity: a measure of how many different species and how evenly they are distributed in the community. Lower diversity is considered a marker of dysbiosis (microbial imbalance) in the gut and has been linked to autoimmune diseases, obesity, and cardiometabolic conditions.

Short-chain fatty acids (SCFAs): fatty acids with two to six carbon atoms that are produced when bacteria in the gut ferment dietary fibers. These are essential for microbiota health as well as our own.

THE ESTROBOLOME: THE GUT-HORMONE CONNECTION

Your hormonal health is also closely linked to your gut health. Your body produces estrogen in various forms, including estradiol (predominant in premenopause), estrone (predominant in postmenopause) and estriol (predominant in pregnancy). Once it's produced, it enters the bloodstream and makes its way to the liver (all blood circulates through the liver), where it is metabolized into inactive forms that are then sent off via bile into the intestine for elimination. Your gut bacteria play an essential role here. There is a collection of gut microbes called the *estrobolome* that can modulate the metabolism of estrogen (as well as other sex hormones) in your intestine through an enzyme they create called *beta-glucuronidase*, which can convert the inactive estrogen back into active forms. So, some of the estrogen that was shipped to your bowels for removal can be reactivated and sent back into circulation.

That's important because an imbalance of the estrobolome can lead to either an excess or deficit of beta-glucuronidase, which in turn can disrupt your hormone balance. Conditions like PCOS (polycystic ovary syndrome) and endometriosis are linked to dysbiosis of the estrobolome in premenopausal women. There is also a huge shift in gut microbiome diversity in our late perimenopause and early postmenopause years that is associated with body composition changes and increased risk for metabolic disease. The reduction of our sex hormones decreases the diversity in our microbiome. But if we focus on maintaining that diversity, it can help with maintaining a healthier balance in our sex hormone circulation.

GROW YOUR GUT FLORA

Okay, so that's a lot to digest (pun intended!). At this point in time, aside from getting tested, you can't really know what your gut flora looks like, but you can take meaningful action to foster the healthiest gut flora possible. Bacteria follow the food you eat. Protein, saturated and unsaturated fats, carbohydrates, and dietary fiber all influence the abundance of different types of bacteria in the gut.

The first step is to eat a balanced diet rich in variety. Individual microbes flourish on different foods and nutrients. If your diet is imbalanced, so will be your gut bacteria, which sets up a vicious and unhealthy cycle where one type dominates over others. You can break this cycle and establish a rich, diverse colony of gut bacteria, including the varieties that are associated with leanness and health, by balancing your diet. At the end of the day, lean people have a richer, more diverse gut colony than those who have obesity. The most essential dietary component for all beneficial bacteria is fiber—so get at least 25 grams, preferably 30, especially if you're in and beyond the menopause transition, a day from a wide variety of foods, especially vegetables and legumes.

The next step is to make sure that your daily diet is rich in specific probiotics and prebiotics. Probiotics are live bacteria and yeasts that, when administrated in a viable form and in adequate amounts, are beneficial to your gut microbiome and overall health. Probiotics come in many different forms, including fermented foods such as kimchi, sauerkraut, soft and aged cheeses, miso paste, sourdough bread, and probiotic heavy hitters such as kefir and yogurt. When choosing a specific probiotic food such as yogurt, look for the Live and Active Culture (LAC) seal. Foods with this seal contain at least 100 million bacterial cultures per gram—the more the merrier for gut health!

These probiotic foods establish a healthy colony of microbes in your gut, which in turn send messages up the vagus nerve saying that everything is A-OK in the intestines, so you can calm down and stop craving sweets. Of course, they also aid with digestion, which in and of itself can yield dramatic benefits. In one particularly revealing study, a group of overweight women and men kept their calories constant but changed their diet to include probiotic-rich yogurt. After just 6 weeks, they lost an average of 4 percent body fat. They didn't eat less or exercise more. They simply improved their digestive health, which in turn boosted their metabolism and led to fat loss and a healthier body composition.

Once you've established a healthy colony, you have to care for it. That's where prebiotics come in. Just as you wouldn't plant a garden and not feed or water it, you can't just pour some kefir on top of a bad diet and expect those beneficial microorganisms to grow and flourish. You need to feed them! Fiber from a balanced diet is one way to nourish your gut microbiome. To really fertilize these colonies, it's even more productive to give them their favorite foods, or prebiotics, which are specialized plant fibers that act like Miracle-Gro for your gut flora. Excellent prebiotic food sources include barely ripe bananas, artichokes, onions, garlic, leeks, asparagus, dandelion greens, oatmeal, and legumes.

PREBIOTICS, PROBIOTICS, AND SYNBIOTICS IN A PILL

As the benefits of gut health and the microbiome become more widely understood, so do the probiotic and prebiotic (as well as synbiotics, which contain both) supplements battling for your attention. It is best to eat foods with prebiotics and probiotics so that you get the bacteria you need. Taking a probiotic supplement in a pill form is iffy because there is no real guarantee that the bacteria are truly functional; you need to be sure it's a high-quality supplement that is specific to the flora you are trying to promote rather than a kitchen sink of bacteria.

HEALTH AND PERFORMANCE BENEFITS OF A PROBIOTIC-RICH DIET

Every day scientists are discovering more benefits of having teeming, diverse gut colonies. Some probiotic health and performance benefits we know for certain include:

Improved energy: Probiotics and a healthy gut flora facilitate good digestion, allowing you to optimally absorb all the vitamins and minerals you need to perform and recover.

Increased immunity: Research shows that probiotics can help fight bad bacteria and fend off and reduce the duration of upper respiratory infections (such as the common cold) and gastrointestinal woes such as diarrhea. One particularly interesting study found that highly trained distance runners (who are prone to falling ill from overtaxed immune systems) had less than half the number of sick days when they pumped up their diets with probiotics.

Heat tolerance: Though more research is needed, it appears that having a healthy level of probiotics also improves exercise performance in the heat. In one study, runners were tasked to run to exhaustion in a series of tests pre- and postprobiotic supplementation (specifically 45 billion CFU of *Lactobacillus*, *Bifidobacterium*, and *Streptococcus* strains). After supplementation, the runners improved their performance by a whopping 14 percent in hot conditions. It is likely that the gut lining is protected from damage, which allows digestion and the cooling system to function optimally.

Lower inflammation: Research shows that probiotics can lower levels of inflammation in the body. This helps prevent numerous diseases and illnesses, including chronic diseases such as cancer, heart disease, and diabetes, as well as inflammation-based conditions such as rheumatoid arthritis, psoriasis, and irritable bowel syndrome.

Improved well-being: Probiotics have been linked to general health benefits of all kinds, including lower cholesterol; lower blood pressure; healthier blood sugar, body weight, and body composition; and even better oral health. Healthy probiotic levels may also improve mood, and some research finds that they may even help treat depression.

PROTECT YOUR GUT DURING EXERTION

Spurred by some powerful advertising from the pharmaceutical industry, far too many athletes take ibuprofen before they exercise to head off the possibility of pain. This is a bad idea for a number of reasons, but from a gut health standpoint, it's an awful practice. The common use of anti-inflammatory drugs such as NSAIDs (ibuprofen, aspirin, and naproxen sodium) and acetaminophen can aggravate gastrointestinal (GI) bleeding and cause leaky gut. This paves the way for nasty bacteria to get into your system and interfere with fluid balance at the level of your kidneys, making it easier to get dehydrated. Research shows it also interferes with recovery. You don't need it. Don't take it.

Heavy training loads can also stress the gut with or without the NSAIDs. One trick to try for gut protection and better performance is to eat a few peppermint Tums (calcium carbonate) about 20 minutes before heading out the door. For high-intensity sessions such as track intervals or a race, have some additional Tums handy to help slow down any GI issues. The calcium works with neuromuscular contractions and muscle metabolism, the carbonate helps to coat the intestinal cells, reducing endotoxin release and the ensuing symptoms, and the peppermint is a homeopathic remedy for GI disturbances.

Low doses (3 to 5 grams per day) of creatine monohydrate are a longer-term "fix" for exercise-induced gastrointestinal issues. It helps enhance the resiliency of the cells, helps reduce inflammation, and modulates the immune system. By reducing the erosion of the gut mucosa, you maintain the natural barrier for a longer period of time, since it can erode in as little as 30 minutes. It works especially well when the gut is stressed from increased body heat and low oxygen/low blood circulation during exercise. Using this each morning of taper week can significantly improve your gut integrity.

HEAR HER ROAR

THE ELITE RUNNER BATTLING IRRITABLE BOWEL SYNDROME

I've worked with quite a few athletes (recreational and professional) who have battled undue fatigue, anxiety, GI issues, and overwhelming food cravings. Standard lab results in all these athletes came back in the normal range, but they still struggled with these aforementioned issues regardless of rest or other treatments. By understanding how different strains of gut bacteria affect physiological and psychological outcomes, we can use individualized plans to reset gut flora and alleviate issues completely.

Here is the perfect example from Kiki Silver, MD, of Boulder Peak Health in Colorado, who specializes in fatigue, digestive issues, and hormone imbalances. I send many athletes to her with excellent results.

Lisa, a professional world-class runner, was referred to me for evaluation of a combination of symptoms commonly shared by other elite female athletes: irritable bowel symptoms including fluctuating loose stools and constipation, abdominal bloating and excessive intestinal gas, food cravings specifically for complex carbohydrates, and difficulty losing weight despite a caloric intake that matched the high volume and intensity of her training.

Lisa was frustrated by her inability to correlate her irritable bowel symptoms with any particular food and was also concerned that her overall symptoms would jeopardize her upcoming races. She had already sought care from her regular primary provider, who told her to train less and work on stress reduction. She, however, was correctly convinced that her symptoms were a manifestation of a deeper issue.

Irritable bowel syndrome (IBS) is a collection of symptoms lasting for at least 6 months and occurring at least three times a month in the past 3 months. IBS always involves abdominal pain or discomfort—which can vary from mild discomfort to more severe discomfort. This pain must be associated with two of these three characteristics to be diagnosed as IBS: relief with defecation, change in frequency of stool, or change in stool appearance. IBS is typically diagnosed after more serious conditions have been excluded through comprehensive tests. IBS is incredibly common; it affects up to 10 to 15 percent of the population and is more common in women (2:1 female:male ratio). Several causes identified in the pathology of IBS include altered gut motility, gut hypersensitivity, inflammation, hormonal changes, and food allergies and sensitivities, as well as alterations in gut flora.

Several large trials have investigated the use of probiotics in GI conditions ranging from IBS to more severe inflammatory bowel disease; in IBS specifically, the trials have pointed toward a potential benefit from probiotics. The trials also suggest that an even greater reduction of symptoms is possible by matching the probiotic(s) used to an individual's specific gut flora (possible with a stool analysis). Probiotics may be able to improve gut permeability, improve gut motility, reduce visceral pain perception, and decrease the bad microbes growing on or attaching to the intestinal lining.

After Lisa had a thorough workup and a confirmed IBS diagnosis, I proceeded to run a more comprehensive stool analysis. The results of this stool test revealed that her gut flora was not only low in relative abundance but also low in diversity—with very low levels of the favorable *Lactobacillus* and *Bifidobacterium* species. In addition, she had low levels of the preferred fuel source that her colon cells needed to thrive. With this extremely helpful information, I was able to advise Lisa on which specific probiotics to take and helped her identify dietary sources of both prebiotics and probiotics.

I also recommended additional dietary sources that would help along with the probiotics to promote gut health and support the integrity of her intestinal lining. Lastly, Lisa minimized the alterations in her overall immune balance associated with her intense training and high stress load. After several weeks with these changes, Lisa noticed a decrease in her IBS symptoms and a reduction in her food cravings. Within 2 months, she had complete resolution of her IBS symptoms and food cravings and was making progress toward a desired and healthy body composition.

This case study illustrates the true symbiotic relationship we have with our gut flora; this relationship needs to be nurtured, especially in women who are prone to IBS, in order to achieve a harmonious coexistence.

GUT BOMBS

A healthy, balanced diet rich in probiotics and prebiotics is the key to developing a thriving, diverse gut colony. But you can't expect your happy and healthy microbiome to withstand the gut bombs many of us throw their way—sometimes every single day. Here are some common enemies of your beneficial bacteria and how to protect your microbiome from harm.

Antibiotics: It's right there in the name—*anti*biotic. There's no doubt that these drugs are an essential part of our modern medical arsenal and have improved and extended lives worldwide. They are also being horribly abused and overused. The Centers for Disease Control and Prevention (CDC) estimates that about half of all antibiotics prescribed are unnecessary since many illnesses are actually viral and therefore will not respond to antibiotics. If you have a cold, sore throat, or other upper respiratory infection, chicken soup (with plenty of garlic) and rest is the way to go. Spare your gut flora the decimation caused by antibiotics. You'll have better immunity in the long run when and if you really need them. In your home, soap and water are just fine for washing hands and cleaning up; avoid antibacterial products.

Anti-inflammatories: This one's important on a few levels. Women often take NSAIDs such as ibuprofen (Advil) and naproxen (Aleve) for menstrual cramping. These medications work by decreasing the production of certain hormone-like substances called prostaglandins that are the culprits behind cramps. There are also prostaglandins that protect the lining of the stomach and intestines. NSAIDs decrease the production of them, too. This leads to erosion of the protective mucosa of the gut, which in turn leads to a condition called leaky gut, where the gut wall becomes too permeable, allowing toxins from your gut to spill into your bloodstream and wreak havoc in the form of inflammation, GI distress, autoimmune disorders, and poor athletic performance.

This issue is especially important if you're active, because your gut is already prone to damage from the stress of exercise-induced hypoxia, where the oxygenated blood gets pumped away to your working muscles, leaving the gut to fend on its own. Probiotics help keep your gut barriers strong, even under these circumstances. Knocking them out with NSAIDs opens the door—and your gut wall—to trouble.

Artificial sweeteners: Recent research shows that artificial sweeteners alter your gut bacteria in ways that produce glucose intolerance. This usually occurs when your body can't cope with heavy sugar loads in your diet, and it sets the stage for obesity and metabolic disease such as diabetes. This is an area of ongoing investigation, but the development of glucose intolerance may be partially why diet soda is linked to overweight and obesity despite having less sugar and calories.

Processed foods: Refined sugary foods cause an explosion of Firmicutes in the gut. When this type of bacteria takes over your gut, weight gain typically follows.

Oral contraceptives: It's something nobody talks about, but it is emerging as a health concern. Birth control pills and other hormone therapies interact with your gut flora in ways that may put you at risk for autoimmune disorders (in a nutshell, when the body's immune system attacks healthy cells). Though more research is needed, evidence indicates that combined hormonal contraceptives may modulate the immune system in ways that increase your risk for diseases like Crohn's disease, lupus, ulcerative colitis, and multiple sclerosis.

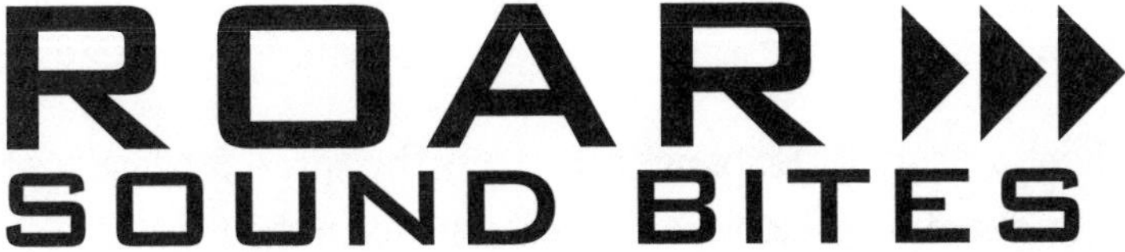

- The bacteria in your gut can impact your mood, cravings, and fat storage. Nurturing a healthy flora is essential.
- Eat a diet rich in probiotic and prebiotic foods to increase the diversity of the gut microbiota.
- Lean people have a richer, more diverse gut colony than those who are overweight.
- Sex hormone metabolism is a key component of a healthy gut microbiome; dysbiosis is linked to endometriosis and PCOS.
- Take antibiotics only when absolutely necessary. They wipe out the good with the bad bacteria.

9

BUILD YOUR BONES

YOU CAN'T BE STRONG IF YOUR SKELETON IS WEAK—HERE'S HOW TO FORTIFY YOUR FRAME

As a woman, you have a higher risk of brittle bones and stress fractures, especially as you age. Women comprise 80 percent of people with osteoporosis in the United States. Half of women over the age of 50 will break a bone at some point in their lives because of osteoporosis, a condition where the bones become brittle. That is some nerve-wracking stuff!

But don't be scared; instead use this information as motivation to be as strong and powerful as you can be. When it comes to bone health, time is of the essence, so you need to start working on this right now. Though they appear to be static structures, like the steel-beam infrastructure of a building, bones are actually in a constant state of remodeling, as your body absorbs old bone and creates new bone to lay down in its place. This modeling and remodeling process yields a net positive gain during childhood and into early adulthood, with women hitting about 90 percent of peak bone mass by their early 20s and making minor accumulations until about age 30. To put things in perspective, 100 percent of the skeleton is replaced in the first year of life, but that decreases to 10 percent upon early adulthood, and the remodeling efforts continue to decline with age.

Testosterone fuels greater muscle development, which in turn leads to bigger bones. Therefore, as a woman, your peak level of bone mass is already lower than a man's. Once you hit your peak, you start to slide in the other direction as the breaking down starts to outpace the rebuilding. Estrogen plays an important role in bone remodeling, so it helps keep the decline in check. Premenopausal women tend to lose bone slowly, about 0.5 to 1 percent a year. That loss accelerates as women enter the menopause transition and estrogen starts to fluctuate and decline. A 2019 study of 173 women and men between the ages of 35 and 50 published in the *Journal of Osteopathic Medicine* reported that 26 percent of the women (and 28 percent of the men) had osteopenia (bone density that is below normal but not low enough to be categorized as osteoporotic). That's something women need to take very seriously, because unless we take action, we can lose up to 20 percent of our bone density during the 5 to 7 years following menopause. That loss slows down and becomes more gradual again after that period, but you're still facing loss.

Whether you are young and still laying down new bone or postmenopausal and on a precipitous slide, the sooner you act, the stronger you can make and maintain your skeleton. As with your muscles, a little loss is inevitable with age, but your diet, exercise, and lifestyle habits can go a long way in helping you hang on to what you have.

MAKE AN IMPACT

Every move you make is the product of your muscles pulling on your bones to make it happen. The more active you are, the more strain you put on your bones. The cells within your bone sense that stress and respond by making your bones denser and stronger. Girls and boys who are physically active generally achieve greater peak bone mass when they grow up than their more sedentary peers. In addition to increasing your bone density, regular exercise can help prevent bone loss—and even replace a bit of lost bone—when you're older. The best activities are those that are weight bearing (force you to work against gravity) and have multidirectional forces through the bone such as jumping (i.e., jump rope, plyometrics), dancing, and tennis and other ball sports, and of course strength training. Bicycling and swimming are excellent for your muscles and heart but not so much for your bones. If those are your primary activities, add cross-training (such as the moves found in Chapter 7) to your exercise routine a few times a week to keep your skeleton strong. Be sure to target your upper body, since women tend to have less muscle mass—and hence thinner bones—in their torsos.

If you've already been diagnosed with osteoporosis or osteopenia, you may need to choose your activities a bit more carefully, but you still can and should exercise to prevent further decline. In general, you want to avoid lots of bending or twisting moves that can put too much pressure on the vertebrae in your spine. Consult with your doctor about plyometrics. Some impact through small jumps like jumping rope may be beneficial if performed and progressed properly. You definitely want to continue strength training 2 or 3 days a week.

Numerous studies have found that postmenopausal women with low and very low bone density see significant bone density gains—improving about 1 percent a year—in their spine and hips, which are areas affected most by osteoporosis, when they participate in a regular strength-training routine. And don't be afraid to lift heavy (with proper training, of course).

SHOULD YOU GET YOUR SKELETON SCANNED?

The recommendations for bone scans have traditionally skewed somewhat older. The US Department of Health and Human Services, for instance, doesn't recommend standard screening for women until age 65 (though they note you can ask your doctor about it if you're younger and have gone through menopause). Many osteoporosis practitioners and researchers are now recommending that women get bone density screening when they reach menopause so we don't miss the opportunity to intervene during the critical window of bone loss that can occur during this time.

Even if you've not yet reached menopause, if you have risk factors such as a family history of osteoporosis, have been using medications such as glucocorticoids (steroids) that are known to impair bone health, or have reasons to suspect bone density issues, such as being prone to stress fractures, you should talk to your doctor about getting a bone density test called a dual-energy x-ray absorptiometry scan (DXA or DEXA) to see a baseline measurement of your bones.

In the 2017 "LiftMOR" study, researchers had a group of over 100 women average age of 65 who had been diagnosed with low bone density either lift heavy (after a period of base training) or do low-intensity lifting for 8 months and found that the heavy lifters consistently showed superior improvements in bone mineral density in their hip and lumbar spine area.

Pay special attention to posture exercises, such as moves for your upper back that strengthen the muscles between your shoulder blades. These can strengthen your spine-supporting muscles and reduce the sloping shoulders and rounding-forward posture older women can get, which places undue stress on the spinal column and can lead to compression fractures.

Improving posture, balance, coordination, and flexibility are key components to lower your risk of falls. Different types of yoga and Pilates can improve all of these, but check with your instructor to avoid poses that may put you at risk for fractures.

Finally, tai chi is an excellent form of exercise for everyone, but especially for women with thinning bones, because it strengthens the entire lower body and greatly improves balance. By improving your balance, you lower your risk of falling, which can be very dangerous for people with osteoporosis.

GOT MILK? IT MAY NOT HELP

The National Dairy Council has done such an impressive job with their advertising campaigns that drinking milk has become nearly synonymous with building bone. Well, it's really not that simple. It is true that calcium is a key ingredient for building bones. In fact, nearly all your body's calcium is stored in your bones and teeth, where it supports their structure and hardness.

However, calcium doesn't just dwell in your bones. Your body uses this essential mineral for numerous functions, including regulating your heart rhythm, transmitting nerve impulses so your muscles can contract, and even blood clotting. When there's not enough calcium to go around, your body borrows some from the bone bank—your skeleton. You need ample amounts of calcium in your diet so you don't weaken your skeleton. Recent studies call into question exactly how much and what the best sources are, however.

Currently the Institute of Medicine calls for women between the ages of 19 and 50 to get 1,000 milligrams a day and women over 50 to get 1,200 milligrams a day. The problem is that research doesn't show that taking that much calcium protects your bones; in fact, it may be detrimental to other aspects of your health.

For example, in large studies by Harvard University of male and female health professionals, those who drank just one glass of milk or less per week were at no greater risk of breaking a hip or forearm than those who drank more. Other studies comparing people taking calcium supplements or placebos found that the calcium supplements offered no protection against fractures. A 2015 meta-analysis of 59 randomized controlled trials reported that increasing calcium from dietary sources or by taking calcium supplements produces small, limited increases in bone mineral density that are unlikely to lead to a significant reduction in risk of fracture.

Further research adds to the confusion, suggesting that taking calcium without vitamin D, which plays a critical role in maintaining bone health, may even increase the risk of hip fractures. Other countries have significantly lower daily calcium recommendations and no greater rate of skeletal disease.

So right now, there's no great evidence to chug a lot of milk. Better ways to get calcium, as well as vitamin D, are to include fish in your diet several times a week. Sardines and salmon are on par with milk when it comes to amounts of calcium (about 200 to 300 milligrams per serving) and vitamin D, and salmon has even more vitamin D than milk. Certain yogurts are also fortified with both bone-building nutrients. If you don't like fish or dairy (and even if you do), consider taking a vitamin D supplement in the range of 1,000 to 5,000 IU (see Chapter 15 for more information on supplements), because research finds many women and men are deficient.

Despite its significant role in bone formation, vitamin K is an underappreciated and little-talked-about nutrient. Low levels of vitamin K have been linked to low bone density. The Harvard Nurses' Health Study found that eating just one serving of lettuce or other vitamin K–rich foods (leafy greens and veggies) a day can cut the risk of hip fracture in half compared to eating just one serving a week. It really doesn't take much to get the recommended 90 to 120 micrograms of vitamin K that you need each day. Just one serving of broccoli, Brussels sprouts, or dark leafy greens does the trick. As a bonus, leafy greens are also a good source of calcium.

Finally, magnesium is looking increasingly important. A 2020 study published in *Maturitas* listed magnesium, along with vitamin K_2 (which is found in cheese, egg yolk, and fermented foods), vitamin D, and calcium, as promising in the management of osteoporosis. High-magnesium foods include dark leafy greens, nuts, seeds, avocados, beans, and fish like salmon, mackerel, and halibut.

STRESS FRACTURES AND WOMEN ON THE RUN

Stress fractures plague so many young female athletes and may be related to estrogen deficiency and menstrual dysfunction, even if the athlete's menstrual cycle seems normal.

For example, Jillian is a competitive age-group triathlete, regularly winning or placing top three in 70.3 and Ironman distance races. She came to me with a stress fracture in her lower fibula (smaller leg bone that doesn't bear much weight) and a weak point in her tibia (mid-shin). She was eager to heal the stress fracture and build bone mass to prevent further fractures, as she had the Ironman championships in Kona in her near future.

Although her menstrual cycle was regular, her doctor told her she was training too much and needed to eat more, as well as think about an alternative lifestyle to long-distance triathlons. When we evaluated her diet and training, there was some room for improvement through upping her overall protein and fat intake, but she had no calcium, vitamin D, or vitamin K deficiencies.

To dig a bit deeper, we ran a series of blood tests to investigate her estrogen, progesterone, cortisol, DHEA, and testosterone levels. The results indicated that even though she appeared to have a normal cycle, her hormonal levels were far from normal. Jillian had low levels of estrogen and progesterone, leading to a short luteal phase. She also had elevated cortisol and low DHEA, all of which indicate a chronic stress response from the hypothalamic–pituitary–adrenal axis and are a sign of REDs. The combination of hormone imbalance and the high training volume with a somewhat inadequate calorie intake caused a reduction in bone remodeling and turnover, which ultimately created lower bone density.

Over the next 6 months, we implemented dietary changes to improve her energy availability. Specifically, we adjusted her energy intake to support her training, took steps to improve her sleep for optimal recovery, and further supported bone development by increasing her intake of calcium, vitamin D, and vitamin K to ensure she was hitting adequate amounts of each. These steps worked together to reset her menstrual-cycle hormones. Jillian's stress fracture healed without any additional complications, and her body composition improved, as did her training, recovery, and performance.

BONE BANK ROBBERS

Just as your diet and lifestyle can help build your bones, they can also break them down. As you've already seen, a sedentary lifestyle is bad news. But I'm not terribly worried about you being sedentary if you're holding this book in your hands. Another big bone robber is smoking. Again, I'm going to assume that this is not a problem for most of you. Nevertheless, I do know some active women who sneak cigarettes on the sly. If that's you, do your bones (and every other part of you) a favor and quit. Among countless other terrible things, smoking has been linked to low bone density.

Alcohol use is also a potential bone robber. While there's a bit of evidence that moderate drinking may protect bones (which is *not* a reason to drink if you don't; the potential cons outweigh the pros here), there's unquestionable evidence that heavy drinking is bad for your bones. So, if you do drink, stick to one drink (12 ounces of regular beer, 5 ounces of wine, or 1.5 ounces of spirits) a day. Also watch your soda consumption, specifically cola, though all soda is problematic. There is evidence that too much soda can weaken bones by altering your body's balance of calcium and phosphorus in an unfavorable direction. The Framingham Osteoporosis Study found that women who reported drinking cola every day had lower bone density than women who reported drinking it less than once a month.

Finally, if you're not getting your period because of the female athlete triad or what is now called REDs, it's imperative that you address the underlying issues. Women who stop getting their periods because of extremely low body weight, inadequate diet, or excessive exercise may lose significant amounts of bone density that is very difficult if not impossible to recoup even after they start menstruating again.

WHEN TO CONSIDER MENOPAUSAL HORMONE THERAPY (MHT)

If you are a menopausal woman who has or are at high risk for osteoporosis, talk to your doctor about menopausal hormone therapy (MHT). MHT is FDA approved for the prevention of osteoporosis. It is not, however, approved for the treatment of postmenopausal osteoporosis. Nonestrogen medications are preferred for treatment of existing osteoporosis. There are other pharmaceutical interventions, such as selective estrogen receptor modulators (SERMs, such as raloxifene) that have been approved for the treatment of osteoporosis.

ROAR ▶▶▶ SOUND BITES

▶ Eighty percent of people with osteoporosis in the United States are women.

▶ Strength train 2 or 3 days a week and do 10 minutes of jump training 2 or 3 days a week to keep your skeleton strong.

▶ There's no good scientific connection between drinking milk and strong bones; consider other ways to improve your bone health.

▶ Stress reactions and fractures may indicate a serious hormonal imbalance.

▶ Can your cola habit. It's bad for your bones.

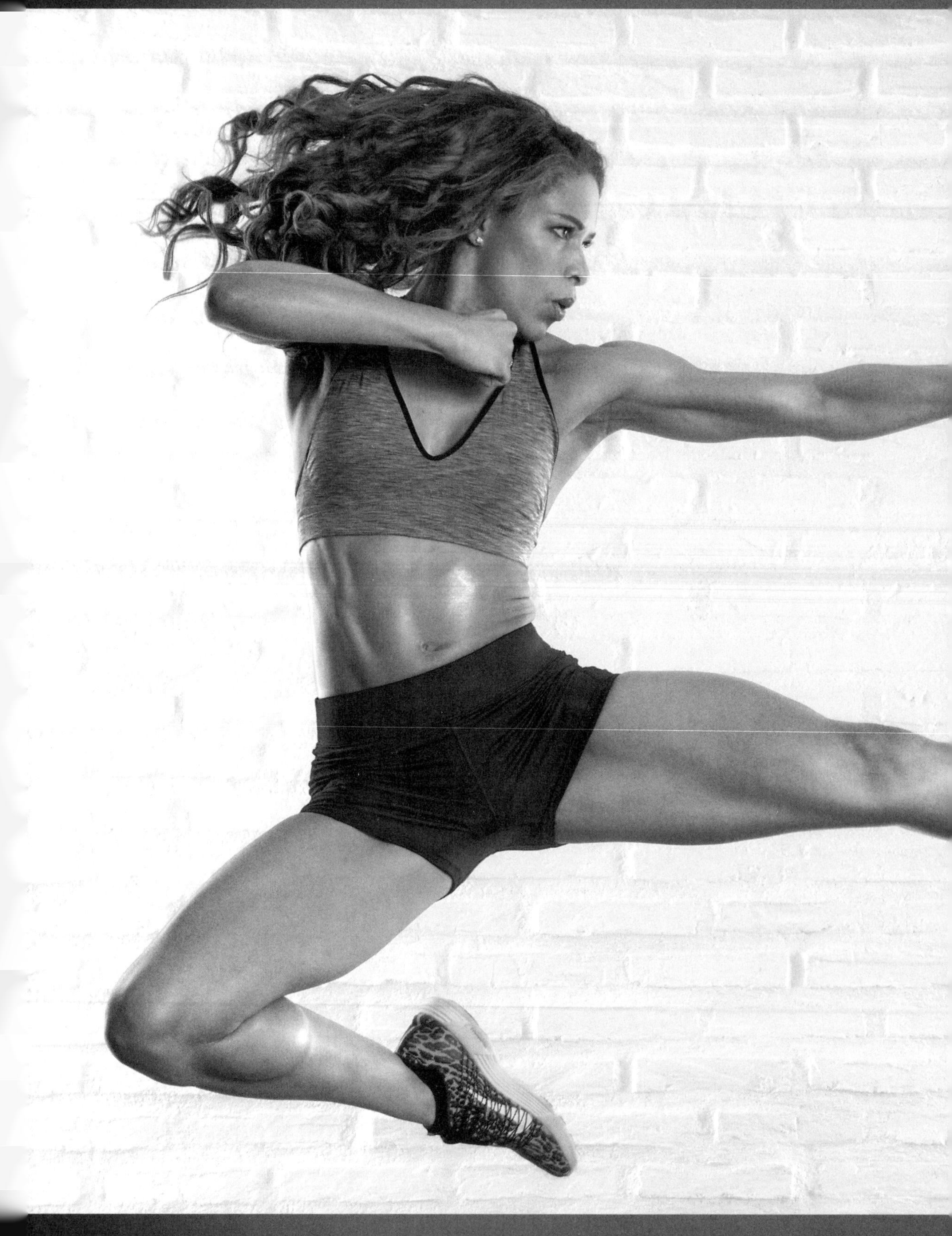

PART III

YOUR PLAN FOR PEAK PERFORMANCE

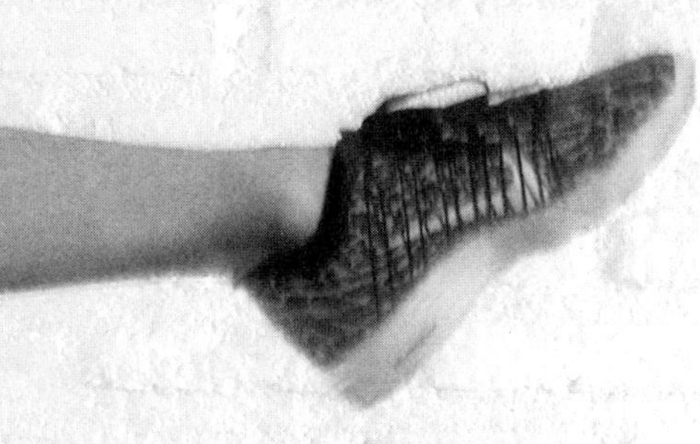

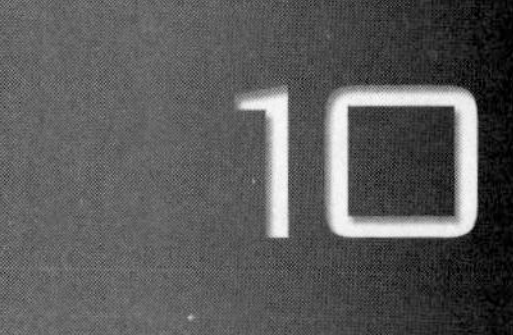

DAILY FUELING

YOU CAN'T OUTRUN A BAD DIET, BUT OPTIMAL NUTRITION CAN HELP YOU ACHIEVE A PERSONAL BEST

With all the conflicting information on what you should and shouldn't be eating, it's difficult to get it right. To be clear, I'm not suggesting there's a 100 percent right or wrong way for any one woman to eat. That's impossible. But I am telling you that there are certain nutrients—both large and small—that every woman does need to feel and perform her best. Here's a look at all the necessary components of an active woman's daily diet.

FIRST: EAT ENOUGH

When women come to me because they're struggling with poor performance, one of the simplest (though not always easiest) and most successful strategies I provide is getting them to eat more. Many women athletes are chronically underfed, whether it's because they're afraid to eat; they're in a constant state of trying to lose weight (aka afraid to eat), or they are unknowingly underfueling themselves because they just don't realize how much energy and nutrition they need.

This is more common in women than men, and a research review published in the journal *Archivos Latinoamericanos de Nutrición* (Latin American Archives of Nutrition) shows the consequences: Women athletes are more susceptible to iron, calcium, and vitamin D deficiencies than their male peers. Iron is essential to produce oxygen-carrying hemoglobin, and calcium and vitamin D are essential for bone and muscle health (among many other things!). The women were also at increased risk for being low in magnesium, which helps with muscle function, blood pressure, bone health, and maintaining blood glucose.

The researchers reviewed 42 studies published between 2013 and 2020 that examined the effects of deficits in total calories, protein, and vitamins and minerals on performance. They found that not only were women more likely to be deficient in these key nutrients, but also between 30 and 70 percent of the women in the studies were energy deficient.

This paves the way for low energy availability (LEA) and REDs (relative energy deficiency in sport), which, as you know, increases your risk for low bone density and injuries like stress fractures, as well as mood disorders and, of course, poor performance and recovery. (See "Understanding the Consequences of LEA.")

Here are just a few examples of how many female athletes in various sports were at risk for low energy availability and the detrimental health consequences it brings, according to recent research:

- Nearly 80 percent of elite female cross-country runners show risk for LEA in one study.
- 88 percent of professional female soccer players had LEA in another study.
- 96 percent of ballet dancers had LEA in another study.
- *100 percent* of synchronized swimmers had low energy availability in one study!

More broadly speaking, a 2022 study of more than 200 female endurance athletes published in *Frontiers in Sport and Active Living* reported that 65 percent were at risk of LEA, 23 percent were at risk of exercise addiction, and 21 percent had disordered eating behavior.

LEA is a problem I see every day. Sometimes women end up in this type of undernourished state because, as I mentioned upfront, they've been restricting food for years (maybe most of their lives) and they are afraid to eat enough. Other times, women can inadvertently underfuel because they start performing more high-intensity exercise, but since they're working out for a relatively short amount of time, they don't register that they need to eat more to support that harder type of training. They also may not feel as hungry right away because their appetite is blunted by the intense exercise. So they go about their day and end up in a hole. So many women barely achieve their resting metabolic rate needs (about 1,300 to 1,400 kilocalories)—the amount of calories needed to just lie on the couch watching Netflix, let alone eat enough for life and training.

As an active woman, you need to eat enough, being sure to consume a well-rounded diet that includes ample amounts of fruits and vegetables and all your macronutrients (protein, fats, and carbohydrates). For most active women, that's well north of 2,000 calories a day. In fact, the range is often 2,300 to 4,000 calories depending on the sport, training block, and body composition.

UNDERSTANDING THE CONSEQUENCES OF LEA

Technically speaking, low energy availability, or LEA, is defined as having limited energy available to support your normal body functions once your energy expended through exercise is subtracted from your total dietary energy intake.

Plainly speaking, that means you're not eating enough to support both your training and your basic biological needs. This is what makes LEA particularly insidious. You may be able to run, swim, bike, lift, and otherwise complete your workouts (at least for a while), but your body doesn't have enough calories and nutrition left over to keep your organ systems operating at optimal levels.

When this happens, your body enters a state of LEA, which my former PhD student and now doctorate specializing in LEA, Dr. Katie Schofield, likens to how your phone goes into low battery mode: It still functions, but the screen goes dim, and some of the apps start shutting down to conserve energy. Only in the case of your body, those "apps" are your organ systems, like your reproductive and endocrine systems!

Prolonged LEA can have serious consequences on your health. As mentioned in Chapter 2, one of the most notable consequences is on your reproductive system. Again, many women still believe that it's "normal" for female athletes to lose their periods when they train. It is far too common. But it is *not* normal! Research shows that when women dip into LEA, it disrupts the production of luteinizing hormone, which plays an important role in ovulation and regulating the menstrual cycle.

One of the downstream consequences of disrupting your hormones with LEA is serious and potentially lasting negative impacts on your skeletal system. Without enough energy, your osteoblasts (the cells that build bone) and osteoclasts (the cells that break down and resorb bone) can't do their job properly, and you end up breaking down more than you build up. The end result is bone stress injuries and stress fractures, as well as an increased risk for osteoporosis down the line.

LEA also can lead to a host of other health disruptions, including irritability, bouts of depression, brain fog, depressed immunity, loss of libido, GI issues like constipation and diarrhea, and can lead to nutritional problems like anemia.

It seems obvious that LEA can also hurt your performance. But here's the problem: Depending on your sport, you might not see decrements and may even see some improvements for a period of time because, remember, LEA is about not having enough energy left over after training, not *for* training per se. So though chronic LEA negatively influences muscular adaptations and muscle protein synthesis, research shows that it may fly under the radar for prolonged periods of time before adaptations stagnate and performance declines. Worse, you may already be damaging yourself, such as bone loss, before you reach that point.

Here are some telltale signs of underfueling. Many trainers and coaches will see these signs and chalk them up to "overtraining." But in reality, they're symptoms that you're not eating enough to support your training.

Decreased training response. One of the first signs of lower energy availability is your performance plateaus or decreases. You can't hit your wattage. You have less strength and power. Your heart rate is off. You're not recovering well.

Irregular periods. One of the reasons I am so adamant about tracking your period (if you usually have one) is that a telltale sign of underfueling is change in your menstrual cycle—bleeding becomes lighter and shorter; you skip a period or two. These are signs that there is not enough fuel coming in to support your endocrine health.

Bone health decreases. Stress reactions and fractures are a major warning sign of low energy availability.

Immunity drops. You end up more prone to infection. So if you're starting to pick up every cold, your immune system is depressed.

Gut distress increases. This one can be tricky because it can mimic symptoms of hormonal fluctuation that women often experience. But low energy availability also can cause IBS symptoms, bloating, gassiness, nausea, and generally not feeling well after eating. That's because your gut microbiome is off from the chronic inflammation that happens when your body is under stress from not having enough energy to perform all of its functions.

Coordination worsens. Without the energy you need, you are more fatigued, which impairs your cognition, reaction time, and coordination.

Chronic hangriness. Low energy availability can make you perpetually hangry. You feel more irritable, anxious, and depressed. Your hunger cues may be gone at this point, so you don't even know that you're "hangry." Or you may feel really hungry at odd times like when you're out running errands or when it's time for bed.

But don't wait for these symptoms to pop up to eat enough! Proper fueling is the number one way to enjoy immediate performance gains. How can you check if you're dipping into LEA, even if unintentionally? If you know your body composition, you can start with using the equation for determining energy availability (EA), which is your dietary energy intake (kcal) minus your exercise energy expenditure (kcal) divided by your fat free mass (FFM) in kilograms (kg). You want the final number (EA) to be over 45 calories per kilogram of FFM; 50 calories per kilogram FFM is a good number to aim for if you train and/or compete regularly. Anything less than 30 calories per kg is defined as LEA, and at that point you can start experiencing health risks like suppression of bone formation after only five days.

Realistically, I know that many women, even with the best of intentions may fail to hit those EA marks. That's why it's important to be very cognizant that you are refueling after your training, within 30 to 45 minutes, to stop the brain from perceiving low energy intake. It's also important to be sure you're not going low-carb/keto because, as research shows, getting adequate carbohydrates may help you avoid LEA even during those times when your EA is lower than is optimum.

THE MACRONUTRIENT MEDLEY

To achieve your energy needs, you must eat the right amount of macronutrients. There are three essential macronutrients every woman (human, really) needs: carbohydrates, protein, and fat. They've all fallen victim to fad diets, and fat in particular was out of vogue for many years. But they are all critical for exercise and recovery as well as for everyday life. In Chapter 11, you'll learn how to specifically fuel yourself before, during, and after exercise. But first we have to focus on daily, not exercise-specific, fueling to best support your active female physiology.

TO CARB OR NOT TO CARB—THAT IS NOT A QUESTION

Back in the old low-fat days, carbohydrates were completely overdone. Stuffing ourselves with starchy bagels and plates of pasta did indeed make us metabolically unhealthy and contributed to problems with overweight. In the years that followed (including current times for many), carbs have become a four-letter word, even among active women, who are grain- and starch-phobic. However, we can't just eliminate this essential macronutrient. Carbohydrates are indeed essential for everyday health.

Let's start with some basic physiology. Your body uses carbohydrates for energy during exercise. They fuel your brain and central nervous system, help your body burn fat (as exercise physiologists like to say, "Fat is burned in a carbohydrate flame"), and help preserve your precious muscle tissue by preventing your body from using protein as a primary energy source.

Remember, too, that your glycogen (stored carbs in the muscles and liver) supply is limited. Fully stocked, you have about 500 grams of glycogen stored in your muscles and about 100 grams in the liver, generally considered enough to fuel a 2-hour run, depending on your pace—the harder you push, the faster you burn through your stores. At the bare-bones minimum, an active woman needs 130 grams of carbohydrates or the equivalent of about 520 calories' worth (the amount in 1 cup of pasta, 1 cup of beans, and a potato). This amount does not support physical activity. This is simply what is required each day in order to support the central nervous system, maintain red blood cell production, keep the immune system running, and fuel the brain. Your brain alone requires roughly 60 percent of your body's resting glucose utilization.

What you eat day to day profoundly impacts how much glycogen you have in the tank at any given time, and this relates to exercise. Whether you're a regular CrossFitter, Olympic/power lifter, swimmer, runner, cyclist, or any other type of exercise enthusiast, it's important that you have enough glycogen on board to get the job done, especially if you plan to go hard or long.

As you'll see in the next chapter on sport-specific fueling, all this doesn't mean your goal is to try to stuff your glycogen stores the night before a big event (aka carbo-load). As women, we rely on blood glucose first, then fatty acids to fuel our exercise efforts. Our need for carbs is less about preventing our glycogen stores from getting tapped out and more about keeping blood glucose available for energy and for burning free fatty acids.

BIG BRAINS NEED CARBS

Understanding how and why we developed such large brains is one of the most puzzling topics in the study of human evolution. It is widely accepted that the increase in brain size is partly linked to changes in diet over the last 3 million years. Increases in meat consumption and the development of cooking technologies have received particular attention from the scientific community. In a new study published in the *Quarterly Review of Biology*, Dr. Karen Hardy and her team bring together archaeological, anthropological, genetic, physiological, and anatomical data to argue that carbohydrate consumption, particularly in the form of starch, was critical for the accelerated expansion of the human brain over the last million years.

With a global increase in obesity and diet-related metabolic diseases, interest has intensified in ancestral or paleolithic diets, not least because human physiology should be optimized for the nutritional profiles we have experienced during our evolution. Up until now, there has been a heavy focus on the role of animal protein and cooking in the development of the human brain over the last 2 million years, and the importance of carbohydrate, particularly in the form of starch-rich plant foods, has been largely overlooked.

Dr. Hardy's team highlights the following observations to build a case for the necessity of dietary carbohydrates in the evolution of modern big-brained humans:

- The human brain uses up to 25 percent of the body's energy budget and roughly 60 percent of blood glucose. While synthesis of glucose from other sources is possible, it is not efficient, and these high-glucose demands are unlikely to have been met on a low-carbohydrate diet.
- Human pregnancy and lactation—which, of course, are specific to us gals—place additional demands on the body's glucose budget, and low maternal blood glucose levels compromise the health of both the mother and her baby.
- Starches would have been readily available to ancestral human populations in the form of tubers, as well as in seeds and some fruits and nuts.
- While raw starches are often only poorly digested in humans, when cooked, they lose their crystalline structure and become far more easily digested.
- Humans have many salivary amylase genes; primates have far fewer—about a third of humans'. We evolved to have more of these genes to increase our ability to digest starch.

Dr. Hardy proposes that the coevolution of cooking and the increase in salivary amylase genes increased the availability of preformed dietary glucose to the brain and fetus, which, in turn, caused the acceleration in brain size.

CARBOHYDRATE CONTENT (G) IN A TYPICAL SERVING

BREAD AND BAKED GOODS	BREAKFAST CEREALS AND GRAINS	VEGETABLES	FRUITS	DAIRY AND DAIRY SUBSTITUTE PRODUCTS	OTHER
½ whole grain bagel (34 g) 2 whole grain pancakes (32 g) 1 multigrain English muffin (27 g) ½ fruit muffin (23 g) 1 small whole wheat pita (16 g) 1 slice sprouted grain bread (15 g) 1 cup pasta (35 g) 1 cup brown rice (45 g)	⅔ cup cooked black rice (34 g) 1 cup cooked quinoa (29 g) 1 cup cooked oatmeal (27 g) ¾ cup Nature's Path Organic Flax Plus cereal (23 g)	1 cup broccoli (6 g) 1 cup potatoes (26 g) 1 cup beets (13 g) 1 cup carrots (12 g) 1 cup corn (25 g) 1 cup yams (35 g)	1 small (1.5 oz) box raisins (34 g) 3 medium dates, fresh (31 g) 1 large apple (30 g) 1 medium banana (27 g) 1 medium grapefruit (26 g) 1 medium pear (25 g) 1 large fresh fig (24 g) 2 kiwifruit (24 g) 1 cup raw cherries (22 g) 1 cup fresh blueberries (21 g) 1 medium orange (18 g) 2 thick pineapple slices (16 g) 1 cup fresh strawberry halves (12 g) 1 medium peach (11 g) 2 large apricots, fresh (7 g)	1 cup fat-free milk (12 g) 1 cup low-fat plain kefir (12 g) 1 cup almond-cashew-hazelnut milk (2 g) 1 cup unsweetened almond milk (1 g) 1 cup Greek yogurt (9 g)	1 Tbsp jam, honey, or maple syrup (17 g) ¼ cup chocolate chips (10 g) ¼ cup broad beans (fava beans) (26 g) ½ cup chickpeas, kidney beans, or black beans (21 g) ½ cup edamame, shelled (10 g)

Now, here is where I'd be remiss if I didn't talk about fat adaptation, because I know there are a lot of low-carb followers out there, and going high fat and super low carb is extremely popular right now. To answer the million-dollar question of whether a high-fat diet can improve performance, the answer, I believe, is no. Here's why.

For one, low-carbohydrate diets increase fatty acid oxidation during exercise and encourage intramuscular fat storage. The body is smart; if there isn't enough primary fuel to support the stress it's under, it'll go for a secondary source—in this case fat—then store more of it for the next time it encounters that stress. But this does not translate into improved performance.

Research shows no real performance benefits from low-carb over moderate-carb diets. In fact, research on elite female racewalkers reports that though the athletes did increase their fat burning after adapting to a ketogenic low-carbohydrate, high-fat diet, they also decreased their economy of movement—they used more effort to maintain the same pace—and performance, as compared to having adequate carb intake and stores. Though some low-carb athletes will "carb up" in preparation for a competition, this study shows that strategy won't work. Even after 2½ weeks of high carb restoration and a taper, their performance didn't rebound.

In women in particular, high-fat, very low-carb eating contributes to increased oxidative stress, which blunts training adaptations both in endurance and strength/power-based sports. Low-carb training has become very popular among CrossFit athletes, which can be to their detriment over time. In a 2019 study investigating overtraining syndrome in these athletes, the authors note, "The most remarkable trigger of OTS [overtraining syndrome] among HIFT [high intensity functional training; i.e., CrossFit] athletes was the long-term low carbohydrate and calorie intake," which increases catabolism and downregulates the endocrine system. In other words, you're eating your muscles and not making more, which is obviously bad for performance. It also hurts your immune system, which is already taxed by exercise stress. It can interfere with iron absorption and lead to iron deficiency. I'll note that there have been small, short-term trials where CrossFit athletes follow a keto diet for a few weeks and lose fat (but don't improve performance). The concern is what happens over time.

Underconsuming carbohydrates also sets the stage for putting you in a state of low energy availability, where your body may have the energy it needs for training but doesn't have enough left for other functions, so you end up with disruptions in menstruation, performance, and bone mass. In the end, a low-carb diet compromises your ability to maintain high-intensity or prolonged periods of exercise and puts your body under exorbitant stress.

That doesn't mean you need to pile your plate high with bread and pasta. As a woman, you become more sensitive to carbohydrates as you age and especially as you enter the menopause transition, because of the decline in your estrogen levels, so eating a diet too high in carbs is detrimental from a blood sugar and metabolism standpoint. Starchy vegetables such as sweet potatoes, yams, and winter squash as well as root veggies such as carrots, onions, and garlic are superior forms of carbohydrate from a nutritional standpoint. You don't need to eat a ton of carbs, but you should eat the right carbs throughout the day (and time them correctly before, during, and after exercise, which we'll cover in depth in the next chapter) for your physiology and fitness level.

What I find works best from both a body composition and performance standpoint among my female athletes is aiming for a daily intake of about 40 to 45 percent whole-food carbohydrates (e.g., veggies, fruit, ancient grains).

CAFFEINE: A POTENTIAL PERFORMANCE-BOOSTING BUZZ

Caffeine is hands down the most popular ergogenic aid in the world. It's found in coffee, teas, sodas, pills, gums, and energy shots. Each of these products deliver varied doses of caffeine. I'm addressing caffeine in the "daily fueling" chapter, because so many of us use it every day—often multiple times a day!—as well as before and during training and competition.

Caffeine is a world-renowned brain stimulant, so it gives you a quick jolt of energy when you're ready to go. Caffeine also increases your power output and time to exhaustion and lowers your perceived exertion. Or more simply: You can run, bike, swim, row, or whatever longer and more powerfully while feeling less tired. It was actually listed on the World Anti-Doping Agency's (WADA's) banned substance list in 1984 but removed in 2004 when they realized that using enough to get popped in a test was extremely difficult (and not exactly performance-enhancing in those huge amounts).

Aside from the stimulating effects on the brain, caffeine also stimulates the release of fatty acids, which helps your body use fat as fuel, so you don't burn through your carbohydrate stores as quickly during endurance exercise. It also improves power and sprinting performance. Caffeine increases the calcium content of muscle, which strengthens your muscle contractions, which is just what you need for banging out the last 200 meters in a race or powering through that final set of pullups.

Caffeine also raises blood pressure, heart rate, and stomach acid production. Some of these effects, particularly those on blood pressure and heart rate, are less pronounced in regular caffeine users.

A study published in 2016 in the *Strength and Conditioning Journal* found minor sex differences in our responses to caffeine. Women had greater blood pressure increases but less heart rate changes compared to men. High levels of circulating estrogen made women feel the effects of caffeine—such as the jitteriness—more, but that didn't change their performance improvements. Research on women hasn't shown the benefits of caffeine for short high-intensity sprints but is most effective for longer, sustained exercise.

The most consistently effective dose according to a 2021 International Society of Sports Nutrition position stand on caffeine and exercise performance is 3 to 6 milligrams per kilogram body mass. Minimal effective doses of caffeine currently remain unclear, but they may be as low as 2 milligrams per kilogram body mass. Very high doses of caffeine (e.g., 9 milligrams per kilogram) are associated with a high incidence of side effects and do not seem to be required to elicit an ergogenic effect, according to the paper.

For reference: A double espresso delivers about 150 milligrams, 16 ounces of strong coffee contains 330 milligrams, and one Red Bull has 80 milligrams of caffeine. Caffeine is easily absorbed by the stomach and intestine, so you reach peak blood levels within 45 to 60 minutes after taking it. The maximum caffeine effect on fat stores can take up to 3 to 4 hours. For optimum benefits, take your caffeine an hour before endurance exercise or up to 20 minutes before high-intensity training.

During exercise, your body clears it much faster than it does when you're sedentary, so when you start using caffeine in an event, you need to keep using it till the end. As with everything else, if you plan to use caffeine during a big event or competition, be sure you train with it first so you know how your body reacts. Don't cut it out completely leading up to an event or you may experience symptoms of caffeine withdrawal.

PRIORITIZE PROTEIN

Protein will likely always be a diet darling in the eyes of most of the public. It's easy to understand why. If you read the media headlines, there's seemingly nothing it can't do. Want to lose weight? Eat protein! Want to reduce blood sugar swings? Eat protein! Make muscle? Protein! Rev up metabolism? Protein! Feel fuller sooner? Protein! Recover from hard exercise? Protein! Protein! Protein!

The fact is, protein actually is a dietary superstar. Unlike carbohydrates and fat, which are primarily fuel sources, protein is structurally essential: It's found in every cell and tissue of your body. The problem is, most active women still aren't eating enough, especially if they're following the current dietary guidelines, which call for eating 0.8 gram of protein per kilogram of body weight (1 kilogram = 2.2 pounds), which generally equals between 45 and 50 grams for a 135-pound adult woman. That amount is to maintain nitrogen balance and prevent muscle loss in sedentary women! It's to prevent deficiency and considerably less protein than active women really need. In fact, a 2022 meta-analysis concluded that adults should be taking nearly twice that amount (1.5 grams per kilogram of body weight) if they want to maintain and/or augment muscle strength along with resistance training. I and many others contend that amount is even higher, closer to 1.8 grams per kilogram of body weight, and with age, that can be closer to 2.0–2.2 grams per kilogram of body weight!

Adequate protein is especially important for women. Our hormonal fluctuations often put us in a catabolic state, so depending upon our menstrual cycle and menopausal status, we may be more inclined to break down than to build muscle.

Women should pay attention, especially after ovulation and during the luteal (high-hormone) phase after ovulation when progesterone rises. Progesterone breaks down protein (as well as carbohydrates and fats) to provide amino acids as the building blocks for the uterine lining. We need slightly higher doses of protein (about 12 percent) in times of elevated progesterone to mitigate those effects and maintain our muscle mass.

During peri- and postmenopausal years, our sex hormones begin to fluctuate and decline, and we lose the anabolic (muscle-making) stimulus that estrogen helped

PROTEIN CONTENT (G) IN A TYPICAL SERVING

LEAN MEAT	EGGS	FISH	DAIRY PRODUCTS	BEANS AND LENTILS	NUTS AND SEEDS*	GRAINS
3 oz lean rump steak (26 g) 3 oz lean sirloin steak (26 g) 3 oz lean bison (24 g) 4 oz lamb chops (23 g) 3 oz chicken (31 g)	2 large eggs (12 g) 3 egg whites (11 g)	3 oz tuna, canned in water (22 g) 3 oz fresh cod (20 g) 3 oz cooked blue mussels (20 g) 4 colossal shrimp (18 g) 6 oysters, raw (5 g) 3 oz salmon (22 g)	1 cup (8 oz) fat-free Greek yogurt (23 g) ½ cup fat-free cottage cheese (15 g) 1 cup (8 oz) low-fat plain kefir (11 g) 8 oz fat-free milk (9 g)	1 cup lentils (18 g) 1 cup shelled edamame (18 g) ½ cup chickpeas or black beans (7 g)	24 raw almonds (6 g) 3 Tbsp sunflower seeds (6 g) 1 oz raw cashews, hazelnuts, or Brazil nuts (5 g) ¼ cup raw walnuts (5 g) 1 Tbsp pumpkin seeds (high leucine) (3 g)	½ cup uncooked amaranth (14 g) ½ cup uncooked kamut (14 g) ½ cup uncooked hulled barley (12 g) ½ cup uncooked quinoa (12 g)

**High good-fat content*

provide. So we need more protein to pick up the slack where our hormones left off. Research also shows that with age, we need more protein for the same training adaptations.

Adequate protein has other health benefits. A Johns Hopkins University study found that a diet with protein levels above current recommendations (about 25 percent of calories coming from lean protein sources) led to a greater reduction in blood pressure, bad LDL cholesterol levels, and triglycerides than a traditional higher-carb diet. Other research shows that people who eat diets with higher levels of protein can fend off obesity, osteoporosis, diabetes, and especially heart disease. The Optimal

Macronutrient Intake Trial to Prevent Heart Disease (OmniHeart) reported that both higher-protein and higher-fat diets improved 10-year heart disease risk better than a high-carb diet did.

How much protein is enough? Broadly speaking, women should aim for 1.7 to 2.4 grams of protein per kilogram of body weight per day (1 kilogram = 2.2 pounds; to determine your weight in kilograms, multiple by 0.455; 128 pounds × 0.455= 58 kilograms). Menstruating women need to hit those higher amounts during the luteal phase. Women in the menopause transition should target the higher end of that range (2.2 to 2.4 grams per kilogram), aiming for the lower end on easier days and the higher end on very heavy training days. Research also shows that higher protein daily intakes (greater than 2.0 grams per kilograms of body weight per day), coupled with heavy resistance training, are important for maintaining lean mass and resting energy expenditure when women are intentionally or unintentionally restricting their calories, both of which are common among recreationally active to elite female athletes. Contrary to some older concerns, high-protein diets (greater than 2.2 grams per kilogram of body weight per day) have not resulted in any adverse effects to bone mineral density or kidney function in healthy women.

Equally important as how much protein you eat is when you eat it. Your body responds best to an even protein distribution throughout the day. I recommend starting the day with a healthy hit of protein—25 to 30 grams at your morning meal, along with your carbs—because you start the day in a catabolic (muscle-devouring) state after not eating all night. A morning protein hit restocks your stores and helps regulate your appetite for the day ahead—critical for both fueling activity and preventing overeating later on. Premenopausal women should aim for 30 grams of high-quality protein within 30 to 45 minutes after exercise, and regular doses of 30 to 40 grams of protein at each meal and 15 to 20 at your snacks. As you reach peri- and postmenopause, your anabolic resistance increases, so you want to aim to have that postexercise protein closer to 40 grams.

By making sure you're taking in regular doses of protein throughout the day, you'll maintain a good nitrogen balance (i.e., the equilibrium between protein intake and losses) for lean mass development. This will help improve your recovery, reduce postexercise soreness, and lower your risk for injury as well.

You also want to focus on getting the right kind of protein from the best food sources as part of your daily diet. This is a key element that many soy-loving women miss. It's easy to get confused, as protein is pretty complex. Let's break it down. Protein is comprised of 20 building blocks called amino acids. Of these, your body makes 11. Because you can manufacture them yourself, these are considered nonessential amino acids. Your body cannot make the other 9, known as essential amino acids, so you need to get them from food sources. Taking it one step further, protein comes in two varieties, complete and incomplete. Complete protein sources are those that contain all 9 amino acids. Incomplete sources contain some but not all, so you have to pick and choose more carefully to get everything you need throughout the day. You can find complete proteins in meat, fish, eggs, and most dairy products. Plant sources, such as nuts, whole grains, and vegetables, are usually incomplete sources.

The good news is that some foods we naturally eat together, such as beans and rice or peanut butter on bread, work together to make a complete protein. No need to stress about combining foods to make a complete protein at every meal. As long as you eat all the amino acids you need within a day, you'll get all the complete protein you need.

What you should pay attention to are key amino acids. The essential amino acid (EAA) content of protein, in particular the leucine content, can dramatically affect muscle protein synthesis. For example, whey protein has distinct anabolic (muscle-building) characteristics and anti-inflammatory properties, both of which help you turn the protein you eat into lean, active muscle tissue. (You need 40 grams of soy to get the same leucine level as just 25 grams of whey.) There are also fast- and slow-releasing proteins. The best option after exercise is a combination of fast-release (whey) and slow-release (casein) for a continuous "feed" of muscle-mending amino acids into your bloodstream.

To make it easy, I tell women to aim to make protein about 30 to 35 percent of their daily calories. A good daily benchmark is between 1.0 and 1.2 grams per pound of body weight, and be sure to stick to the high end if you're very active.

To sum it up, you may need more, maybe a lot more, protein than you've been consuming. When women hear how much protein they need, their eyes often get big and they say, "How?? How can I get that much protein?" It's actually easier than you think. Animal-based protein (chicken, beef, or pork) provides about 30 grams per 4-ounce (palm-sized) serving. One cup of 2% cottage cheese is also about 30 grams, as is one 3.5-ounce can of tuna. Low-fat Greek yogurt contains about 20 grams per cup; adding nuts and seeds brings you to about 30 grams.

If you are plant-based, you can meet your protein needs with foods like tempeh and edamame, as well as nuts and seeds (and nut and seed butters) and beans and legumes. A blender is also your friend here. You can blend 3 to 4 ounces of tofu with nut butter, frozen cauliflower, and hemp and chia seeds to get a completely vegan 30-gram protein hit.

ROAR DAILY DIET CHEAT SHEET FOR ATHLETES

As a general guideline, your daily nutrient intake should consist of about 40 percent carbs, 30 percent protein, and 30 percent fat. To keep your energy levels high for workouts and daily life, it is important to have enough carbohydrates and protein in your diet and to not be so strict about restricting fats. These are obviously broad-brush recommendations. And these recommendations may evolve as more research is done on female athletes, taking into account phases of the menstrual cycle, contraceptive use, menopausal status, and more. Here's what to know:

CARBOHYDRATES

Your stored glycogen (carbs) is very limited. Did you know:

- When muscle glycogen stores are used up, exhaustion occurs.
- Muscle glycogen depletion occurs after about 2 hours of continuous low-intensity training but occurs within 15 to 30 minutes of high-intensity training.
- When liver glycogen is depleted, you cannot keep blood glucose levels normal. This is when you hit the wall and cannot continue.
- With low blood glucose levels, your body has to rely on fat for fuel; however, this is a very slow process and will slow your performance.
- Signs and symptoms of low blood glucose include light-headedness, lack of coordination, weakness, inability to concentrate, blurry vision, and feeling spacey.

HOW MANY CARBOHYDRATES DO YOU NEED IN A DAY?

- For extreme intense training of 5 hours or more per day (Ironman or multisport events), you need 2.7 to 3.2 grams per pound (6 to 7 grams per kilogram).
- For a light or active recovery day, aim for 1.15 grams per pound (2.5 grams per kilogram).
- For short, intense days (like CrossFit training), aim for 1.15 to 1.4 grams per pound (2.5 to 3 grams of carbs per kilogram).
- For moderate- to high-intensity training lasting 60 to 120 minutes, you need 1.4 to 1.6 grams per pound (3 to 3.5 grams of carbohydrates per kilogram).
- For endurance training involving 2 to 5 hours of intense training per day (distance running, cycling, swimming), you need 2 to 2.7 grams per pound (4.5 to 6 grams of carbs per kilogram).

My activity per day is: ____
My weight in pounds or kilograms is: __________________________________
My carbohydrate need is (weight in pounds or kilograms) × (grams of carb for activity level):
____

PROTEIN

For general muscle growth, repair, and strength adaptations, protein is the key for success! Did you know:

- In activities lasting 2 hours or more, amino acids (the building blocks of protein) can lend up to 5 to 10 percent of the fuel necessary to keep going.
- Hydration is key with any endurance activity, and the amino acids of protein are an effective rehydration mechanism.
- An endurance athlete needs upward of 1 gram of protein per pound of body weight a day for optimal muscle repair, growth, recovery, and fat mobilization.
- Protein is also necessary to facilitate fat loss, as it keeps the muscles repairing and rebuilding, which allows carbohydrates to refuel the muscles and liver, thus allowing fat stores to stay empty.
- Whey isolate, pea protein isolate, and casein protein powders are very simple means of increasing your protein when you are on the go and need something quickly.

HOW MUCH PROTEIN DO YOU NEED IN A DAY?

- For strength/power phases of training, you need 0.9 to 1.0 gram of protein per pound (2 to 2.2 grams per kilogram) of body weight per day.

- For endurance phases of training, you need 0.8 to 1.0 gram of protein per pound (1.8 to 2.2 grams per kilogram) of body weight per day.
- For optimal recovery, aim to consume about 30 grams or 0.15 to 0.17 gram of protein per pound (0.32 to 0.38 gram per kilogram) of body weight within the first half hour post-event/training session.

My phase of training is: ______________________________

My weight in pounds or kilograms is: ______________________________

My protein need is (weight in pounds or kilograms) × (grams of protein for phase of training):

____

FAT FROM FOOD DOES NOT EQUAL BODY FAT

Let's start with a round of applause for the demise of low-fat food recommendations and celebrate the fact that the federal government finally dropped the restrictions on total fat consumption in the official Dietary Guidelines for Americans in 2015, a full 35 years after they first started cautioning everyone to be fearful about fat.

Since its introduction to popular culture beginning in the 1970s and ramping up through the 1990s, fat restriction proved to be a national health disaster. Ditching fat—and very often replacing it with starch and sugar and low-fat processed products such as Snackwell cookies and crackers—was a disaster for our metabolic health.

Yet we were so thoroughly indoctrinated with the idea that fat from food equals body fat that we simply couldn't let it go. But we must. I will say it again. Low-fat, high-carb foods are not good for you. It's too much sugar without enough satiety. You don't feel full. If you keep eating all those carbs without enough fat, your insulin levels shoot up, which causes your cortisol levels to skyrocket. The combination makes you store belly fat and puts you at risk for metabolic disease such as diabetes.

Fat is an essential source of fuel for aerobic exercise and life itself. It protects your inner organs and allows estrogen to function properly, so you have regular menstrual cycles, which in the long run not only protect your fertility but also preserve your bones. When we pull fat from our diets, we also lose the essential fatty acids necessary for immune and nerve cell function. A little fat makes everything better—flavor, nutritional value, and satiety. Try cooking with these healthy fats: olive oil, rice bran oil, nuts and seeds, nut butters and oils, avocado and avocado oil, as well as fish and fish oil.

What about saturated fat? Surely there has to be some bad fat? The only truly bad fat is one that we human beings have to process ourselves (the word *process* is the root of most dietary evils)—trans fats. Trans fats are often disguised as partially hydrogenated oils, so avoid anything that has that phrase on the ingredient list and you'll be golden. Like fat itself, saturated fats have been unfairly demonized. Saturated fats, alternatively, are not such a bad thing in moderation. In fact, landmark research from the University of California, Berkeley, in 2010, which involved more than 20 studies and nearly 350,000 people, proved there wasn't sufficient evidence to link saturated fat to heart disease. The Women's Health Initiative had found the exact same thing in a smaller study 4 years earlier.

In fact, some saturated fats, such as stearic acid, may have health benefits, and others such as lauric, palmitic, and myristic may not be all bad or have a neutral effect. There's even evidence that saturated fats may help balance cholesterol levels and lower inflammation. The key—and this is important—is getting saturated fats from whole, natural, and unprocessed sources. That means grass-fed beef; organic foods such as chicken, eggs, and dairy; and rich dark chocolate. It does not mean you can consume processed lunch meats, cakes, cookies, and sweets with abandon without health consequences. You still need to eat wisely.

For women, it is advisable to get more dietary fat from unsaturated fats, especially omega-3 fatty acids (found in fish such as salmon), which are natural anti-inflammatories, and omega-6 fatty acids found in walnuts and seeds. There is some debate regarding the health benefits/risks of high amounts of omega-6 fatty acids (which are also found in vegetable oils, so we tend to get a lot in the modern Western diet), because they may trigger the body's production of proinflammatory substances. So I generally encourage women to focus on getting more omega-3s and to get most of their omega-6s from whole foods rather than processed foods made with high amounts of oils. The omega-3s in fish oil (1,000 milligrams a day) have also been shown to quell common menstrual problems such as cramps and back pain.

I recommend getting about 30 percent of your calories from fat by eating healthy, whole foods to keep your body functioning at its best. Fat is slower to digest, so you need to be careful about how much you eat immediately before and during exercise. We'll cover that in detail in the following chapter.

HEAR HER ROAR

THE ENDURANCE ATHLETE'S DEFICIENT DAILY DIET

Sometimes even those who know better don't know better. Take my coauthor, Selene Yeager. As a certified trainer with the National Academy of Sports Medicine, a USA Cycling licensed coach, and a longtime ultraendurance athlete whose accomplishments include a trip to Ironman Kona, a medal at Leadville 100, and multiple-stage race wins around the world, she, by her own admission, botched her nutrition many times. After years of practice, she thought her training and racing nutrition was (mostly) dialed in at the time of this book's original publication (2016), but some extensive blood work done while training for a massive month of nearly back-to-back stage races revealed that her daily diet was anything but. (See Chapter 17 for a complete overview of Selene's blood work and how you can do the same test.)

Selene's glucose levels were stubbornly high, as were her blood lipids. Her bilirubin, a product that is formed when old red blood cells are broken down (this can indicate hemolytic anemia), was high, too. Her iron level was low, as was her vitamin B_{12} (definite indicators of anemia). Even though she generally felt pretty good, she would find herself wandering into the kitchen at random times—usually midafternoon and late evening—seeking a jar of Nutella, honey, Greek yogurt, cheese, or wine.

Selene had made a mistake I see in many of my athletes. She was eating enough food, but she wasn't eating enough of the right kinds of food—specifically carbohydrates—for her female physiology. Tired of the sugar rushes and crashes she experienced while following a high-starch, carbohydrate-based (bread, pasta, and grains) diet years ago, she pared down her cereals and grains when she wasn't riding and relied on veggies and fruits for her carbs instead. Because foods such as Brussels sprouts and broccoli are so high in fiber, she was full before she got the nutrients her very active body craved. She also wasn't providing her brain with the fuel it needed to do her job as a writer as well as an athlete, which left her feeling fuzzy headed when she wanted her mind to be sharp.

I advised her to keep 2 days of dietary records, from which I made the following ROAR makeover recommendations:

Day 1

6:30 a.m. Wake up

7:45 a.m. Breakfast

4 oz orange juice

2 cups coffee

2 eggs scrambled with goat cheese and chili peppers

½ toasted flatbread with butter

ROAR MAKEOVER NOTES: Within 30 minutes of getting up, have a bit of protein (10 to 15 grams) and a bit of carbohydrates (20 to 30 grams) to bring your blood glucose up, but not to spike and drop it. Remember, your body has been without food all night. The idea is to boost blood fuel levels so that your cortisol level drops (it peaks early morning, mostly because of low blood sugar; you want to keep cortisol down, as it has adverse effects on bone formation, the immune system, and body fat). Also stay isocaloric. Consider stirring a few tablespoons of fat-free Greek yogurt into your juice to reduce the blood sugar spike and limit any insulin response to the pure sugar in the juice. Add a couple of egg whites to the whole eggs to boost protein without too many additional calories. Replace butter with almond butter for more omega-3s.

10:30 a.m. Snack

4 oz Greek yogurt with honey

ROAR MAKEOVER NOTES: This is a lot of sugar. The Greek yogurt is a good source of protein, but change to 0 to 2%. Some fat is okay, but in yogurt less fat equals more protein, because when fat is removed during production, there is a greater concentration of protein. Add blueberries for flavor instead of honey. These simple changes will provide more protein, fiber, and antioxidants and have a less severe effect on blood sugar.

12:00 p.m. Lunch

½ whole grain flatbread with mixed veggies and spicy Thai tuna

Handful of baby carrots with hummus

Wild berry seltzer water

ROAR MAKEOVER NOTES: Good.

2:45 p.m. Random kitchen invasion

White tea, brewed with a bit of honey

While the tea is brewing, I eat a couple of tablespoons of cold vegetable soup out of the container in the fridge, nosh on a small piece of blue cheese, and eat about eight almonds and a square of dark chocolate infused with cayenne pepper.

ROAR MAKEOVER NOTES: This tells me you need food. Plan ahead for snacks in the afternoon. Most everyone has a lull around 3:00 p.m.; it has to do with our circadian rhythm, which causes a dip in core temperature. The body's perception is that you need a boost of carbohydrates to wake up. Some good-quality protein (15 to 20 grams) will do the job. Enjoy your tea as usual.

5:30 p.m. Snack

Bowl of vegetable soup

ROAR MAKEOVER NOTES: Okay, but you need a boost pretraining (see below).

6:30 p.m. Core workout and pool session

ROAR MAKEOVER NOTES: A protein load before and after training will boost muscle adaptations. Your preworkout snack could be a scoop of whey isolate protein powder and espresso mixed with water (iced protein latte!). The caffeine and protein will boost your training session, allowing you to get more power and adaptations. You have a 30-minute window for protein postworkout and up to 2 hours to restock your carbohydrates. Six to 8 ounces of low-fat chocolate milk for protein and carbs with some almonds (for extra protein) is an ideal recovery snack. It helps with the slow release of protein throughout the day to maximize muscle synthesis and reduction of body fat.

8:30 p.m. Dinner

Arugula salad with beets, olives, blue cheese, crushed nuts, and tuna. One glass of wine.

ROAR MAKEOVER NOTES: Add a greater variety of veggies to your dinner. Look for a bright rainbow on your plate. Make the salad and veggies the base layer of your meal with the tuna as a second protein layer (30 to 40 grams of protein). Blue cheese is okay as a topping, but don't look at it as a great protein source. Also consider an evening snack with about 150 calories' worth of protein and carbs about 30 minutes before bed. Most of your repairs happen while you sleep, since this is when you get a peak of human growth hormone. A bit of protein (15 grams) right before you head to bed helps the building blocks (amino acids) assimilate and repair.

Day 2

5:30 a.m. Wake up 6:30 a.m. Pre-swim

½ banana and 1 cup coffee

ROAR MAKEOVER NOTES: Add some protein, such as ¼ cup fat-free Greek yogurt. Fat-free is best before and after training for more rapid gastric emptying, which circulates the amino acids faster. Two percent at all other times is ideal for protein and satiation.

8:00 a.m. Pre-ride breakfast

Waffle with butter and honey, strawberries, 2 veggie sausages, and 2 scrambled eggs

ROAR MAKEOVER NOTES: Swap the waffle for a whole grain variety. Substitute the butter and honey with a drizzle of almond butter or tahini. You can also top the waffle with fat-free or low-fat ricotta cheese thinned with unsweetened vanilla almond milk with strawberries mixed in.

Also consider a protein pancake with strawberries and ricotta rolled in the middle. These modifications will boost your overall nutrition profile by taking out excess sugars and replacing null fats (butter) with beneficial ones (omega-3s).

10:00 a.m. to 2:30 p.m. Mountain bike ride

Ate one bar and drank a bottle and a half of an electrolyte mix. Felt lousy on the second half of the ride.

ROAR MAKEOVER NOTES: You want to consume about 200 calories per hour. Remember to keep food in your pocket and hydration in your bottle.

3:00 p.m. Lunch

Large glass of almond milk, mixed roasted veggies with oil and vinegar, and a chunk of dark chocolate

ROAR MAKEOVER NOTES: This is severely lacking postworkout protein. Aim for about 20 grams within 30 minutes of completing your ride.

6:30 p.m. Dinner

A bowl of coconut soup with tofu. A large serving of Thai green curry with beef, peppers, and Asian veggies. Two glasses of wine and one glass of water.

ROAR MAKEOVER NOTES: To boost your overall nutrition profile, minimize the coconut milk (in the soup and curry) and add wheat berries, amaranth, quinoa, or basmati rice for healthy carbohydrates. Have a prebedtime snack such as fat-free hot chocolate with 15 almonds.

ROAR MAKEOVER SUMMARY: Without enough daily carbohydrates to help restock her stores, assist with recovery after hard rides, and just perform daily functions, Selene's body went into semistarvation mode and started using more fat and protein for everything from repairing muscles to fueling her immune function. This led to a stressful situation for Selene's body as she created high levels of cortisol and low levels of growth hormone DHEA, which in turn triggered sugar cravings, limited fat burning, and increased fat storage. As a result, her circulating sugar and fats were out of whack and her weight fluctuated seemingly overnight. Because of the lack of sufficient carbs, her body was breaking down red blood cells and using up her precious amino acid stores to do the work. It also explains her occasional late-day fridge and pantry raids.

ROAR MAKEOVER SOLUTIONS: In a nutshell, we bumped up her protein intake a bit, kept her fat intake pretty much the same, and added some starchy carbs back to her plate. "I was shocked how little it actually took to appease my body and make me feel so much better," she recalls. "Just one-half cup of starchy carbs at my meals, and I felt clearer and stronger."

It was important for Selene to front-load her calories in the day. The body is primed for carbohydrates, along with protein, in the morning but leans more toward protein as the day wears on. This has to do with hormonal perturbations (cortisol peaks in the morning and reduces insulin sensitivity). She also introduced foods that benefited her immune system and helped to drop cortisol, such as omega-3s and a bit of magnesium postworkout.

I also recommended that Selene optimize her nutrient timing by fueling with a bit of protein 30 minutes before and after each training session. She started taking one high-dose iron tablet per week to help support the integrity of her red blood cells so they wouldn't break down as quickly, which also made the liver's job easier and aided in the reduction of bilirubin. To top off her newly optimized nutrition, Selene supplemented her diet with a probiotic for maximum gut health and nutrient absorption, magnesium to help with glucose control, and vitamin D to increase bone health.

Her follow-up blood work iced that carb cake. Just 4 weeks later, her glucose had fallen below 100 for the first time in years; her lipids were back in a healthy range; her vitamin B_{12} levels stabilized; and though her iron was still low, it was trending in the right direction. With her macronutrients in balance, so was her body. That meant better performance, energy (mental and physical), and overall health both on and off the bike.

Even more telling? A few years later, she started slipping into old habits. Her blood sugar, lipids, and key vitamins and minerals followed suit, shifting into unhealthy territory. But she knew what to do to nip the issues in the bud and get her blood work back in line before they harmed her health. Remember, no matter how fit you are, there's no outrunning improper nutrition!

ROAR ▶▶▶ SOUND BITES

▶ Most fad diets fail for women because of our different hormonal responses to restriction as compared to men's.

▶ Carbohydrate sensitivity changes over the course of a woman's life span, but carbs are still essential. Don't cut them out completely.

▶ Quality and timing of protein work with your body's natural biorhythms to help with body composition, reparation, and sleep.

▶ Ditch the notion that "low fat" is better—there is room for fat in your diet, especially from avocados, nuts, seeds, and dairy.

▶ Eat low on the food chain: The closer it is to the natural form, the better it is for your body (we are not as smart as nature!).

11

SPORT-SPECIFIC FUELING

HOW TO EAT FOR WHAT YOU DO

When's the last time you grabbed a jug of milk from the fridge and sauntered out to the driveway to dump it into your car's tank before heading out on a road trip? Never—because cars don't run on milk. They run on gasoline, and depending on the car, not just any gasoline. High-performance cars are even more finicky about their fuel and demand high-grade gas at the pump for optimum performance and miles per gallon.

You, as a human being, follow the same fueling principle. First and foremost, you need to fuel yourself with food. Second, the higher performance you demand from your body, the more finely tuned your food choices need to be. Finally, as a woman, your nutrition needs are even more specific. So while you could complete your next workout on gummy bears and Kool-Aid, you really shouldn't.

Whether you're going for a long run, heading to your regular CrossFit box, or rolling out for an all-day charity bike ride, what you eat can make or break your experience no matter how fit or prepared you are. The longer and/or harder the workout on tap, the more important your nutrition is. Nutrition can make or break a race, but you don't have to race to reap these benefits. Eating to enhance your exercise—whatever exercise you do—should be a priority so you can maximize the results of your time and efforts. Here's what you need to know.

TOPPING OFF YOUR TANK: WHAT TO EAT BEFORE EXERCISE

Ideally, you're eating a balanced diet the majority of the time (as per the advice in the previous chapter), so you're pretty much ready to go whenever you want to hit the gym or head out for an easy workout. When preparing for a harder, longer, or more intense bout of physical activity, however, you need to top off your tank. As mentioned earlier, timing of nutrient consumption around exercise directly influences performance, recovery, fat oxidation, and energy expenditure. Evidence indicates that for women specifically, exercising in a fasted state can blunt fat oxidation, whereas exercising in a fed state will result in a greater total daily energy expenditure and increased fat oxidation, potentially improving body composition.

In a nutshell, you want that preworkout snack to accomplish three goals. One, provide fuel so you go into your workout fully energized. Two, help minimize the muscle breakdown that occurs during your workout while maximizing the training adaptations (getting fitter and stronger) you want. Three, make you feel good mentally and physically. You never want wild energy swings, cramping, or gastrointestinal (GI) distress when you're out there trying to perform your best. Note: I'm not just talking to endurance athletes here. Strength and CrossFit athletes also have more robust performance and muscle protein synthesis when they go into a workout properly fueled.

Meeting all three of those goals means eating the right stuff, obviously, but also at the right time. Generally speaking, if it has been 2 or more hours since you last ate, you want to aim to eat a balanced snack that contains about 150 to 200 calories, 30 to 45 minutes before starting to exercise. You definitely want some carbs, but women particularly should pay attention to pre-exercise protein, aiming to get about 15 to

20 grams of protein before hard efforts. Research shows that pairing protein with hard exercise sessions can improve your body's ability to make muscle out of the protein you eat (an ability that diminishes with age) as well as boost how well your muscles adapt to your training efforts. The end result is that you hang on to the muscle you have and perform stronger and faster for years to come.

Good examples of well-balanced preworkout snacks include a little high-protein cereal with a milk alternative (almond, oat, hemp) or a slice of low-fiber bread (low fiber is typically not recommended for daily consumption—but it is before exercise) with a slathering of nut butter and a sprinkle of salt.

Now the GI issue. Again, women are more prone to stomach issues than men because of our hormone fluctuations. But certain sports also lend themselves to belly trouble more than others—particularly jostling activities such as running. I recently gave a talk to a room full of runners, some experienced marathoners, others just starting to get into the running scene. The one thing that they all had in common was GI issues. Regardless of planning, they still couldn't get over the fear and real occurrence of GI disturbances.

Different types of upper- and lower-GI symptoms occur in about 45 to 50 percent of runners. The physiology of digestion—especially during activity—is complex, so the fuel and fluid you put into your system can have an enormous impact. As you'll see in the following section, what you eat and drink during activity is particularly important, but this also holds true for what's already in your digestive system when you start.

During intense exercise, your body redirects blood flow from your gut to your working muscles. This makes your gut a bit hypoxic (low in oxygen), since it's not getting the oxygenated blood it needs to do its job, so it starts shutting down, and it becomes harder for fluids and nutrients to leave the intestine and get into your bloodstream where you need them. The result: Delayed gastric emptying (extra pressure in the stomach—or the slosh factor), intestinal cramping, diarrhea, and some bleeding of the stomach and colon may occur (which is why some people may see a bit of blood in their urine or bowel movements afterward).

CAN I TRAIN FASTED IF I WANT TO LOSE WEIGHT?

I hear this all. the. time. An athlete wants to perform well, but they also want to lose weight. Despite my advice, they believe the solution is using their workouts to create a calorie deficit and lose body fat.

Whether you call it bonk training, fasted training, or fat-adaptation training, the strategy of going out and doing a training session often first thing in the morning on no food has been around for a long time and has come into favor again. Most women I see who want to try this approach are doing it because they believe it will help them get lean more quickly. It nearly always backfires from a performance standpoint, and research shows there is not a greater improvement in body composition when training fasted. Moreover, women do better in a fed state with regard to improving exercise-induced adaptations to the muscles.

Here's why. When you go out and exercise in a fasted state, you're putting your body under added and possibly undue stress. This is particularly bad in the morning because your cortisol levels are already elevated. If you go out and exercise first thing, your body wants to pump out more cortisol but needs the right ingredients to manufacture it, which are your sex hormones—testosterone, estrogen, and progesterone. So your body steals those hormones to make more cortisol. Now your cortisol is very elevated, which stimulates fat storage, not muscle fat storage. In short, you're storing more of what you're trying to lose!

Research shows this in well-trained and professional athletes. When researchers at the University of Georgia tracked the hourly and daily energy intake of a group of female professional cheerleaders to determine the impact on body composition, they found that higher daily energy intakes (kilocalories per kilogram) were significantly associated with lower body fat percentages and that participants with fewer hours in a negative energy balance had a lower body fat percentage and higher lean body mass percentage. Likewise, longer periods with low to no food intake were correlated with greater percentages of body fat.

Even across heavy training blocks, if energy intake is not dialed around training, research shows there is an increased risk of endocrine dysfunction and body fat gain, despite the heavy training loads, *even among men*.

Low fuel in and around training sessions will inhibit your adaptive responses; reduce your body's ability to lose body fat and gain lean mass; and increase your risk for stress fractures, poor blood glucose control, poor sleep, mood disturbances, and ultimately poor performance. In short, if you want to achieve your best performance and body composition, it is imperative that you fuel your workouts!

Whether or not you succumb to GI issues, either upper as with heartburn and nausea or lower as with gas and diarrhea, depends on how hard you're exercising, how much food you had in your system when you started, and what that food was. Drinks count, too. Acidic drinks such as coffee and orange juice (or a heaping dose of both, something I see far too often) can exacerbate symptoms. For those people who tell me, "I eat and drink this way before hard training bouts and I never have problems, but I always do come race day," please remember the nerve factor. Anxiety messes with your digestion and can mean multiple bathroom stops before you even start. Also, as a woman, you're five times more likely to have diarrhea, intestinal cramping, and side aches as compared to men, but men tend to have greater risks of vomiting and nausea. Most of this increased lower-GI-symptom risk is due to the fluctuations of estrogen and progesterone, with a greater incidence of lower-GI issues during the 5 to 7 days before you get your period (the high-hormone phase of the menstrual cycle).

If GI issues plague you, you need to pay extra-special care to your pre-event fueling. Use the taper week to top off your glycogen and electrolyte stores, not the night before or the morning of the event. Remember, it is the day before the race that matters most for fueling, recovery, sleep, and so forth. One of the most common mistakes athletes make on race day is to gauge the size of their prerace meal on the distance of the event. This faulty reasoning can lead to a host of GI problems, as excess amounts of food will tax your body, demanding blood flow to the stomach while muscles in your arms and particularly legs are screaming for fuel. If you know you have GI issues, and morning race nerves exacerbate them, a top-up, pre-event meal is best to keep GI distress at bay.

This light pre-event or race meal should be low fiber, carb based, and low fat, and it should have a moderate amount of protein. Skip anything like dairy and fructose that might take your gut longer to digest. A growing body of scientific literature is showing that the maximum amount of fructose anyone should have is 50 grams a day, but I recommend limiting yourself to 25 grams of fructose. For reference, one banana has about 7 grams of fructose and ¼ cup of raisins has about 12.5 grams; however, berries are relatively low, coming in with about 3.5 to 4 grams per cup. A common go-to race breakfast for my GI-inclined athletes is as simple as two pieces of gluten-free toast (GF because it is quick to digest) with almond or regular butter, salt, and an easy-to-digest protein drink (whey protein or vegan protein with 5 grams of branched-chain amino acids [BCAAs] added). Yes, this seems light in calories (about 500) for an event longer than 4 hours, but it is topping off, not loading up.

QUICK REFERENCE FOR ENDURANCE EVENT AND TRAINING NUTRITION

	GOOD	OKAY	NOT GOOD
NIGHT BEFORE A MORNING EVENT OR MORNING OF AN AFTERNOON EVENT	Waffles Pasta Whole grain pancakes and bread Oatmeal Quinoa Fish Poultry Salad (be careful with fiber)	Real food that you normally have for dinner/breakfast	High-fat, high-protein meal (no more than 35–40 g protein) Anything fructose based
1–3 HOURS BEFORE	Bananas Grapes Oranges Berries Toast with almond or other nut butter	Sandwich PB&J or lean protein wrap (for example, grilled chicken with avocado; light on fibrous veggies, so skip lettuce)	Apples Grapefruit Anything high in fiber
0–1 HOUR BEFORE	10–15 g protein 30 minutes before heading out Fat-free* unsweetened yogurt Almond butter and jam sandwich on low-fiber bread Almond milk with protein powder	Low-fiber toast and jam English muffin with low-fat spread Small handful of nuts and a banana	Anything fructose based Anything high fat or high protein

	GOOD	OKAY	NOT GOOD
DURING	30–40 g carbs per hour of exercise lasting longer than 60 minutes Salted new potatoes Sandwich bites Low-fat* muffin Pretzel bites Jelly beans or Swedish fish	Uncoated protein bar (190–210 calories, 6–10 g protein) Exercise-specific blocks/chomps/chews Trail mix, depending on the intensity of exercise	Fruit-based bars (too high in fructose) Gatorade and other drinks that are 5–8% carbohydrate Gels and GUs
AFTER/ RECOVERY* (LOW TO NONFAT PRODUCTS TO FACILITATE GASTRIC EMPTYING)	Restock protein within 30 minutes 25–30 g high-quality protein (e.g., 25 g whey isolate, 30 g pea protein isolate, hitting 3–3.7 g leucine) Restock carbs within 2 hours (sources rich in glucose are ideal) PB&J or turkey and cheese sandwich Lean protein, starchy veggies, root veggies Smoothie of frozen banana or mango with whey protein powder, fat-free Greek yogurt*, and almond milk	Wraps (veggie, lean protein, hummus) Small bean and rice burrito with salsa (no guacamole or sour cream) Low-fat or fat-free* mocha with low-fat muffin or bagel with low-fat spread	Any processed sugar, candy, or engineered nutrition—the only exception is protein powder, be it whey isolate, casein isolate, pea protein isolate

**Low- and fat-free items are recommended in and around training only to facilitate faster gastric emptying; higher fat options are fine for all other times.*

KEEP ON KEEPING ON: WHAT TO EAT DURING EXERCISE

An entire multimillion-dollar sports nutrition industry has been built on this very topic. Long before there were bars, gels, blocks, and chews, there was food—yep, real stuff such as sandwiches, bananas, and even cookies (which, when you think about it, is all most bars really are). Then somewhere along the way, we decided that prepackaged, scientifically engineered foods were better. Now I see clients who don't eat or drink anything remotely resembling food, and we're not better off for it.

For one, athletes are often eating when they should be drinking, and they think they're bonking when they're really getting dehydrated. So, keep that in mind here. When you're out there feeling the wall approaching, it's very often because you have a big drop in total-body water and your blood is turning thicker, not because you don't have enough fuel to burn. You have enough stored carbohydrates to run for about 2 hours (depending on pace, intensity, and fitness levels). The main goal of eating, particularly carbohydrates, during long or more intense exercise is to keep your blood sugar concentrations topped off so you have a steady stream of energy to keep going. How much you need is the big question that everyone wants to know.

That depends on a lot of things. How fit are you? How long have you been working out, training, or racing? How hard are you going? How much did you eat going into your exercise bout? How old are you? Are you a woman or a man? As you might expect, many of the laboratory studies on this topic have been performed on young, well-trained men. Those guys were able to burn through and hit optimum performance at about 78 grams (312 calories) an hour of carbohydrates from mixed sources (meaning a combination of sugars rather than just one kind; the body absorbs a combination better).

The results from these studies trickle down and leave many athletes with the impression that more is better. The more calories you can consume, the better your performance will be and the longer you'll be able to go. That's not really true. If you're reading this book, chances are you are not a man. I know some women who can approach that 300-calorie-an-hour mark, but not many, and even then only through years of practice and training, because they compete in super-ultraendurance events. For women, all those calories shouldn't be in the form of carbs.

I think women (and men) are better off aiming for a calorie count rather than a specific range of carbohydrate grams every hour because it works far better with your physiology. Inside your small intestine are specific receptors that assist with the digestion of carbohydrates, protein, and fat. So it's best to feed your body a steady stream of mixed macronutrient foods to avoid overloading any one macronutrient receptor at one time, which so many people do when they keep dumping in carbohydrates the whole time. Carbohydrate overload makes you feel bloated, gassy, and uncomfortably full—not good for performance. A better range for most active women is 0.9 to 1.15 food calories per pound (2 to 2.5 food calories per kilogram) of body weight per hour running or 1.3 to 1.6 food calories per pound (3 to 3.5 food calories per kilogram) per hour while cycling or participating in another nonjostling sport.

Contrary to what you may have heard, when in doubt, err toward the lesser amount. It is very common for athletes to overeat during training and racing, with the thought that they are supplying their muscles with needed carbohydrates. But, in reality, you're consuming more than your gut can absorb, so the excess just remains in the stomach or intestinal tract too long, causing nausea, pain, and discomfort (which, of course, impairs performance).

I'm going to drill the point home here. The solution to staying strong and delaying fatigue is taking care of hydration first and foremost—reducing your loss of blood volume—and topping off your stores with small amounts of carbohydrates from real food when possible, not the kind you drink or slurp (see "The Trouble with Gels" on page 208), and simple sugary treats when it's hard to eat on the fly.

Remember, too, that if you're going to be participating in big special events, you need to train your nutrition, keeping in mind that your nerves will be sending a flock of butterflies into your belly during the actual event, and whatever you eat needs to be familiar and very easy to digest. The goal is to eat food that provides fuel for the muscles without causing GI symptoms. As a rule, these types of foods should have a blend of simple sugars such as glucose, dextrose, and sucrose to speed the delivery of the sugar from the stomach, through the intestinal wall, and into the bloodstream.

Be a label reader. With stiff competition on the sports nutrition shelves, more and more companies are moving toward all-natural products, which usually contain dried fruit, evaporated cane sugar, or agave nectar. Cane sugar is fine, as it is sucrose. Products that contain fructose should be avoided, as fructose is not rapidly absorbed through the GI tract but has to go to the liver to be metabolized. Try to get a little protein into your system as well. Amino acids can provide up to 10 percent of your total energy during a long run, ride, or other cardio exercise bout. If you don't get enough through what you eat, your body will take what it needs by breaking down your muscles, which makes it harder to recover as well as make gains in your training. You don't need much, just about 7 to 10 grams of protein per hour, but for long, higher-intensity exercise, it really helps. The foods found in "Put a Rocket in Your Pocket" on page 210 will do the trick.

The Trouble with Gels

I've ruffled a lot of feathers over my 20-plus years in the sports nutrition field (including what I wanted to study—namely women's physiology—getting there!). But the topic that tends to rile people up the most is my stance on energy gels, which in a nutshell is NO. I understand that energy gels are a super-convenient, calorie-dense, easy-to-put-in-the-pocket fuel source. They are also one of the most detrimental fuel sources for performance.

To understand why, consider the nutritional breakdown of a standard gel (to be clear, I am speaking about gels—blocks, chomps, and chews contain different ingredients and do not pose the same risks). One packet generally ranges from 100 to 120 calories per serving, typically about 20 to 40 grams of carbs, and is comprised of maltodextrin and fructose with a bit of sodium, potassium, flavorings, and preservatives. If you read the label, you'll see that most directions state that a gel must be consumed with 2 to 4 ounces of water. Do you know why? Because a gel is a very concentrated carbohydrate (specifically, a 73 percent solution). By recommending water, the companies are trying to water down the concentration of the solution so your body can effectively get it out of your stomach and into your gut, where it can be absorbed for energy.

It's all about osmolality (the concentration of dissolved particles such as electrolytes in your blood plasma). The higher the carb concentration, the higher the osmolality, and the slower it leaves your stomach and your intestines. By nature of how concentrated the gel is, it will sit in your stomach and increase osmotic pressure, drawing water into the stomach to bring down the pressure and allow the solution to exit your small intestine. This backward flow of fluids from the bloodstream into the gut can effectively start dehydrating you. Even when you drink the amount of water recommended on the label, the maltodextrin or fructose combination of sugars remains unchanged and outside of the range of osmolality for fluid absorption.

The second problem is the blend of carbs that most gel manufacturers use. Research shows that a combination of two sugars is absorbed through the intestinal wall and into circulation faster than a single source. This happens because you can activate more transport mechanisms. Gels pair the worst offenders: fructose and maltodextrin.

Many people gravitate toward ingredients like fructose, because they associate it with fruit and the label often promotes it as "natural." A little dried fruit is okay because it's generally lower in fructose than a gel, and the fructose is wrapped in fiber that keeps the fruit's entire fructose load from spilling into your gut at once. It's important to remember that a large amount of fructose in the intestines pulls water in, flooding the intestines, and leaves you with major GI distress. That's because your gut has fewer shuttles for fructose, and fructose takes longer to absorb, which draws water into the gut as your body tries to dilute what is sitting there. Water going into your gut is never a good thing when you're exercising. You end up with what I call goo gut: bloating, gas, diarrhea, and general GI discomfort.

This problem is compounded by maltodextrin, which is made with the building blocks of glucose rather than straight glucose. Maltodextrin is used because it doesn't affect osmolality the same way as the simple sugars glucose, fructose, or sucrose do. So a gel can actually contain quite a bit of maltodextrin and still get shuttled out of the stomach quickly. Sounds appealing. There's just one problem. Maltodextrin can overload a key "gate" in the small intestines; thus, it creates the same high-osmolality environment as fructose—complete with the same increased lag time and undesirable results.

In the end, you don't get the fuel you need, you compromise your hydration, and your belly is upset to boot. I'll note that this can happen with the new generation of isotonic gels, which are designed to deliver quick carbs during exercise and can be consumed without water. Though they are isotonic, they are still high in carbohydrates (i.e., 22 grams, mostly from maltodextrin, in 60 milliliters of fluid), making them roughly a 13 percent solution, which will still impact gastric emptying.

Of course, the human body is not an algorithm, and there are definitely outliers within physiology. I won't disregard that I have had many athletes tell me that they have success on liquid calories (which we'll talk about in the next chapter) and gels without any GI distress. There are very talented, elite, and pro athletes who do get by on gels and water. But as we dig a bit deeper into these success stories, it becomes evident that these athletes do not use just gels; they use them in collaboration with other racing foods.

While I do caution against gels, I understand that they are needed in certain situations. My coauthor will put some gels in her pockets to use for fuel on a long day, but she, like most, cannot get by with just gels and water. I want you to understand how physiology works so you can make the best choices for optimum performance, but I won't condemn you if you do pull out an emergency gel for a blood sugar lift, especially if you've run out of glucose tablets (which you'll see in a moment is my first go-to for quick energy).

PUT A ROCKET IN YOUR POCKET

Repeat after me: Food in your pocket and hydration in your bottle. And by food, I mean food—edible goodness that looks like food, tastes like food, and is recognizable by your grandma (or perhaps great-grandma, depending on how old you are) as being real food.

If you've relied on prepackaged bars for years, the prospect of putting real food in your pocket can be daunting, I know. I've seen it firsthand. Many athletes genuinely don't know what to eat during exercise if it doesn't come in a wrapper with the word *energy* on the label. Relax, it's easy.

Real in-exercise performance food comes in many forms. It can be ⅓ cup low-fructose fruit (figs or dates) with 1 tablespoon of nuts, or a handful of small potatoes (cooked and salted), or three or four rice balls (basmati rice, honey, and tamari or soy sauce), or a homemade bar that isn't sugar based, or protein bites. You can simply try sandwiches cut up into smaller bites (peanut butter and jelly on white bread, cheese on focaccia, even a turkey-and-cheese panini). Some of my athletes like low-fat muffin bites, low-fat brownie bites, or cookies. Turkey jerky is great for a bit of salty, nonsweet food on longer, lower-intensity rides or runs. Just wrap it up in something easy to open, and you have energy in your pocket!

It is often hard to eat during high-intensity rides and runs. Think back to your childhood. What was your favorite gummy candy? Swedish fish? Jellybeans? Mike and Ike candies? All these supply quick hits of sugar that your body can easily digest. Just make sure that the primary sugar is not fructose or high fructose corn syrup. Glucose and/or sucrose are better options, while brown rice syrup is best. Here you can also turn to engineered nutrition in the form of blocks, chomps, chews, and the like. First, these products are generally not made of maltodextrin and fructose, so you won't run into problems. Second, chewing small bits of carbohydrates slows the distribution of the load on the digestive system and allows for better absorption than swallowing a big bolus of gel. In the last hour of a ride, run, or race, when all that matters is keeping blood sugar up for pace, use glucose tablets (they start to be absorbed in the mouth).

Steer clear of anything that contains sucralose and other sugar substitutes such as stevia or sugar alcohols. These compounds are not very well absorbed and can cause GI distress pretty quickly. They also can alter your gut bacteria in unhealthy ways.

Finally, it is true that it's difficult to eat in certain sports—such as mountain biking and trail running. But with a little planning, it can be done, and your performance will improve. The best strategy is to get familiar with the course ahead of time and plan your feeds in transition zones such as the base of a technical climb or when you pop out on the road for a stretch. It's a matter of planning your eating strategies according to the course profile, not time on the clock.

HOMEMADE BAR

- **¾ cup brown rice syrup**
- **⅔ cup natural almond or peanut butter**
- **1½–2 cups crisped rice cereal or other flax-flake, low-sugar, high-protein cereal such as Kashi**
- **1–2 crushed vanilla beans (or dried vanilla bean powder) (optional)**
- **¼ cup raisins (optional)**
- **⅓ cup crushed pretzels (optional)**
- **Dash of sea salt**

In a microwaveable bowl, microwave the brown rice syrup on high for 1 minute 20 seconds, or until it bubbles. Stir in the nut butter until well combined. Then stir in the cereal and any optional ingredients. Pat the mixture into an 8" × 8" pan and sprinkle with salt. Chill for 30 to 45 minutes, or until firm. Cut into 2" × 2" bars.

SALTY BALLS

- **½ cup natural chunky almond or peanut butter**
- **½ cup brown rice syrup**
- **½ cup vanilla protein powder (vegan or dairy)**
- **¼ teaspoon ground cinnamon**
- **1 teaspoon espresso powder (optional)**
- **2 tablespoons unsweetened Dutch-processed cocoa powder or coconut or almond meal (for rolling)**
- **Dash of sea salt**

In a microwaveable bowl, combine the nut butter and brown rice syrup. Microwave on high for 1 minute, or until the syrup boils. Note that the longer it boils, the harder the finished ball will be. Stir until combined. Add the protein powder, cinnamon, and espresso powder (if using), stirring well. Use a tablespoon or melon baller to roll into bite-size 1" balls. Roll in the cocoa or coconut or almond meal to coat and sprinkle the sea salt on top. Store in an airtight container in the fridge for up to 2 weeks.

CHOCOLATE-ALMOND POWER COOKIES

- **¼ cup spreadable light butter**
- **2 tablespoons natural almond butter**
- **⅓ cup plus 2 tablespoons brown sugar**
- **3 egg whites (or egg replacement)**
- **¼ cup almond or dairy milk (optional)**
- **2 teaspoons vanilla extract**
- **1 teaspoon dried vanilla bean powder (optional)**
- **¼ teaspoon ground cinnamon**
- **2 teaspoons espresso powder (optional)**
- **⅔ cup old-fashioned oats**
- **½ cup quinoa flour**
- **½ cup almond meal**
- **¼ cup plus 1 tablespoon unsweetened dark cocoa powder (Dutch processed or Hershey's Special Dark)**
- **1 teaspoon baking soda**

Optional add-ins:

- **Mini dark chocolate chips**
- **Raisins**
- **Dried cherries**

Preheat the oven to 375°F. Cream the butter and almond butter with the brown sugar. Stir in the egg whites, milk (if using), vanilla, vanilla bean powder (if using), cinnamon, and espresso powder (if using). Mix well. In a separate bowl, stir together the oats, flour, almond meal, cocoa, and baking soda. Slowly stir the dry ingredients into the wet ingredients. Stir in milk if needed for consistency. Sprinkle in a few tablespoons of optional add-ins if desired. Drop by tablespoons onto a cold cookie sheet or baking stone. Bake for 10 to 15 minutes, or until golden brown.

CAN (AND SHOULD) WOMEN CARBO-LOAD?

As I mentioned in the previous chapter, women don't tap into and empty out their glycogen stores the same way men do during exercise sessions, so though women absolutely need carbs and perform best in a fueled state, the traditional practice of carbo-loading isn't as effective for us.

Carbo-loading—the practice of "topping off" your muscle, blood, and liver glycogen (carbohydrate) stores by consuming high amounts of carbs in the days leading up to a big event—was developed in 1967 by Swedish scientist Gunvar Ahlborg, who discovered a positive correlation between the amount of glycogen in the body and endurance performance. He conducted a series of experiments showing that by intentionally depleting glycogen over a series of days and then loading up on carbs, athletes could experience "glycogen supercompensation" and increase their endurance.

Over time, the cumbersome (and often problematic) multiday carbo-loading system transformed into a carbo-loading protocol without any special "depletion phase." Athletes will just dial up their dietary carb intake during their taper week, so they're exercising less and skewing their carbohydrate intake from the usual 55 percent to 70 percent of total caloric intake 3 days out from their event.

Many athletes will boil this all down to just 1 day, ramping up their day before, the morning of carbohydrate intake—à la prerace pasta party—which research has found can improve endurance performance in novice marathoners by about 4 percent.

But it doesn't work quite as well in women. As discussed in the previous chapter, we rely on blood glucose first then fatty acids to fuel our efforts. If we're premenopausal, the phase of our menstrual cycle also influences our ability (or lack thereof) to access and replace liver and muscle glycogen. Our bodies don't respond the same way to these deliberate attempts to stuff our glycogen stores days ahead of time and have extra glycogen at our disposal when it's time to go.

We saw evidence of this back in the '90s, when Canadian researchers reported that not only did women burn more fat than men during endurance exercise, but they also stored less muscle glycogen in response to carbo-loading than their male counterparts. In fact, men increased their muscle glycogen concentration by 41 percent in one study while women increased it by zero. The men also improved their performance at lactate threshold by 45 percent while the women eked out only a 5 percent improvement in performance.

Granted, the wrinkle in this research is that the studies were focusing on what percentage of carbs the women and men were consuming while not evaluating if the women were eating enough to begin with. The team followed up with a study in 2000 that not only increased the athlete's relative carbohydrate intake but also boosted their total caloric intake by 34 percent. That worked better. The women were able to increase their muscle glycogen stores by about 17 percent, which was still smaller than the men's 23 percent increase, but an improvement.

But the real issue this study shed some light on is that women really need to eat enough, including carbohydrates, before, during, and after their training and competing on a regular basis rather than trying to cram carbs in the days or night before. Increasing overall calorie intake, including adequate carbohydrates, especially in the luteal phase, when your body is pulling more blood glucose to build up the endometrial lining, improves your carb availability for exercise. That should be your standard operating procedure as a female athlete.

Instead of worrying about piling enough pasta on your plate the night before a big event, eat enough to meet your energy needs. The easiest way to be properly fueled is to be sure you're eating enough carbohydrates to fuel the work at hand. Here are the ranges I recommend.

- For a light or active recovery day, aim for 1.15 grams per pound (2.5 grams per kilogram).
- For short, intense days (like CrossFit training), aim for 1.15 to 1.4 grams per pound (2.5 to 3 grams of carbs per kilogram).
- For moderate- to high-intensity training lasting 60 to 120 minutes, you need 1.4 to 1.6 grams per pound (3 to 3.5 grams of carbohydrates per kilogram).
- For endurance training involving 2 to 5 hours of intense training per day (distance running, cycling, swimming), you need 2 to 2.7 grams per pound (4.5 to 6 grams of carbs per kilogram).
- For extreme intense training of 5 hours or more per day (Ironman or multisport events), you need 2.7 to 3.2 grams per pound (6 to 7 grams per kilogram).

RESTOCKING YOUR STORES: WHAT TO EAT AND DRINK WHEN YOU'RE DONE

First, let's be clear on one thing: You don't need any special recovery strategies after a casual run, ride, or trip to the gym. You can just go about your day, and you will replenish yourself through your daily diet. I see too many recreational athletes drinking high-calorie recovery shakes and eating protein bars when they don't really need them. How do you know when you need recovery fuel? When you finish a really hard workout or event that leaves you feeling like you've really done something. You're a little wrung out and depleted. That's when you know you need to put some nutrients into your system to stop muscle breakdown and replenish your glycogen stores.

What should you eat? For years, sports nutritionists have recommended a snack or drink that has 3 grams of carbohydrate for every 1 gram of protein because protein assists with restocking glycogen as well as muscle repair. But that's not what women really need. We need protein, and we need it fast. Remember, progesterone exacerbates muscle breakdown in women. So you need more protein to protect those muscles and come back stronger. Women recover faster with 25 to 30 grams of protein (with about 3 grams leucine) within 30 minutes of a hard workout. (Note peri- and postmenopausal women should aim for 40 grams of protein to help with recovery.)

This is important for both endurance and strength workouts, but it has particularly potent effects following a strenuous weight-training workout. When you combine those amino acids with intense power moves such as Box Fitness resistance training and fast intervals, it significantly increases the quality of your muscles and slows down age-related muscle decline. Research shows that postexercise protein intakes of about 0.32 to 0.38 grams of protein per kilogram of body weight are recommended for beneficial adaptations in recreational and competitive female athletes. That's about 22 grams for a 64-kilogram/140-pound woman.

That's not to say you don't need those carbs, too. You do. Do not skip the postworkout carbs in an attempt to shave weight—something I see far too often among even top-level pros I've worked with. They believe that if they delay food postworkout, they will prolong their fat burning (since the body has nothing else left to burn) and lose weight more effectively. In fact, the opposite happens. They gain weight. By withholding recovery fuel, they actually put their body in a catabolic state that stalls their recovery, dims their metabolism, and increases their fat storing because the body is afraid it is in a state of famine (see pages 174–175 on Low Energy Availability and REDs).

Always have carbohydrates along with your protein. For one, they work like magic together to increase your glycogen storage rates. The results are quite dramatic. In one study of cyclists who completed a 3-hour cycling bout, those who recovered with a carbohydrate-protein recovery drink restocked their stores four times faster than those who replenished with carbs alone. Research also shows that taking in carbohydrate and protein together postexercise helps to reduce inflammation and can boost immunity.

Remember again that, as a woman, your recovery window to take advantage of all these benefits is pretty short—about 30 to 45 minutes. As the minutes tick away, your insulin sensitivity declines, so it takes your muscles longer to absorb the glucose from your bloodstream. As a result, your overall glycogen storage is lower. In fact, just 2 to 2½ hours later, your glycogen storage rate drops by 50 percent. Eating immediately after hard exercise delays this decline in insulin sensitivity. If you have a recovery snack or meal within 30 minutes, you can then extend your ability to rapidly store glycogen up to 8 hours by simply eating a little carbohydrate every couple of hours.

What are the best carbs for recovery? Many people believe the best postexercise carbs are grain based, like oatmeal, pasta, bread, and cereals. But that isn't exactly true. The best carb sources are those that are richer in glucose, because they shoot straight into your system. Starchy veggies such as white potatoes, peas, corn, winter squash, and root veggies such as parsnips are not only richer in nutrients, but they also provide greater amounts of carbohydrates overall. Compare the carbs in a cup of mashed potatoes (45 grams) with a cup of cooked oatmeal (27 grams), quinoa (39 grams), or the ever-popular cooked pasta (38 grams), and there's really no comparison!

HEAR HER ROAR

THE GI-DISTRESSED TRIATHLETE

When I first met Sonja Wieck, now 35, she was in peak form and entering the prime of her racing career. Unfortunately, she wasn't able to reap the rewards of all her years of hard work because her nutrition kept getting in her way.

In 2012, Sonja had qualified for and was competing in the coveted Ironman World Championships in Kona. She came off the bike in fifth place ready to contend for a podium position and started the run. Before long, her gut began to revolt, sending her to the Port-a-Johns and slowing her to a shuffle. In her words, "It just killed my day."

She brushed it off as a bad day, as so many athletes do. But then during her first race in 2013, the Oceanside 70.3, she had another major nutritional malfunction. This time, instead of GI distress, she simply bonked and hit the wall. Frustrated, she came to me for help. I have to admit, it was a pretty easy fix. Sonja was hydrating with drink mix tablets that contained sorbitol—a natural laxative—as the main sweetener, so by the time she got to the run, well, she had to run.

She was also drinking Coke too early in her races. (Flat Coke is common in extremely long endurance events such as Ironmans and ultramarathons.) Ingesting too much sugar not only contributed to her GI distress but also stalled out her energy supply because her gut was a mess. Coke is a wonderful lift when you need it. But once you start drinking Coke (or consuming caffeine in other forms), there's no going back because of the active receptors in the brain.

We cleaned up her entire nutrition plan by swapping all the sugary, artificial crap for more natural choices. Here's what it looked like before and after:

BEFORE THE ROAR MAKEOVER: One gel right before the start. On the bike, three bottles filled with Nuun (electrolyte-enhanced drink tablets), gummy energy chews, and gels for fuel. On the run, 4 to 5 cups of Coke and more energy chews.

AFTER THE ROAR MAKEOVER: Sonja was ingesting so much sugar and sorbitol and caffeine—no wonder she was a wreck. Prerace, she ditched the gel and ate a small, white-bread sandwich with jam and salt. On the bike, she drank OSMO (which is what I recommended for her at the time, but other light-carb drinks will do); three Picky Bars (all-natural, gluten-free energy bars), eating one every hour for the first 3 hours; then Honey Stinger chews the last hours on the bike. On the run, she added green tea extract to her OSMO bottles to give her a steady influx of caffeine without the ups and downs of Coke. She popped a few chews here and there as she needed them.

Sonja smoked the next race. In her words, "I went to Saint George 70.3 regional championship and won my age group and the amateur race. My energy was consistent, and I felt full and steady throughout the race. My fitness was finally able to shine through because nothing else was in the way. I took this same nutritional strategy into my next full Ironman race in Brazil and won my age group, won the amateur race, and for the first time broke 10 hours in an Ironman distance!

"Since the first time I tried the nutrition plan that Stacy wrote for me, I have not had a nutritional issue in training or racing. I now think very little about whether or not my nutrition plan will work. I know it is what I need. It is solid and consistent."

As are Sonja's results. She most recently won Ironman, Tahoe. Amazing what happens when you work with your physiology rather than fighting against it.

What not to refuel with is fruit. Yes, it's high in simple sugar, but that simple sugar is most often fructose (there are some exceptions, such as bananas and grapes). Your liver loves fructose and will soak it up at the expense of your muscles. Better to stick to veggies, which are made up of long chains of glucose and are more efficient at restocking your stores.

ROAR ▶▶▶ SOUND BITES

▶ Improving training to improve your performance (be it a race, your body composition, or your general health) depends on fueling your body to adapt.

▶ Compared to men, women are 5:1 more likely to experience GI distress. Avoid fructose and maltodextrin during exercise to work with your gut's physiology instead of against it.

▶ Avoid using NSAIDs in and around exercise: They can predispose you to leaky gut and GI issues.

▶ Hydration in the bottle, food in the pocket! Don't rely on a typical sports drink or liquid sports supplement to do both; use a low-carbohydrate, higher-electrolyte drink and eat real food.

▶ Women have a smaller window for recovery than men do. Maximize muscle adaptation and repair by eating for recovery within 30 to 45 minutes postexercise.

12

HYDRATION IS POWER

WHAT TO PUT IN YOUR BOTTLE FOR PEAK PERFORMANCE

"I used to treat my bottles as another vehicle for getting calories," recalls professional cyclist Tayler Wiles. "So, I'd fill my bottles with sugar-filled, carb-dense liquids in races and use them to wash down gels and wonder why I'd end up with a horrible, rotten gut feeling. Worse, even though I was drinking, when I'd use 'pee sticks' to check my hydration levels, I was actually seriously dehydrated!"

Tayler is an amazing athlete. A soccer star growing up, she came into cycling and fell in love with endurance sports in college. By her own admission, she had a lot to learn in a short amount of time to allow her to reach her lofty goals of qualifying for world championships and ultimately competing in the Olympic Games. As a former medical student, she was also a complete sponge for information, soaking up every last syllable and putting all my advice into action. The biggest, and simplest, piece of advice I gave her is what I give to everyone, and you have read it here numerous times: Food in your pocket, hydration in your bottle. The results were immediate.

"I started eating real food like paninis, rice cakes, and homemade bars on the bike and drinking just functional hydration in my bottles rather than carb-dense sports drinks. I started feeling so much better. I started eating more and hydrating better during training because I no longer had that horrible gut rot. Once I made this change, I saw a huge improvement in my level of training."

Tayler ended up making the long team for the Rio Olympics (but ultimately was not selected for the games) in 2016. She won her first World Tour stage at the Euskal Emakumeen Bira in 2019. And she then narrowly missed the selection for the pandemic-delayed Tokyo 2020 games in 2021, after becoming a rider *Cycling News* deemed "one of the most respected domestiques in the peloton."

HYDRATION GONE WRONG: WHEN YOUR DRINKS DEHYDRATE YOU

Hydration should be such a simple thing. You exercise, you lose fluids, you drink, repeat. But many sports drink manufacturers have made it very complicated and in the process less effective. Most of the commercial sports drinks on the market not only won't hydrate you as well as they claim, but they might actually impede your performance by effectively dehydrating you.

In most cases hydration is more important than what you eat while you exercise, and if you mess it up, you mess up your fueling as well. I learned this the hard way as an athlete and saw it firsthand as a scientist working with ultraendurance cyclists, runners, and triathletes. Athletes would have GI problems, muscle cramping, and difficulty recovering, but they couldn't understand why, because they were supposedly doing everything right. To figure out why, I tracked the hydration status, GI comfort, power output, and overall training stress on Tour de France riders. Ultimately, I found that by changing what they were drinking, we could reduce dehydration, increase power, prevent cramping, and eliminate GI problems.

I performed the same testing on elite female athletes, and guess what? Their hydration needs were different from men's. This was because of the hormonal impact on blood plasma volume, core temperature, and sodium retention and loss. Even more so than men, these women really benefited from simplifying their hydration.

How can sports drinks actually dehydrate you? Picture this: It's the last 10 kilometers of a bike race or hard ride. You're in a break and hammering along with the front pack, taking pulls in a rotation, and all is going your way, until you feel it. Your legs are getting heavy, and that dreaded flatness starts creeping in. You assume that you haven't eaten enough, so you reach into your pocket for a gel, tear it open, and slurp it down, chasing it with a hit of your sports drink. Three minutes later you feel a rush of energy, but then 4 minutes later your legs still feel flat and dead. The finish line is getting closer, and you are beginning to think damage control. You find a bit of recovery until about 2 miles to go, at which point you hit another gel, hoping for a lift to get that last bit of power for your final kick. You try to kick it up, but your legs just don't respond. You finish far from where you would like to be.

What went wrong? You thought you were eating and drinking enough, but the fatigue and borderline cramping crept in and knocked you off your game. It's a relatively easy fix. It's not a calorie thing, but a blood volume thing. Basically, you're dehydrated.

Even if you drank a bottle an hour ago, was that really enough? In my experience, athletes are so focused on calories that they don't pay attention to the fact that what they are drinking contributes to fueling, not hydration. Let me explain.

The main point of hydration is to keep your body-fluid levels high enough to continue functioning properly. You use the water in your body to get rid of the heat you produce and cool you down while you're exercising. When everything is working properly, it's an amazingly efficient process. Your blood circulates to your muscles to deliver fuel and nutrients as well as sweep up the waste and heat your muscles produce while they're working. The blood then circulates to the skin to dump the heat through evaporative cooling (sweating).

Sweat works by pulling water (which comes from the plasma) from your blood through your skin, where it can evaporate and cool you down. The more you sweat, the more your blood plasma volume drops. So your body needs to pull water from other spaces to try to keep your blood volume high enough to continue sweating. If you slack on your hydration, you don't have enough fluid in your body to keep your blood volume high enough to sweat efficiently and cool yourself. With less water in your blood, the blood is more viscous, so your heart has to work harder. Your heart rate goes up. Your power goes down. Your core temperature rises. All of that leads to fatigue, reduced performance, and the dreaded power decline at the end of a hard workout.

This whole scenario sets up a serious competition between your muscles and your skin. As soon as you start to exercise, your muscles and your skin fight for your blood to keep your muscles pumping and your body cool. As body water drops, this competition becomes fiercer. Ultimately, your muscles win this round (though as you'll see in a second, they don't really win the fight) and less blood goes to the skin so more fuel can reach your working muscles. With less blood to the skin, there's less sweat to keep you cool, and your risk of heat illness goes up.

Obviously, this situation can't continue indefinitely. Eventually your working muscles and cooling systems will both need more blood than your cardiovascular system can supply. When your body reaches this point, you can't keep your temperature in check, and your muscles start shutting down when they reach the tipping point of 102°F (38.8°C). When your core temperature reaches 104°F (40°C) to 105.8°F (41°C), your central nervous system sounds the alarm that you need to slow down to save yourself. So it's not just core temperature that hinders your performance, but the overall heat stress and limited blood circulation.

This perfect storm of hot skin, low body water, and high core temperature makes it impossible for your muscles to perform the job at hand, whether it's pedaling, running, rowing, or whatever you want them to do. This situation is even more pronounced in women. A 2021 mini-review published in the *Journal of Applied Physiology* found that compared to men, women had a higher core temperature and increased cardiac strain in response to exercise-induced dehydration at a lower percent body mass loss (just about 0.5 percent to 1.0 percent!). In plain language, that means we store more heat, have a harder time offloading it, and we often reach that tipping point sooner than men.

The researchers hypothesized that this may occur because the average female may have less body water in relation to their mass than males (approximately 31 vs. approximately 44 liters or about 49 percent of body weight vs. about 58 percent), because we naturally have a higher percentage of fat tissue (aka hips and breasts), which doesn't hold as much fluid as skeletal muscle. So, the same percent body mass loss represents a larger portion of their total body water. Our body temperature also increases faster and challenges our thermoregulatory system earlier when we start exercising, because women typically sweat less than men. Our sweat glands are less sensitive to stimuli, we have lower fluid output per sweat gland, and our sex hormones can promote fluid retention depending upon the phase of our menstrual cycle.

As a specific example of this in action, the mini-review cites research showing that when women and men cycle at 65 percent of their VO_2 peak, women's core temperature starts rising just 30 minutes into the session, at which point they've sweated out only about 0.5 percent of body mass. The men's core temperature, on the other hand, doesn't become elevated until an hour into the bout, at which point they've sweated out three times as much (1.5 percent of body mass). Echoing these findings, another study showed that when women and men experienced the same level of dehydration—about 1.2 to 1.8 percent—during intermittent exercise, only the women experienced an elevated core body temperature.

As the mini-review points out, our sex hormones also come into play, as our resting and exercising core body temperature goes up about 0.3 to 0.5 degrees Celsius during the luteal phase of our menstrual cycle.

You assume that drinking will help with all this, but that is not always the case, especially if what you're drinking is contributing to making you dehydrated. The mass hydration market out there has saturated the general public with the message that when you drink a typical Gatorade-like 5 to 8 percent carbohydrate solution with sodium (roughly 12 to 19 grams of carbohydrate with about 52 to 110 milligrams of sodium per 8 ounces), you are taking care of your hydration, sodium, and fueling needs. The focus is always on carbohydrate availability and calories. I've done extensive research and been dismayed to find that the focus of hydration research is far too often really about carbs as liquid calories. As a physiologist who specializes in hydration, thermoregulation, and performance, I consider this message misleading and incorrect.

PUMP UP THE VOLUME

Now that you understand the basics of hydration, let's take a look at how fluid gets from your bottle into your bloodstream. It starts in your gut, specifically your small intestine, where 95 percent of all fluid absorption happens. The small intestine is very sensitive to water and sodium and acts like our lady of justice in the body, trying to keep the two in balance so your blood plasma has just the right level of osmolality. Normal blood plasma osmolality is between 275 and 295 milliosmoles (mOsm). I don't expect you to remember that, but it will help you understand how hydration works.

To make sure the fluid you drink makes its way into your bloodstream swiftly and efficiently, the fluid you're pouring down your throat and into your belly should be of lower osmolality than your blood (ideally between 210 and 260 mOsm; water, for reference, is zero). Why? Basic science. If blood is more concentrated than the fluid you drink, the cells in your small intestine will let that fluid through the intestinal walls to add water to the bloodstream and lower the concentration levels.

On the flip side, if you take in fluid that is too concentrated, your intestinal cells will reverse course and pull water from the vascular spaces of your body to dilute the higher osmolality in your gut. In other words, water leaves the spaces where you want it and goes into your digestive system to dilute the fluid sitting in your gut. As you might imagine, the last thing you want is to have water pouring into the small intestine when you're trying to hydrate. The end result is that you have effectively dehydrated yourself and may have triggered GI distress to boot.

The composition (as well as the concentration) of the fluid you're drinking is also important. For optimum hydration, your body also relies on what are called fluid cotransporters, essentially molecular pilots that carry fluid across your intestinal cells and into the water spaces of the body.

Sodium is a top-gun-level pilot for hydration and works best when it has a good copilot—glucose is the copilot of choice. Sodium is absorbed into your cells by a few mechanisms, but mostly it hitches a ride with glucose. Without glucose, the constant flow of sodium and water into your bloodstream slows down. This is why sports drinks that actually hydrate (don't just sit in the stomach and cause sloshing, bloating, and discomfort) contain a small amount of sugar (glucose and sucrose) as well as sodium for optimal absorption and hydration.

But sodium isn't the only electrolyte that facilitates hydration. The most important electrolytes for fluid balance are sodium (as mentioned) and potassium. Often you see magnesium with calcium added, which helps with muscle function (including the intestines!). One important, and often overlooked, consideration of the electrolyte profile is the compound to which a given electrolyte is bound. To avoid exacerbating GI issues, you need to look to minimize the chloride ion. So, look for sodium citrate, potassium citrate, magnesium carbonate (not magnesium citrate—the citrate form is used as a laxative prior to colonoscopy!), and calcium carbonate. When you're at rest, chloride is a key ion in this absorption process. But during exercise, there is a reabsorption mechanism in the sweat glands (independent of blood concentrations), reducing chloride excretion. Ideally, for maximum fluid absorption, you want to drink a 1.5 to 3.5 percent glucose plus sucrose solution with sodium citrate (to reduce gut issues that can come from too much chloride) and potassium chloride or citrate, magnesium, and calcium.

Some of my athletes will say that they just put water in their bottles when they're not doing activity that is hard and/or long. But you still want proper hydration. And plain water isn't optimum for hydration. It contains no drivers and, like a fluid that is too concentrated, may just slosh around for a while before it gets where it needs to go. Plain water also can cause a volume response—signaling your body to pee out more than you've taken in.

If you don't have a sports drink handy, you can make your own simple hydration drink using a pinch (about $\frac{1}{16}$ teaspoon) salt and a teaspoon of maple syrup in 500 milliliters (16 ounces) of water. That yields a 250-milligram sodium, 4-gram (about 1.5 percent) carbohydrate solution for easy hydration.

HOW MUCH FLUID DO YOU NEED EACH DAY?

There has been a wave of internet influencers promoting the miraculous health benefits of drinking a gallon of water every day—that's twice the usual recommendation to drink eight 8-ounce glasses (which also doesn't have any scientific bearing).

Unfortunately, a specific recommendation is not appropriate, as fitness status, environment, training history and plan, as well as sex differences all influence how much fluid you need. Generally, if your urine first thing in the morning is relatively pale yellow, you are off to a good start. Throughout the day, eating watery fruits and veggies, drinking tea, water, low-carbohydrate electrolyte drinks will help keep you hydrated. The afternoon (around 3 p.m.) tiredness often is due to low body water and a drop in core temperature, thus drinking a warm drink (tea, coffee) will help hydrate and bring up the core temperature, reducing the fatigue.

The Institute of Medicine (IOM) reports that most women meet their hydration needs consuming about 78 ounces (2.3 liters) of total water per day from both beverages and food.

THE WINNING (AND NOT WINNING) SOLUTION

So what's the winning solution for hydration? Not the ones so many recreational (and even professional) athletes use. Here are the nutritional aspects of a typical *nonwinning*, carb-heavy sports drink:

- 5–8% carbohydrate solution (12–19 g carb per 8 oz)
- Osmolality of around 300–305 mOsm
- Sugars: maltodextrin, fructose, sucrose
- Sodium: 52–110 mg per 8 oz
- Examples include Gatorade, Powerade, Tailwind, UCAN, Hammer (HEED, Perpetuum)

That sports drink does, of course, provide some carbohydrates, but not in the levels you need to sustain long-term endurance exercise. Sports drinks often contain maltodextrin and fructose, which you know from Chapter 11 are notorious for causing GI distress. Instead, you want to seek a sports drink that supplies some glucose, sodium, and other key cotransporters as described above. A *winning* solution contains the following per 8 ounces:

- 3–4% carbohydrate solution (7–9.4 g carb per 8 oz)
- Sugars: 7–9.4 g from glucose and sucrose
- Sodium: 180–225 mg
- Potassium: 60–75 mg (another fluid cotransporter that can help sodium)
- Examples include Nuun Endurance hydration powder, SOS Hydration, Skratch Labs hydration mix

Now let's go back to the initial race scenario, but this time with a different hydration strategy. You're in a break, and your legs are starting to feel a bit heavy. Instead of reaching for gels for calories, you realize you need hydration and reach for your bottle. This time your drink is lower in carbs, higher in key minerals, and less dense than your blood. Then *you* attack, *you* push the power, and BAM! You finish where you want to be—in the front of the pack.

SALT SWEATERS AND SHAKERS

Now you know that sodium is important for healthy hydration, but unfortunately, a lot of athletes get stuck on the issue of salt. I counsel a lot of Kona-bound triathletes, and nearly everyone will ask if they need to take salt tablets, pour more salt in their drinks, or take sodium-based electrolyte supplements. It's understandable. Hawaii is hot, you sweat a lot when it's hot, and you lose a lot of sodium when you sweat a lot, especially if you're a salty sweater (that's you with the white streaks on your helmet straps, running cap, or face).

The short answer is an emphatic *no*, you do not need salt tablets! Even as a salty sweater, your body has ample sodium stores, and you will consume plenty of sodium from the foods you are eating and (if you chose your hydration source wisely) drinking. You're not trying to replace sodium; you are taking in sodium to work with your physiology under exercise stress conditions. In the human body, fluid is composed of water and electrolytes; the key electrolyte that allows fluid to move freely is sodium.

Even if you sweat a lot, you do not lose enough salt to warrant dumping in high loads during exercise. Salt tablets can contribute to GI distress. The chloride ion of sodium chloride (common table salt) can contribute to increased intestinal permeability, allowing gut bacteria to leak into your body, which in turn causes an abnormal water flux and severe diarrhea. Furthermore, when you ingest a high dose of sodium, you end up with a bit of reverse water flux. If you have a high concentration of sodium in the digestive tract, water will leach into your GI tract to try to dilute the salt rather than be absorbed into the blood. This contributes to dehydration and that awful feeling of gut sloshing. Realize, too, that the normal reaction to exercise is for blood sodium levels to increase, not decrease. That means as you lose more water from your blood through sweat, your blood becomes more "concentrated" with solutes such as sodium.

In a nutshell, you do not need salt tablets, and taking them can actually impair your performance. What you do need is a physiologically sound sports drink that supplies around 350 to 450 milligrams of sodium per 16 ounces. In this day and age, the typical diet has plenty of added sodium, but if you eat a very minimally processed diet, go ahead and be more liberal with your saltshaker. You can also eat more sodium-rich foods such as anchovies, smoked salmon, pickles, and salted nuts to keep yourself well hydrated, especially when you're exercising a lot in the heat.

Before we leave sodium, many athletes ask if they should get their sweat tested to see how much sodium they're losing when they sweat during exercise. I go into this in Chapter 17, but the short answer here is no, you do not need sweat testing. The issue with sweat testing is that the results are lab-valid but not real-life valid. The values you get in a lab test are not indicative of what your true sweat capacity is. Also, it is not recommended to try to match sweat rates with fluid intake (90 to 100 percent of sweat losses), as this is a primary trigger for water intoxication (more on that in a bit).

Also, sweat composition is not an accurate reflection of what your body needs. For example, if you are in the high-hormone phase of your menstrual cycle, you will have a different sweat rate than when you are in the low-hormone phase. If you had a salty meal the day before, your sweat sodium concentration will reflect that dietary intake; and if you are in the high hormone phase, progesterone stimulates the body to release more sodium (hence a more concentrated sweat). Save your money and follow the recommendations for good hydration formulas here instead.

WATER INTOXICATION: DRINK ACCORDING TO THIRST AND SENSE

For far too many years, endurance athletes—especially those who were exercising for many hours, such as marathoners, Ironman triathletes, and long-distance cyclists—were urged to drink before they were thirsty to prevent dehydration. The implication was that more was better, and that had some grave consequences in the form of hyponatremia, also called water intoxication, or dangerously low blood sodium. In fact, one study conducted on participants in the 2002 Boston Marathon found that 13 percent finished with hyponatremia, the majority of whom were women.

Yes, you can drink too much, and hyponatremia is a real risk. More recently researchers, trainers, and coaches are pushing back and advising athletes to drink according to thirst. This is okay as a very general starting point, but the message can be taken too far, and you end up not drinking enough. Sometimes your thirst is not an accurate indicator of your hydration level, and here is why.

There are a few issues with drinking to thirst, and one is that the basic science behind it has been done on men. There is a significant sex difference (and age difference for that matter) when it comes to thirst sensation. Let's go back to those two key female hormones, estrogen and progesterone. Both affect your hypothalamus—the part of the brain that regulates fatigue as well as fluid balance hormones. When we are in the high-hormone phase, our baseline setpoints are reset, so we have lower plasma osmolality, lower plasma volume (up to 8 percent), and a lower setpoint for AVP (arginine-vasopressin) release. Our thirst is muted because of these resets, so we don't go crazy with the drive to drink during the high-hormone phase. If we do drink to thirst, there is a bigger chance of dehydration (and if people drink on a schedule but just plain water, they are likely to develop clinical hyponatremia because of the plasma osmolality shift). This can become more pronounced during perimenopause as your hormones start to fluctuate, sometimes dramatically. This lack of thirst also gets worse as you get older.

SIGNS AND SYMPTOMS OF HYPONATREMIA

- Nausea and vomiting
- Headache
- Confusion
- Loss of energy and fatigue
- Restlessness and irritability
- Muscle weakness, spasms, or cramps
- Seizures
- Coma

Your body can also, in nontechnical terms, go a bit haywire from the heat. You can lose enough water to disrupt your body's systems and signals, like your thirst reflex, so you're not getting the message to drink. You may have experienced this after hot workouts. For instance, have you ever done a tough workout on a warm or hot day, and when you get home, you feel a bit sick but not all that thirsty? Physiologically, you are dehydrated, but the systemic dehydration has kicked in and lessened your desire for water and food. In this instance, your body is not telling you to drink, and you may feel like you don't want to drink, even though that is exactly what you need.

So how much should you drink during activity? If you tend to drink to thirst, and that has worked for you, you can start there, but also use sense. We're far better off using sex-specific guidelines to reduce the risk of heat illness as well as hyponatremia. Everyone is an individual, so your fluid needs may be very different from your teammate's or training partner's. The old recommendation was to drink to replace body-weight loss during exercise (you have likely heard the advice to weigh yourself before and after exercise to determine how many ounces you lost), but this can contribute to overdrinking and does not take into account body-weight loss from fuel burned (glycogen) or any residual fluid or food left in your gut consumed during exercise.

To maintain hydration and hence power during exercise, I recommend women take in fluids at the rate of 0.12 ounce per pound (about 8 milliliters per kilogram) of body weight (that's about 17 ounces for a 140-pound woman/500 milliliters for a 63-kilogram woman) per hour in temperatures 75°F (24°C) and below, and 0.16 ounce per pound (about 10 milliliters per kilogram) of body weight (roughly 22 ounces/600 milliliters for the same woman) per hour in temperatures above 80°F (27°C). Smaller individuals may need less, and larger ones may need more.

In Chapter 17, I'll show you how to totally dial in your personal hydration using pee sticks. In the meantime, use the guidelines below to determine whether you should drink to thirst or if you are better off following a hydration schedule.

Drink to Thirst During Exercise If:

- You have prehydrated prior to the training session or race; otherwise, dehydration can predispose you to tissue injury, decreased motivation during exercise, and poor recovery (adaptations, sleep, rehydration).
- You are heat acclimated.
- You are adequately trained (after significant time off with lower fitness levels, dehydration and exercise stress can exacerbate thermal strain and decrease your performance metrics).
- You have a history of exercise-associated hyponatremia or have a syndrome of inappropriate antidiuretic hormone secretion.

Drink on a Schedule During Exercise If:

- You are a junior athlete and have not gone through puberty.
- You have two or more heavy training sessions in a day, to avoid systemic dehydration.
- You are not acclimated and training at altitude.
- You have a history of heat illness.
- You are a late peri- or postmenopausal woman.

After training and exercise that leave you a bit dehydrated, slowly rehydrate over the course of 2 to 3 hours. Guzzling fluids in large amounts quickly may cause a pressure response to make you pee out more than you absorb. Options for rehydration include your protein drink; watery, lightly salted fruit (e.g., watermelon); and/or more of your functional hydration drink.

EVERYONE CAN HYPERHYDRATE

I'm also a big proponent of prehydrating. Starting the night before a big event, especially if you're in the high-hormone phase or if you're postmenopausal and have noticed your thirst isn't kicking in like it used to, you can hyperhydrate by drinking sodium-rich fluids such as chicken broth or miso soup. There are sport nutrition products that are sodium-based hyperhydration mixes as well as non-sports-related products that work well as a hyperhydration drink, such as Ural (a urinary alkalinizer used for cystitis and urinary tract infections), that are high in sodium. Prehydrating helps you have more fluid on board at the start line so you can better keep your cool and power your way to the finish.

It's one of the single most effective strategies I've used with endurance athletes such as Ironman competitor Hailey Manning. She sums it up: "I have become hugely passionate about properly hydrating! I know if I have a big workout coming up and it's hot, that if I preload my system, I have a great workout. I watch my friends who don't bother, and they just don't perform as well. It may just be one workout, but it all adds up to that magical 1 percent improvement that will make a difference on race day."

LIGHT SPORTS DRINKS: BUYER BEWARE

Some sports drink manufacturers now offer low-calorie, "lighter" mixes (likely in response to the low-carb trends). But buyer beware. For starters, they do nothing to shepherd fluid through the intestinal wall. A bit of glucose and sodium is needed to work with the physiology of the small intestine and pull fluid in (remember the glucose-sodium cotransport system).

Some of these products contain sugar substitutes, which you absolutely don't want. Certain types of sugar substitutes (sugar alcohols such as sorbitol, mannitol, and xylitol) pull water into the GI tract and out of the blood. These ingredients are more commonly used as laxatives and strongly linked to GI distress—that's the opposite of what you're looking for! Likewise, stevia (which is currently very popular in commercial sports drinks) can cause gastrointestinal side effects in some people, including gas, nausea, and bloating.

Other sugar substitutes can actually cause your blood sugar to crash. For example, when you consume sucralose, your body perceives the sweetness and releases insulin in anticipation of the sugar to come. But there is no sugar; thus, your existing blood glucose gets taken up, causing a drop in blood glucose and a bit of hypoglycemia. This signals your body to release more glucose into the blood, which, in turn, causes more insulin to be released, and around and around it goes. During exercise, insulin doesn't play a large role in blood sugar control, but ingesting products with sucralose can make your blood sugar bottom out more quickly (kind of like taking in lots of caffeine), thus increasing the need for carbohydrates.

Again, look for drinks that contain 3 to 4 percent carbohydrate solutions (3 to 4 grams per 100 milliliters/about 7 to 8 grams per 8 fluid ounces).

ROAR ▶▶▶ SOUND BITES

▶ The goal of hydration is to keep your body-fluid levels high enough to get rid of the heat you produce and cool you down while you're exercising.

▶ Do not worry about matching your sweat sodium losses. You just want to make sure you are consuming fluid and food with sodium in it.

▶ Separate your fueling from your hydration.

▶ Do not depend on a typical sports drink for hydration. These sports drinks are about 5 to 8 percent carbohydrate with a low level of sodium and other key electrolytes. This carbohydrate concentration provides some energy for exercise, but it comes at the expense of hydration, because it's too high to maximize fluid absorption in your gut.

▶ An ideal sports drink for *fluid* absorption (aka a functional hydration beverage) should contain 3 to 4 percent carbohydrates (from glucose and sucrose) with sodium and potassium.

▶ You are more predisposed to hyponatremia (water intoxication) during the luteal (high-hormone) phase of your menstrual cycle. Ensure there is sodium in the food and drinks you consume, and be conscious not to overdrink.

13

GOING TO EXTREMES

HOW TO THRIVE IN SOARING TEMPERATURES, FREEZING COLD CONDITIONS, AND THE HIGH MOUNTAINS

By now you fully get the message that (say it with me loud and proud) women are not small men. But as you've seen, sometimes size does matter, and our relatively smaller size can work either for or against us, depending on the task at hand. These advantages and disadvantages become all the more pronounced when we start exercising in extreme environments.

Most, but not all, of the issues we have in extreme conditions come down to thermoregulation—the ability of the human body to maintain its core temperature within a few tenths of a degree of normal (97.7°F/36.5°C to 99.5°F/37.5°C). To fine-tune your temperature so precisely, your body picks up signals from your core as well as your periphery and relays them to the hypothalamus in your brain, where it integrates the information and signals the appropriate coordination of regulatory responses.

Obviously, you are neither a cactus nor a polar bear, so it's not like you can go out into any temperature and expect your body to be able to continue regulating. When the conditions get too extreme, the regulators eventually conk out and you get hyper- or hypothermic (too-high or too-low body temperature, respectively). That's not only bad for performance but also downright dangerous. Fortunately, there are many steps you can take to help your body adapt and perform in various extreme conditions.

Here's a look at how to acclimate to and perform at your best when dealing with extreme heat and cold, as well as high altitude—a unique challenge all of its own. Note: Along with the challenges that thermoregulation presents, there are ways that you can hack into the thermoregulatory system to deliberately elicit specific health and training benefits through cold and heat exposure. We'll address those as well!

BEAT THE HEAT

When the temperature soars, so does our internal system, especially if we're exerting ourselves outdoors. To prevent us from overheating, our bodies dissipate heat by sending blood to our skin to off-load the heat from our core and, of course, through sweating, which leaves a layer of moisture on our skin that cools us as it evaporates.

It'll come as little surprise to you that women and men thermoregulate a bit differently under heat stress. As you saw in the hydration chapter, women sweat less. Our sweat is also more diluted. Though we generally have a higher sweat gland density than men, we have lower output per sweat gland. Though both sexes see their core body temperature rise when they get dehydrated during exercise, women's cores may get hotter at a lower level of dehydration because they start out with a lower volume of body water than men do.

Not only do we sweat less, we also start sweating later than men. We vasodilate first, then sweat, meaning that our internal temperature that kick-starts sweating is higher than men's. Men's overall higher sweating capacity can be an advantage in hot and dry conditions, where sweat evaporates and helps keep you cool quickly, but it is a disadvantage in hot and humid conditions, where they end up with what's called "wasted sweating," where you're pouring sweat, but it's not evaporating or cooling you. Women, who have and use more sweat glands, but generally sweat less and "waste" less sweat, are better equipped to tolerate hot and humid conditions.

And, of course, sex hormones matter. Women have different heat-loss responses across the phases of our menstrual cycle (and a fluctuating internal temperature because of the changes in estrogen and progesterone), which change yet again at the onset of menopause. Skin temperature and blood flow are lower in the high-hormone phase, meaning we are less sensitive to triggers to dissipate heat when our levels of estrogen and progesterone are high. With the onset of menopause, heat-loss responses are significantly inhibited, although they can be improved with increased endurance fitness.

To perform well in the heat, staying on top of hydration is essential. You'll find everything you need to know about hydration in Chapter 12, but to recap—body water is your natural engine coolant. As you sweat, you lose water from your blood (as the plasma volume drops, the body pulls water from other spaces to try to keep blood volume up); if you are slack on your hydration, you compromise your blood volume, which in turn negatively affects your blood circulation and leaves you with less fluid for sweating.

It's important to note here that it isn't just your core temperature that dictates how you perform, but your overall thermal stress and your blood availability. The most difficult situation for your body is the perfect storm of hot skin, low body water, and elevated core temperature. When you're exercising in the heat, the biggest burden your body faces is trying to keep blood flowing to the skin to keep you cool. Skin temperature is affected mostly by ambient temperature, while core temperature is affected by exercise intensity and is largely independent of environmental factors—that is, *when your thermoregulatory system can effectively off-load heat.* With hot skin, there is less cooling available to return to the body, and low body water impacts blood volume, which reduces your capacity to sweat and off-load heat. This situation will increase heat stress, increase heat storage, and in turn increase the overall strain on your body.

Hyperhydration (see "Everyone Can Hyperhydrate" on page 232) is an excellent strategy for dealing with extreme heat, because you have more fluid on board to start with, and that allows more wiggle room for loss. If you're going to be participating in a lot of events in high temperatures, I also recommend doing some work to acclimate to the heat, which includes a little "permissive dehydration."

ACCLIMATING TO THE HEAT

Acclimation is just as it sounds—it's training your body to perform its best in certain environmental conditions. Heat acclimation allows your body to better tolerate exertion in high temperatures. Your total blood volume increases (the watery component and red blood cells), so the blood flow to your muscles and skin is improved and your heart rate and skin and body temperatures are lower at any given exertion. You start sweating earlier and sweating more, so you can better cool yourself. The composition of your sweat also changes, so you lose fewer electrolytes (up to 50 percent fewer) as you sweat. All are key adaptations for sustaining exercise in the heat.

This is particularly important in situations where you're going between extremes, which many recreational athletes do. For instance, you live and train in New England, but you've signed up for a marathon in Florida in the spring. You get to the race and cook, dropping out with the dreaded DNF (did not finish) because all your training was done in the cold, and suddenly you're trying to maintain an 8:30 pace when it's above 80°F.

If possible, get to your destination 14 to 21 days ahead of time. (I know this isn't going to be possible for many people; bear with me, plan B is coming.) This is the amount of time in which the vast majority of heat acclimation occurs. Then just start exposing yourself to the heat on a daily basis. Start small, maybe a ½-hour jog in the mornings, and work your way up to doing some efforts in the heat of the day (especially important if that's the time when your event will take place). You should not feel drained from these bouts. If you are, you need to dial back your effort and do more precooling (more on that in a second).

Two of the biggest mistakes some of my Kona-bound athletes make are attempting key workouts in the heat of the day when they first arrive on the Big Island and not using air-conditioning when they sleep. Why are these mistakes? Trying to train in the heat of the day without proper preparation will cause an incredible amount of thermal stress and jack up your core temperature (we often hear this described as elevated metabolism). This increase in core temperature causes a cascade of effects that reduce your ability to recover and sleep (when all your repair and recovery take place). By not sleeping in a cool room courtesy of your air-conditioning, you reduce your body's ability to fall asleep, stay asleep, and recover.

Make It Hot at Home

If you can't afford the time and expense to acclimate in the actual environment you'll be competing in, mimic the heat the best you can where you are. There are several easy ways of stressing your body's thermoregulation system to kick-start the heat dissipation responses.

One easy way is to simply wear more layers. A hat and gloves go a long way in trapping in some heat. Just be sure everything is breathable and don't overdo it. You want to simulate a hot environment but not give yourself heat illness. You can also use indoor training for heat acclimation. My coauthor, Selene Yeager, trains through cold Pennsylvania winters and needs to be prepared for suddenly hot spring races. She wears more clothes and uses fewer fans than usual when she rides on the indoor trainer. She says it's very uncomfortable at first, but as you'd predict, it works.

Another, stronger stimulus is to elevate heat stress above the sweating threshold of exercise by using hot yoga or a sauna. Just heading into a hot yoga class or sitting in the sauna can help you acclimate by a small degree. A strategic combination of passive dehydration and high-heat conditions (also known as short-term heat acclimation) is the best way to capitalize on the physiological responses of heat acclimation. In a nutshell, you head into a hot place without rehydrating (we are all somewhat dehydrated at the end of the day or after a workout) so that you have a low blood volume and your body is already under thermal stress.

This combination decreases the partial pressure of oxygen at the kidney. Sensing this low-oxygen situation, your body increases its production of EPO (erythropoietin) and subsequently red blood cells, as this hormone controls red blood cell production; but physiologically, you need more water to carry the red cells in the blood, so your body pumps up its total blood volume. The heat stress with dehydration also affects the body's feedback mechanism of getting rid of heat and reducing heat storage; therefore, you start sweating earlier and your sweat is more diluted (you hold on to more of your sodium) to allow your body to cope with the heat stress. Heat exposure like sauna (especially postexercise) also resets your thermoregulation thresholds, so hot temps feel less overwhelming, and improves your performance at high altitude, where the mountain air is dry and dehydrating. Research also finds that heat acclimation improves performance in temperate and cool conditions as well.

Obviously, this doesn't happen overnight. Though women and men are equally responsive to heat acclimation strategies, research shows that females need to do about twice as many heat adaptation sessions (nine as opposed to four) to get the same magnitude of adaptations as their male peers. In fact, a study published in *Frontiers of Physiology* found that women who followed a 4-day heat-training protocol did not show improvements in performance during a 15-minute cycling time trial in a 95°F (35°C) environment. However, women who followed a 9-day heat-training protocol improved their mean power output by 8 percent, their speed by 3 percent, and went 3 percent farther during the same time trial. (See "Sauna Training Protocol," page 248, for specific protocols.)

Again, this works best with some permissive dehydration. This naturally happens with exercise, as we really do not replace all the body water we lose. Drinking to thirst is one of the most effective means of creating permissive dehydration (remember from Chapter 12 that thirst is not an accurate indicator of hydration and often leaves us with low body water). So ideally you would do a workout, do your heat-acclimation work, then slowly rehydrate over the course of 3 to 4 hours. The adaptation process won't work if you gulp down fluid immediately after heat exposure.

Once you're heat acclimated and raring to go, you can implement a few cooling strategies to improve your comfort and performance even more.

Precooling Techniques

Before you start an event in high temperatures, you can do a few things to precool, which effectively reduces your core temperature at the start of the event so you have a longer time before you reach a critical core temperature and the onset of fatigue.

Lie low. A lower resting core temperature gives you an advantage heading into a hot event. So don't exercise hard, get into a sauna, or do anything to drive your core temperature up in the 24 hours before your event.

Take a dip. Immerse yourself in a body of cold water for 10 to 15 minutes. Take a dip in a pool, lake, or ocean if possible. Or, if all else fails, you can take a cold shower. This drops your core and skin temperatures so you don't feel as hot when you start exercising.

Drink a slushy. Drink an icy beverage to lower your core temperature and create a heat sink so you store less heat and you store it more slowly. By doing so, you can tolerate a higher core temperature during exertion and delay the onset of heat-induced fatigue.

Drape cool towels over your neck. Cool your skin with moist towels. Just don't take this too far and start packing yourself in ice. Ice on the skin is too cold and actually constricts your blood vessels, forcing hot blood from the skin back to the core, driving up your core temperature.

Cooling During Exercise

In an ideal situation, you'd be sucking on cold Popsicles throughout the race. But that's not realistic in most scenarios. You can delay the onset of fatigue with some of these in-exercise cooling techniques.

Stash ice-cold beverages. Try to stash some frozen bottles along the course so you can have a cold drink midway. This works well in races where you stock your own feed zone. Ask your friends to cheer at a specific location and hand you a cold bottle. You can also do this when you're out training by planning your routes around convenience stores, where you can go in and get something ice cold—or even just some ice for your bottles. Do not, however, pour ice water on your head! Ice water is too cold for your head, which is very vascular. The extreme cold will constrict those vessels and send hot blood back to your core. It is fine to dump cool water on yourself because it will help pull heat away from your core as if you were sweating (and evaporating) buckets. Cool water on your forearms is an effective technique.

Wear sunblock and/or use sun sleeves. Protect yourself from getting sunburned, which amplifies the heat stress. UV-protectant arm skins not only prevent sunburn, but you can also pour cool water on them, and they'll hold that water against your forearms to help keep you cool. Remember, keeping the skin cool helps reduce overall thermal strain, meaning you can exercise harder and longer in the heat!

FEND OFF THE FREEZE

In cold temperatures, your body tries to hang on to all the heat it can by shutting down blood flow to your skin and shivering to keep warm. And once again, women are a bit different in how we respond when the temperatures drop.

I don't have to tell you this if you're a woman who's ever lived with a guy. You've likely noticed that you might be a Popsicle compared to him—cold hands, cold feet, and all bundled up in cable knit while he's comfortably sporting a T-shirt. What gives? As mentioned earlier, but it bears repeating here, as a woman, you maintain a higher core temperature—about 0.4°F higher on average (97.8°F/36.5°C versus 97.4°F/36.3°C)—and you're actually better at conserving heat when the weather turns cold, but we tend to have cooler skin. Women's hands are nearly 3°F colder on average than men's (90°F/32.2°C versus 87.2°F/30.7°C). That's important when you're trying to stay warm, because when your skin feels cold, you feel cold.

Women are better at conserving body heat and maintaining core temperature because women have about 10 percent more fat, which acts as insulation. That fat is also more thickly and evenly distributed under your skin than a man's. So when it's cold, your body pulls warm blood into your core to protect vital organs. That warm blood is kept warm by the fat layer. But your skin, sitting on the outside and exposed to the elements, feels colder, especially in the extremities, such as the hands and feet.

And of course your hormonal fluctuations also affect your core temperature. Your body runs hottest—hitting a peak of 99.3°F/37.4°C—during your high-hormone phase compared to a low of 98.4°F/36.9°C when hormone levels drop. As such, premenopausal women will also be more sensitive to the cold during certain times of the month.

You can get in trouble if you're not careful about keeping yourself sufficiently warm when exercising outdoors in low temperatures. In cold weather, your body can lose heat faster than you produce it, especially if it's wet and/or windy. When that happens, you're at risk of hypothermia, which is abnormally low body temperature that can cause uncontrolled shuddering and confusion and can leave you physically uncoordinated. Mild cases can be treated with relative ease by going somewhere warm. But extreme cases can be serious, even fatal. Some activities leave you more vulnerable to hypothermia than others. Sports such as running, where you're generating a lot of heat, leave you less susceptible compared to those like cycling and skiing, where you're exposed to a lot of airflow and your body is relatively still for long periods of time. We're also more susceptible as we age, because it becomes harder to maintain normal body temperature.

COLD HANDS?

Women are more likely than men to suffer from Raynaud's syndrome, which is a condition that causes an extreme vasospasm, or narrowing of the blood vessels, in response to the cold, usually in the fingers. But it can also affect the toes or rarely the nose, ears, lips, and nipples. The skin can briefly turn white or blue as blood flow constricts and then becomes red and throbs and burns as blood flow returns. It's relatively rare, occurring in about 5 percent of the general population. However, among women between the ages of 15 and 40, that number appears to be as high as 15 percent.

Estrogen seems to be the culprit. It influences how our vascular system reacts to cold temperatures, and research has found that women taking estrogen therapy (unopposed by progesterone) are more prone to Raynaud's than their peers who don't take the hormone.

People with Raynaud's syndrome are more prone to chilblains—painful swelling of small blood vessels in your skin—when cold skin is warmed too quickly. These can cause itching, redness, swelling, and even bumps or blisters on fingers, toes, nose, and ears. They usually go away on their own or with topical corticosteroid creams. But it's best to try to keep your extremities warm and prevent them!

Wearing gloves obviously can help, but many women feel they need additional help, especially when doing activities like cycling and skiing in the cold. In those cases, you can tuck a chemical heating pack against your inner wrist, as keeping the arteries in your wrist warm will help keep your hands warm. (You can also stick them in your shoes if you'll be riding in the cold.)

That's not to say you should avoid exercising in the cold. Fresh air and sunshine are good for fighting off colds as well as seasonal depression, so there are good reasons to get out there. You just have to be smart. Here's how to warm up to those cold-weather exercise bouts.

Warming Techniques

You can do a few things to keep your body warm when exercising in cold temperatures. These strategies can help you fend off hypothermia and keep your core temperature stable so you can comfortably perform even in the harshest conditions.

Warm up from the inside out. Have some coffee, hot chocolate, or even some steamy chicken soup before heading out. By getting some warm liquid in your belly, you can help keep your body temperature up when you get outside.

Layer up. Resist the urge to throw on all the clothes you own. If you're perfectly toasty when you step outside or on the starting line of a cold event, you're going to be positively baking once you get going and start generating heat. You want to be a little chilly to start. Also, wear layers so you can shed clothes if you get warm and put them back on if you get cold. Start with a light base layer. Add an insulating midlayer (fleece is a great option), and top it off with a breathable outer layer that protects against wind and moisture.

Most important, whatever you wear should be moisture wicking. It's imperative that you stay dry when it's cold. If you get soaked in sweat (or precipitation for that matter), you're going to be chilled to the bone in no time, especially if you need to slow down and stop. Invest in exercise clothes made from technical fabric or merino wool that will wick moisture away from your skin and dry quickly.

Ease into it. It takes longer for your muscles and metabolism to get going in the cold. Do a short warmup inside to jump-start the system, then give yourself extra time to ramp up your effort once outdoors. Standing around waiting for the race to begin can give athletes a rigor mortis feeling called *afterdrop*, where body temperature drops significantly once you start moving because of nerves and wind chill. Others experience a shift in blood circulation, and some just can't warm up at all. If racing, get in a good warmup as close to the starting time as possible and keep moving until the gun goes off.

Cover your head. You do not lose 50 percent (or more, as some myths go) of heat through your head. It just feels like all your heat is leaving through your noggin because you're wearing clothes on the rest of your body. If you stood outside with bare feet and a hat, you'd feel like all the heat was leaving through your feet! But just as you wouldn't go barefoot when it's cold, you shouldn't leave your head unprotected either.

Get a neck gaiter. Covering your neck—and maybe chin and mouth—can make even the coldest conditions more bearable. Some athletes like to use their neck gaiters as a bit of a cold-air-breathing barrier when it's *really* cold by pulling it up over their mouth and taking a few breaths of warmed air to give their throat and chest a break from the sting of the cold.

Protect your hands and feet. Remember, your body is going to protect your organs first and foremost when it's cold. That means the furthest points from your core get the short end of the blood supply. Your fingers and toes are very vulnerable to the cold. The right gear for your extremities can make or break your outdoor exercise experience. Thermal socks, shoe covers for cyclists, really good gloves, and hand and feet warmers that you slip into your gloves and shoes can go a long way.

Eat and drink. Because your body has to work harder when it's cold, you're burning more calories, so it's important to fuel properly. Many athletes blow their nutrition during cold-weather races and workouts because they don't feel like eating or drinking. For short events, this is okay. Training or racing outside in cold weather for less than 2 hours doesn't usually present a problem in terms of nutrition. On long days, the combination of heavy clothing and high-intensity exercise can lead to increased sweating and the possibility of dehydration. You may not feel as thirsty in cold weather because your body chemistry impairs your brain's ability to tell you when to hydrate. Cold weather can also move body fluids from your extremities to your core, causing you to pee more, which can further increase your risk of dehydration. Of course, you won't drink as much in the cold as you do in the heat, but be smart about your hydration and nutrition to keep your performance where you expect it to be!

THE REASON YOU'RE ALWAYS FREEZING AT THE OFFICE

Ever notice that women tend to carry sweaters to work in the middle of July? That's because the air-conditioning temperatures of indoor spaces are based on research performed on men. It's a bit off topic regarding exercise performance, but very relevant to the topic that women are not small men.

Air-conditioning and heating standards in office buildings were set by researchers in the 1960s based on the resting metabolic rate of the average 40-year-old man weighing 154 pounds, which may overestimate the average female metabolic rate by up to 35 percent. It's not only a discomfort for half the population, who research shows prefer temperatures that are about 6 degrees warmer than what men prefer, but also an enormous waste of energy, money, and resources, not to mention lost productivity.

Using Heat and Cold for Long-Term Health Benefits

Admittedly, preparing your body to exercise in extreme heat and/or cold can be a bit of a pain. But once you understand your thermoregulatory system, you also can take advantage of it for health as well as performance benefits by deliberately exposing yourself to extreme temperatures in the form of heat/sauna sessions and cold plunges.

As mentioned earlier, the human body sits in a very tight range for temperature control, and to maintain that tight control, your brain (specifically the hypothalamus) picks up signals from your core and periphery, so it knows what it needs to do to keep the temperature where it needs to be. But where is it getting those signals from? The first line of signaling comes from thermoreceptors, which we have internally and, importantly for our purposes here, in our skin.

It makes sense that the organ that wraps around our entire body would be brimming with thermoreceptors, because that's literally our first contact with the world. Our physiological and behavioral responses are largely based on input from the skin. Interestingly, our face is four to five times more sensitive than the skin on our arms and legs. So if you increase the temperature on your face by 7°F/4°C, you increase your general sweating by 50 percent.

Likewise, rapid cooling of your facial skin initiates a two to five times stronger physiological response as compared to the same rapid cooling of your arms and legs. That's why cooling your face is so effective when you're feeling overheated. It's also why, when swimmers and/or triathletes dive into a cold body of water, it can be hard to get your heart rate up to race, even if you're in a full wetsuit. The initial shock of cold water on your face triggers a cold shock response, which includes high heart rate, a respiratory gasp, hyperventilation, and that sudden panicky feeling you get when you dive in. Then, you get a "vagal response," where the cold stimulates the vagus nerve, which is part of the parasympathetic nervous system, connects our brain to our organs, and counteracts the stress response. So you have a parasympathetic response and your breathing and heart rate decrease, which is the opposite of what you're looking for in a race situation (but can have benefits outside of competition, which we'll get to in a bit).

Deliberately exposing your skin to heat and cold can enhance longevity and our ability to handle stress.

HEAT EXPOSURE

Cultures around the world have used saunas for health benefits for thousands of years with good reason: A 2018 research roundup reported that sauna use was linked to a reduction in high blood pressure, cardiovascular disease, and stroke, as well as pulmonary disease and neurocognitive diseases like dementia. It may improve insulin sensitivity and therefore lower fasting glucose. It also appears to alleviate pain associated with inflammation and arthritis. Other research finds it reduces the risk of early death.

Sauna training is almost like "passive exercise," as your body responds to sauna the same way it does to moderate- to high-intensity exercise: Your heart rate goes up by about 30 percent, your body temperature rises, you break a sweat, and your body produces hormones like noradrenaline and growth hormone. So, you get health benefits similar to a good workout. The benefits are even better for people who exercise regularly. The study found that having high fitness levels from regular exercise plus regular sauna treatments provided extra cardiovascular benefits.

When you have rapid exposure to high heat, you also have a rapid shift in your blood flow, going from your central organs to your periphery. So your general endothelial function improves, helping lower your blood pressure. It also improves your heart rate variability because your cardiovascular system is trained to be more quickly responsive.

Heat exposure like sauna also increases the production of heat shock proteins (which were first described in relation to heat, but we now know they're also expressed during exposure to other stress, including cold). When your body is exposed to a stress, the proteins in your cells can unfold and then refold misaligned, which can pave the way for disease. Heat shock proteins are like your body's molecular EMTs that go in and refold those proteins damaged by the cell stress. They also monitor your cell's proteins, carrying out old proteins and helping newly synthesized proteins fold properly, so they're good for your overall health!

So to sum it up, with heat exposure, you get better blood vessel control, better cellular protein function, better blood glucose control, decreased oxidative stress, improved cardiovascular function, and better exercise performance (especially in the heat and at altitude). Sauna training can be especially helpful for peri- and post-menopausal women whose blood vessels are becoming less compliant and who have less tolerance to the heat. Some menopausal women also find it helps reduce hot flashes that can occur during exercise in the heat.

SAUNA TRAINING PROTOCOL

Sauna training is an excellent secret weapon for both heat and altitude acclimation. But use it wisely. Traditional saunas heat the surrounding air to about 185°F (85°C), while infrared saunas heat to approximately 140°F (60°C). The general guideline is for 25- to 30-minute sessions where the temperature doesn't exceed 165°F. I don't recommend going into the super-high territory that you may see celebrities like Gabby Reece do unless you're *very* experienced with sauna treatments. Also, you should stay in only for as long as you feel comfortable. (No sauna or spa available? Don't sweat it. Hit six to eight 90-minute hot vinyasa yoga classes over a 14-day period and reap the benefits of heat adaptation.)

SAUNA SPECIFICS: Go into the sauna within 30 minutes of completing a workout. Do not rehydrate in these 30 minutes (your protein recovery drink is okay, but no other fluid).

- Try not to drink while in the sauna. If you feel too hot but want to build up tolerance, pour water over your neck or take a cool shower and get back in.
- Upon exiting the sauna, slowly rehydrate over the course of 2 to 3 hours. Gulping down fluid in large amounts after sauna bathing will cancel the heat-stress response to the kidneys.
- Do not use the sauna if you recently consumed alcohol, as it increases the risk of a heart attack or stroke. Alcohol can further impair your judgment, coordination, and balance.
- If you have any muscle or joint aches, swelling, redness, or tenderness at rest or with light exercise, do not use the sauna.
- Do not use the sauna if you have any exuding bruises or sutured wounds.
- Remain in the seated position while in the sauna.

- Leave the sauna if you start to feel uncomfortable.
- Take a warm shower after leaving the sauna. If you want to take a cold shower, wait at least 10 minutes to prevent light-headedness from sudden, dramatic changes in temperature.
- Resting heart rate will be high (around 140), so during the sauna week, you want to decrease intensity; plan for more of a recovery or endurance week to prevent overtraining.

Note: The optimal heat training plan for women is also affected by which hormone phase we're in. In the low hormone phase, which is right before, during, and right after your period, your body needs a 5- to 10-minute "primer" of heat exposure before the full session. So go into the sauna and heat up. Then get out for 5 to 10 minutes before starting your actual session. If you're in the high-hormone phase, your body has already shifted to a higher thermoregulatory threshold, and no primer is needed.

Follow this practice for 9 days in a row for optimum results. The first day you may only be able to tolerate 5 to 10 minutes, but by the ninth day, 25 to 30 minutes should be attainable. The best way to monitor hydration is with pee sticks. (See Chapter 17 for more information on pee sticks.) If you need to accelerate your heat adaptation, follow a shorter 4- to 5-day protocol, using a primer before the true sauna session. That can help push those adaptation responses along a bit more quickly.

COLD EXPOSURE

Like sauna, there's also a long history of using cold water exposure for general health benefits. Many believe it is a tool for health and longevity.

One of the most obvious benefits of cold exposure like a cold-water plunge is that it reduces inflammation, which can help prevent and alleviate pain in muscles and joints. That's why you'll see athletes immersing themselves in a tub of ice-cold water after competitions (though not necessarily after training, since it can blunt important adaptations, which we'll talk about later). But there are other benefits that come from using controlled cold exposure.

As mentioned earlier, cold exposure (especially on the face, but also in the case of submerging in a cold body of water) increases our parasympathetic drive. So you have more time in that rest-and-digest state. Your cortisol is lower. You have better focus and improved sense of psychological well-being (research shows that cold plunges can help relieve depressive symptoms). It increases thyroid stimulating hormone, so it improves thyroid function. The oxidative stress of cold exposure also improves your body's antioxidative adaptation, so you become more equipped to fend off free radical damage. In fact, a study on winter swimmers (13 women and 23 men) from 1999 found that they had improved antioxidant protection and therefore better tolerance to environmental stress over their peers who did not participate in cold-water swimming.

When you expose yourself to the cold, your body also triggers cellular and metabolic reactions to increase heat to warm you. The obvious one is shivering thermogenesis. You have involuntary muscle contractions to produce heat. Cold exposure also activates your brown fat, which is used to rev up your metabolism to help keep you warm (we're born with lots of brown fat as babies and lose it as adults as we develop the capacity to shiver and move to stay warm). Research shows that cold exposure may also transform the type of fat that we form in our bodies to be more predisposed to brown fat, which can help increase metabolism.

The long-term effects of cold exposure are similar to exercise with a decrease in heart rate and better vascular control. And, of course, by regularly exposing yourself to the cold, you build a tolerance to the cold, which improves performance in the cold.

For women in the menopause transition who need help with thermoregulation, especially around sleep, I recommend cold exposure like a cool shower before bedtime to help bring down the core temperature and lull you to sleep. Start with the water on warm (so you don't shock your system) and gradually turn the hot water down until the temperature is cool and you feel chilled. Then get in your PJs, curl up in your sheets, and feel the pleasant tiredness wash over you.

COLD PLUNGES

Anyone who has seen their Instagram feed filled with athletes, celebrities, and social media influencers submerging themselves in portable ice baths knows that cold plunges have become very popular.

If you're interested in incorporating cold plunges into your regular routine, remember that women do not need as cold a plunge as men. Women start shivering at a higher temperature than men and feel colder and less comfortable than men during the same cooling protocol. The research into specific protocols is still sparse, but in general, cold-water immersion is exposure up to the shoulders or neck to water between 32°F and 60°F (0°C to 15°C). Immersion times range from 2 × 30 seconds with 2 minutes between at the lowest temperatures to 6 × 3 minutes at 60°F/15°C.

Note: We'll talk about this more in the next chapter on recovery, but these types of cold plunges are not designed for general exercise recovery but can help with times of high inflammatory responses like multiple event/training days, new heavy blocks of resistance training, and recovery after intense workouts. These work by constricting blood vessels and reducing inflammation and thus pain. But in times when we want to invoke inflammation for adaptation, like during day-to-day training, cold exposure can be a hindrance to recovery and slow adaptations. So when you're in general training, I recommend doing cold plunges twice a week and timing them so they are not close to your training, especially immediately after training.

There are also sex differences. Again, cooling your body works by tricking your body into redistributing the blood from the skin back into circulation through the muscles. Men don't necessarily need this, because their blood vessels naturally constrict postexercise to push blood away from the skin and back into the central circulation. Women, on the other hand, tend to vasodilate after exercise, meaning our blood tends to pool in our skin, dropping blood pressure and reducing blood flow to the damaged muscle. Cool-water immersion for women can help speed up vasoconstriction after hard exertion, to get blood back centrally helping to increase blood pressure and circulation into the muscles. We'll get into when you should—and shouldn't—use cold or cool immersion for recovery in the next chapter.

HEAR HER ROAR

TAKE YOUR ENDURANCE HYDRATION AND NUTRITION TO EXTREMES

It can be challenging enough just sightseeing in extreme conditions, let alone competing in high-intensity sports such as mountain biking in them. Both cold and hot weather—especially hot weather—demand special fueling.

Let's talk heat first, because that's where most athletes run into trouble. As discussed earlier, when you exercise, your heart rate rises to increase cardiac output. Your working muscles need oxygenated blood; you need blood flow to the skin to offload heat, and you need blood flow to keep your organs functioning. With blood flow demands increasing in all those places, your body decreases blood flow to your gut and liver by almost 80 percent. This scenario makes it challenging to avoid GI distress and maintain energy while racing in the heat.

Your top priority here is hydration to keep your blood plasma levels high and allow for cooling so you don't overheat. The critical thing is that the concentration of carbohydrates in your drink needs to be no more than 4 percent (about 1.2 grams of carbohydrates per fluid ounce), especially in the heat! Remember, your gut's ability to absorb fluid and nutrients is significantly compromised from the heat and the lack of blood flow. The more concentrated your fluid, the longer it sits in the intestines, increasing the osmotic pressure. The body's response to this is to pull water into the intestines to help reduce the pressure. This is a surefire way to perpetuate dehydration and GI distress.

Because your appetite and thirst are muted from exercising in hot conditions, it is best to have a reminder (alarm) to sip across the hours that you are racing. This becomes more important as the hours race on, because you are able to only slow the rate of dehydration with key hydration strategies, and your thirst sensation really takes a hit the longer your race goes on.

Choose foods that are easy on the gut. Fat slows gut transit time, which is compounded in the heat. Concentrated carbohydrates can cause GI distress, as we talked about with gels and liquid calories. Eat small amounts of glucose-rich foods often. Amino acids can also help with gut integrity. Also, go easy on caffeine during your event. It can increase core temperature and promote GI permeability.

One of the benefits of sauna sessions and heat acclimation training is that the heat shock proteins help your intestines adapt to the heat stress. So once you've adapted, your body will respond to temperatures above 80°F (27°C) as if you were racing in temperatures around 60°F (16°C).

Cold weather is somewhat easier to contend with nutritionally because your gut isn't as compromised by need for blood flow to offset heat. But it's not without challenges. When it's very cold, it can be physically harder to eat because you have to dig it out with gloved hands, and it's easy to fall behind on your hydration because you're not sweating as much and can simply forget to drink. So you still need a plan.

To illustrate how all this looks in action, here's a sample nutritional plan I devised for Cammie and Kelsey Urban, the awesome mother-daughter racing duo I mentioned earlier. Cammie used it to secure a victory at a master's world mountain bike championship, and Kelsey is using it to work up the ranks as a UCI junior racer traveling the world, where she'll be greeted by climate conditions of all kinds.

COLD TEMPERATURES (50°F AND BELOW)

Prerace (for an event 90 minutes or longer):

- Be well fueled and eat about 150–250 calories 20–30 minutes before the race starts. This is in addition to your usual meals.
- Drink something warm, such as hot chocolate. The warm fluids will help keep your body temperatures up at the start. They will also help you avoid the dreaded afterdrop phenomenon.

During the race:

- Calorie needs after 45 minutes: 1.3–1.6 food calories per lb (3 to 3.5 food calories per kg)
- Fluid needs per hour: 0.12–0.16 oz per lb (8–10 ml/kg) but not to exceed 27 oz/hour
- A mix of protein, fat, and carbohydrates goes further than carbs alone in maintaining even energy in the cold.
- Have unwrapped bites of food in your pocket, and start eating these 35–40 minutes into the race. Small bites of sandwiches, bars, energy chews, and jelly beans are all great options.
- During the last 45 minutes, have a quick hit of sugar in the form of glucose tablets—one every 7–10 minutes.

Postrace:

- Have a recovery drink with almond or rice milk within 30 minutes of stepping off the bike and a real meal within 2 hours. Have another serving of the recovery drink 2½ hours later.

WARM TEMPERATURES (75°F AND ABOVE)

Prerace (for an event 90 minutes or longer):

- Finish your meal at least 2 hours before your race. Eat another 150–250 calories 60 minutes before the race starts.
- Drink 0.12 oz/lb (10 ml/kg) of a prehydration drink 20–30 minutes before the start of the race.

During the race:

- Calorie needs after 45 minutes: 1.3–1.6 food calories per lb (3 to 3.5 food calories per kg).
- Fluid needs per hour: 0.12–0.18 oz per lb (8–12 ml/kg) per hour of a very cold hydration drink, with sodium in the fluid.
- The more cold things you can ingest, the better.

Postrace:

- It is critical to double up on your cold recovery drink. Have a cold recovery drink with almond or rice milk within 30 minutes of stepping off the bike and a real meal within 2 hours. Have another serving of the recovery drink 2½ hours later.

SUCCEED AT ELEVATION

If you've ever run, biked, hiked, or skied in the Rockies, European Alps, the Himalayas, or anywhere high above sea level—especially above 8,000 feet (2,400 meters)—you know performance drops as the air thins. That's because oxygen levels are lower at high altitudes, so your cardiorespiratory system has to work harder to deliver oxygen to your working muscles than it does at sea level.

Your menstrual phase and/or hormonal status also impact your response to altitude. Research shows that premenopausal women who aren't on hormonal contraception have a higher hypoxic ventilatory response at exercise (HVRe), which is the ability to increase breathing to help meet your oxygen needs during their early luteal/midluteal phase than in the early follicular phase. On the surface, that sounds like a positive, but it's important to bear in mind that women's respiratory rates are already elevated during this high-hormone phase, so women may be more predisposed to asthmatic issues and higher respiratory distress. Postmenopausal women have similar HVRe as premenopausal women, though hypoxic cardiac response at exercise (HCRe), which is your cardiovascular system's ability to increase output, is lower postmenopause, likely due to age-related changes.

Sure, you can adapt to altitude (more on that in a second), but even among mountain dwellers, max VO_2 decreases as altitude increases. Research shows max VO_2 begins to decrease significantly above 5,200 feet (1,600 meters). For every 3,200 feet (1,000 meters) above that, max VO_2 drops by about 8 to 11 percent. That's why some athletes and coaches swear by the train low, sleep high philosophy. You get the adaptive benefits of being at altitude and can still push hard during training.

True adaption to high altitude takes weeks, sometimes months, as your body learns to make the most of the limited available oxygen. At high altitudes, your body makes more red blood cells to carry oxygen, and those blood cells become more efficient at delivering that oxygen to your tissues. At the same time, your cells' mitochondria (energy-producing furnaces) multiply to take in as much oxygen as possible.

Interestingly, men and women acclimate a bit differently from one another. In a study of 16 women who were traveling from sea level to Pikes Peak, Colorado, which sits at about 14,100 feet (4,300 meters), researchers found that after acclimation, the women burned fewer carbs and more fat for exercise fuel. Alternatively, research shows their male counterparts tended to use more carbs for fuel at altitude. Since women have more body fat and are better fat-burners at altitude than men, they might be better suited for exercise at high elevations. However, intense exercise may be harder for women because estrogen demands the body's spare carbs (which are needed for hard efforts), and progesterone increases breathing rates (which are already increased at altitude).

Altitude Acclimation Techniques

What's a lowlander to do if she has a big event or mountain adventure planned? Ideally, get out there early—like really early. Fourteen to 21 days are ideal. Obviously, that's not realistic for most of us. Research (on men) has found that 6 days of partial acclimation can help, but again, that's a lot of time and expense most women don't have. Many women will opt to try to go out just 2 to 3 days ahead of time, but research finds no performance benefit to such a short period of time, and in some cases, you may end up feeling worse before you feel better after 3 days.

If you're in a position where you have to hit the ground running at high altitudes, you're at risk for developing altitude sickness, which can happen when you exercise at high altitudes when you're not adapted. Mild forms cause headache, fatigue, and lack of appetite. You can avoid going into the red at altitude by recalibrating your heart rate zones for high altitude (figuring that at about 6,500 feet [2,000 meters], your heart rate will increase about 10 percent over your sea level rate) and using those adjusted values during your event.

You can also help prepare your body for the challenges of altitude by performing heat acclimation training ahead of time.

Altitude Performance Strategies

Once you're on the ground at your destination, these strategies can help you feel and perform your best during your high-altitude event.

Stay hydrated. Ever notice that you pee more at high altitude? Increased urinary output is a very common response to being at altitude, as your kidneys sense low levels of oxygen and kick into high gear, releasing erythropoietin (EPO), which triggers your body to produce more red blood cells so you can carry more oxygen. They also prompt you to pee more to decrease your blood plasma and make your blood thicker and hemoglobin more concentrated. That's a productive process, but you don't want to tip into dehydration. Increasing your fluid intake by about a liter a day will help you stay hydrated as you acclimate and help increase that ever-so-important plasma volume. Avoid plain water; you need some salt in your fluid! Instead sip on a functional hydration beverage (about 7 grams sugar with 190 milligrams sodium per 8 ounces) and increase your intake of watery foods.

Eat more carbs. Though research shows you burn more fat, especially in the high-hormone phase due to estrogen's and progesterone's effects on sparing carbohydrate, you still need more carbs when you're exercising at altitude. When at altitude, the body uses less exogenous carbohydrate (carbs you eat!) as a fuel during exercise and relies more on liver glycogen, regardless of menstrual cycle phase. Eating a higher amount of total dietary carbohydrate helps keep your metabolism kicking for intensity. The additional carbon dioxide that carbs produce kicks up your breathing response a notch and helps prevent altitude sickness.

Open your vessels. Some athletes say they have success with using beetroot juice before events at high altitudes, which can help blood vessels relax and widen, but also know that research on women is lacking here.

Avoid alcohol. Skip the chardonnay and/or IPA. Alcohol is a dehydrating diuretic, and it depresses the normal breathing response to high altitude. Overall, alcohol increases the risk of altitude sickness and can exacerbate symptoms.

BEAT JET LAG

You can acclimate at home all you want, but if you feel like hell from jet lag, all that work will be for nothing. With the globalization of racing and the relative ease of travel, it's hard not to pick a destination race. But the dreaded time-lag toll on the body can seriously hinder how we feel and perform. You may experience swollen ankles or dead legs in the first hours the day after a long flight, as well as extreme waves of tiredness and lethargy. How do we, as athletes, thwart the dreaded jet lag so we can race well and enjoy the trip?

First note that jet lag itself is different from travel fatigue. Travel fatigue can usually be solved by a good meal, rehydration, and a good night's sleep. Jet lag is a temporary disruption of your normal circadian rhythm caused by high-speed travel across several time zones. Typically, your circadian rhythms align with daytime and nighttime where you live, so your core body temperature, hormone production, and melatonin levels rise and fall to help you be alert come morning and during the day and sleep at night. When you travel out of your time zone, especially across three or more time zones, you experience jet lag: Your body's internal clock becomes out of sync with the local time of your destination. This leaves you feeling disoriented and fatigued and can disrupt your sleep patterns, which can make the fatigue worse. It can also throw off digestion, leaving you constipated, queasy, and without your normal appetite. Jet lag affects everyone, but this time lag can take a bigger toll on women because our circadian rhythm influences the release of hormones like estrogen and progesterone, which impact our menstrual cycle, appetite hormones, and blood glucose control. Disturbing your circadian rhythm can disrupt the release of these hormones, leading to a change in your period.

Interesting fact: Women who work shift work can experience the same phenomenon without ever stepping foot on a plane. In fact, the circadian rhythm disruption and sleep-wake disorders caused by working odd hours is sometimes called "social jet lag."

This can all wreak havoc on our core temperature, hormone production, melatonin levels, and of course performance. It is interesting to note that it takes longer to reset the circadian clock following an eastward flight more so than a westward flight, primarily because the human clock is slightly longer than 24 hours, so we have a natural tendency to drift slightly later each day.

HOW TO MANAGE CIRCADIAN RHYTHM DISRUPTION

Whether you're flying across the country or halfway around the world, you can take steps to shift your internal clock and feel and perform better. Here's how to take the sting out of jet lag.

When Flying . . .

- Adjust your sleep/wake times. You can help mitigate jet lag by adjusting your sleep/wake times ahead of your travel.
- For a week preceding your flight, load up on the antioxidant quercetin (1 gram per day) and aspirin (100 milligrams per day) if you are not contraindicated to aspirin. Both act as a low-dose anticoagulant, reducing DVT risk.
- Limit caffeine. On your travel day, limit your caffeine intake to your normal morning hours (between 6 a.m. and 11 a.m.) of your home time zone.
- Avoid alcohol. You don't want anything that will further disrupt your sleep architecture, and alcohol definitely does. Plus, it dehydrates you, which is the last thing you need during air travel, which is already dehydrating.
- Get outdoors. If you land during the day, go for a walk outside without sunglasses to use sunlight to reset your body clock. This will help you adjust to your new time zone.
- Stay hydrated. Before, during, and after your flight take regular sips of a low-carbohydrate electrolyte drink (it can be as simple as a sprinkle of salt and ½ teaspoon of sugar in 16 ounces per 500 milliliters of water) to stay hydrated, which will also help with digestion as you travel. For very long flights, every 6 hours, take one baby aspirin (80 milligrams) if you are not contraindicated to aspirin. This combination will help with dehydration and prevent deep-vein thrombosis (very important if you are a woman traveling in the high-hormone phase of her menstrual cycle—we tend to have 8 percent less plasma volume and a greater tendency for blood clots during this phase).
- Keep the blood flowing. Get up every 90 to 120 minutes (if you're not sleeping) and walk around or do some isometric exercises in your seat.
- Wear compression socks or calf sleeves to increase the circulation in your legs.
- Snack lightly. Nibble on some fresh fruit, high-fiber crackers, or trail mix to keep your GI tract moving along as you travel.
- Upon landing, drink a sodium-heavy beverage or soup. This will rehydrate you and expand your plasma volume.

- On the day you land, get out for a walk (not a jog!) to bring your heart rate up and help alleviate any swelling. Running will be more damaging after a long-haul flight of sitting, because of the sudden impact on the muscles.
- Traveling west to east: Jet lag tends to be a little more pronounced when you fly west to east. In the 4 days before your trip, drink 4 ounces of tart cherry juice (for natural melatonin) with 200 milligrams of L-theanine (a nonprotein amino acid that increases the alpha waves of the brain) about 30 minutes before bed. Go to bed and wake up 1 hour earlier than usual. Expose yourself to bright light, preferably sunlight, which has a powerful effect on your circadian rhythms, as soon as possible after waking. When you arrive, try to avoid bright light exposure. Wear sunglasses if the sun has not set, and seek dimly lit environments to signal your body that it is time to wind down and sleep.
- Traveling east to west: It's easier to adjust your circadian rhythm flying west because your body adjusts more easily to a longer day. If your work schedule allows, make the adjustment easier by pushing back your bedtime and wake time by about 30 minutes for the 2 to 4 nights before your flight. Expose yourself to bright light, preferably sunlight, which has a powerful effect on your circadian rhythms, as soon as possible after waking. When you arrive, help your body reset to the later start of the day by exposing yourself to bright light (sunlight preferably), and do not wear sunglasses the first few days in the new location, all to help your internal clock make the shift.

With these tips, jet lag isn't a necessary evil. Simple techniques to reset your circadian rhythm before you go and upon landing can significantly help. It is kind of like packing your bike box for a destination race—a pain in the butt, but well worth it!

ROAR ▶▶▶ SOUND BITES

▶ You start sweating later and sweat less than your male counterparts, so it's important to use other strategies to keep cool when it's really hot.

▶ Sauna training can help you acclimate to the heat as well as to high altitude.

▶ It's not your imagination; your hands and feet *are* colder than a man's.

▶ Endurance exercise at altitude may be easier for women than men because women burn more fat while men burn more carbs in the rarefied air.

▶ Flying is even more dehydrating during the high-hormone phase of your cycle (when your blood plasma volume is already low). Prepare accordingly by packing some hydration powder for the flight.

14

RECOVER RIGHT

HOW TO REFUEL, REPAIR, REBUILD, AND GET STRONGER IN YOUR SLEEP (LITERALLY!)

When it comes to getting fit, hard work is only half the equation. Rest is the essential and all-too-often overlooked other half. When you hit the weights or bang out a hard ride or run, you place stress on your muscles and cardiovascular system. In order to come back stronger and faster for the next session, it is imperative to recover. If you continue to pile on stress without adequate rest, you'll just get slower, tired, and possibly even injured.

We've talked a lot about what to eat after exercise for prompt recovery. But there's more to making muscle and building fitness than protein, carbs, and hydration. It's important to understand the difference between acute recovery (immediately after a hard exercise bout) and long-term recovery (how you recover and get stronger and fitter over the course of your training), as well as active (gentle movement) and passive (i.e., sleep, nonsleep deep rest [NSDR], food, compression socks) recovery and how they all can work or not work for you. Recovery, like training, is also (surprise!) different for women than it is for men in a few key ways. Here's what you need to know.

THE COOLDOWN FACTOR

If you've ever been coached in a sport or taken an exercise class, you know that intense workouts are always followed by a nice cooldown—easy spinning, slow jogging, chill strokes in the pool. There's a reason for that, and it's not just because it feels good (though that's a *very* good reason to cool down; it leaves you in a happy mood after a hard workout). By continuing to move at a gentle pace, you allow your body to quickly return to resting blood lactate levels. When you stop dead in your tracks and do nothing, the blood pools in your legs, which can make you dizzy. A cooldown is the first step in what is known as active recovery, helping your body bounce back and rebuild with gentle exercise to stimulate circulation. Cooling down is beneficial for both sexes, but even more essential for women since we experience a greater decrease in arterial blood pressure after exercise than men. When you skip your cooldown, your blood flow drops so low that it limits your ability to get key nutrients into your hard-worked cells. Active recovery prevents this drop in blood flow by maintaining the blood flowing back and forth from your muscles, which enhances nutrient exchange and muscle repair. Active recovery is especially advantageous when you have two workouts in one day, as many triathletes do, or when you have an evening session followed by an early-morning workout the next day.

After exercise, there are normal changes in blood pressure and blood flow fluctuations, and it takes longer than usual for core body temperature to return to normal—especially in women, who have a harder time off-loading heat postexercise. Progesterone keeps your core warmer and delays your sweat response. With a hot core, your body diverts more blood to your skin—and away from your muscles—to try to cool you. With less blood circulating to and from your muscles, you remain in a prolonged stressed state with more metabolic waste lingering in your muscles, increasing inflammation.

As mentioned earlier, cooling your body by immersing yourself in cool water or wearing a special cool-water-infused recovery vest can trick your body into redistributing the blood from the skin back into circulation through the muscles. You may have heard that diving into a cold pool can not only stall your recovery but also increase muscle soreness. Men may indeed get more soreness because their blood vessels naturally constrict postexercise to push blood away from the skin and back into central circulation. When men take a postexercise plunge into cold water, they can start shivering and get microspasms in their already-fatigued muscles, which can equal soreness and stalled recovery. This is not the case for women, who need assistance speeding up vasoconstriction after hard exertion. A cool water immersion (but not an ice bath—that's too cold—more on that in a bit) can help accelerate that process as needed.

ACTIVE RECOVERY IN ACTION

A postexercise cooldown is just one step in an active recovery. Active-recovery techniques are also useful in the day(s) following hard workouts when you wake up feeling like someone poured cement into your muscles. You may not feel like moving, but getting the blood circulating through active recovery will make you feel better.

A few active-recovery techniques can be helpful in the hours or days following hard exercise bouts or races. A 2018 meta-analysis of recovery techniques found that techniques like active recovery, massage, compression garments, and cold-water immersion can help manage perceived fatigue after hard workouts. Massage was also found effective for recovering from delayed-onset muscle soreness (DOMS). Here's a quick rundown on these and other popular recovery methods.

Gentle movement: Simple, gentle movement similar to the cooldown, but not necessarily sport specific, is key for active recovery. Whatever you do has to be really, truly, actually very easy. Your muscles can't recover fully if you continue to challenge them, and far too many people go harder than they should when they're supposed to be going easy. The goal is to increase your circulation (which will help repair your muscles) without challenging your muscles. Take a walk, go for a very easy spin, do some slow laps in the pool, or perform some gentle yoga. Keep it short and sweet; about an hour is all you need.

Massage: There's a reason professional athletes have massage therapists—it really works. Massage flushes your muscles, so you push out the fluid that carries the waste products of muscle breakdown and encourage fresh, nutrient-rich blood to come in and help repair and rebuild. Massage also breaks up adhesions (knots) that can form from overuse, so your muscles work more smoothly and painlessly. The results are scientifically shown to be pretty dramatic.

In one study, researchers had volunteers crank out enough reps on the leg press machine to make their quads and hamstrings cry uncle. Afterward, half the group got a massage while the other half hobbled home. The researchers checked in on the exercisers for 24 hours after the experiment. Amazingly, the massage group reported no soreness just 90 minutes later while those in the exercise-only group were still hurting 24 hours later. The researchers also measured the general blood flow in all the participants, as exercise-induced muscle injury is known to reduce blood flow. The massage group had improved blood flow for up to 72 hours after their rubdown. The exercise-only group had hampered circulation for that same 72 hours, after which it returned to normal.

Why suffer for 72 hours? Even if you're not a pro and can't afford a massage every time you need or want one, there's no need to suffer for days. With the right tools and techniques, you can do a pretty good job yourself. Massage guns like Theragun and Hypervolt work like a charm. (They've also gotten more affordable in recent years, with portable, travel-friendly versions available.) You can also do easy, inexpensive self-massage with rubber balls and foam balls. See "Work Out the Knots" on page 269 for self-massage techniques you can perform with a few simple recovery tools. For the best results, do these moves as soon as you can after a hard workout.

Compression pumps: These are zip-on leg sleeves (often with feet) that attach to a motorized pump. They systematically inflate in a way that provides compression and release deep into your muscles. A deep squeeze from your feet to your groin pushes fluids out and reduces blood flow in. Then the blood flows back into the muscles when the sleeves release. This flood significantly increases tissue oxygenation, nutrient exchange, and metabolic waste removal.

You can find these leg compression machines from companies such as NormaTec, RecoveryPump, Elevated Legs, and Game Ready. A few, such as the Game Ready system, combine the pneumatic compression with circulating cool water. The cooling-compression combination is particularly good for women, as it can help counteract the vasodilation response women experience and enhance blood flow to the muscles. Cooling-compression is also ideal for joint inflammation or soft-tissue injury that involves swelling, regardless of sex. Because a woman's blood flow naturally takes longer to normalize postexercise, women should use compression pumps within 30 minutes of finishing a workout or race, whereas men can wait a bit longer (60 to 90 minutes) to garner the benefits.

Electrical muscle-stimulation devices: Electrical muscle-stimulation (EMS) devices allow you to get the benefits of active recovery without you actually moving a muscle (though your muscles will move!). They work on the principles of electrostimulation; that is, they apply a simulated neural input to contract a muscle. In short, you place electrodes on your muscles, turn on the machine, and watch your muscles contract without doing a thing. It's pretty freaky at first, but very effective and widely used by professional athletes of all sports. There are various EMS devices on the market, including Marc Pro, PowerDot, and Compex. The Compex and PowerDot use a traditional EMS program that delivers a strong, static contraction with a sudden release. The Marc Pro employs a moderate contraction with a slow release. Both are great at stimulating active recovery and enhancing blood flow to tight, bound areas of muscle, but some experts believe that the Marc Pro may be more suitable to muscle recovery (or to those with chronic pain) because it allows fluids to flow in and out of the muscle cells without undue fatigue that some people experience with traditional EMS systems.

Pneumatic compression and muscle-stimulation products carry a fairly high price tag. But if you're an athlete who already invests in a coach and regular massages, it could be worth a look. Your local physical therapist may also be able to provide these services at a lower cost than purchasing the equipment yourself.

Compression garments: You don't need expensive equipment to get some of the benefits of compression. You can get some tired-muscle relief from compression tights and/or socks as well. Worn by nurses for decades and popular among endurance athletes like triathletes, distance runners, and cyclists, compression garments accelerate the flow of blood back to the heart, which can improve blood oxygen levels and subsequent recovery. The science isn't definitive on how well these garments work, but research suggests that they can help lessen swelling, fatigue, and muscle soreness after intense exercise. One study published in the *Journal of Strength and*

Conditioning Research reported that women and men who wore compression socks for 48 hours after running a marathon improved their performance on a treadmill test 2 weeks later.

WHEN TO DELAY RECOVERY

So now that I've impressed the importance of recovery upon you, I'm going to throw in a bit of a curveball. There are times when what is good for fast, immediate recovery may actually interfere with the long-term adaptations you get from exercise. Ice baths fall into this category as do, surprisingly, antioxidants.

Again, let's talk ice baths and cold plunges. If you've just finished a long, hard event like a marathon, ultra, or strength competition and just want to relieve some of the swelling and soreness you know is coming, they are fine. But, again, outside of those circumstances (and cold plunges for health, vagal response training, as discussed earlier), I don't recommend them as a routine part of a training/recovery protocol. The constriction from icy water causes too much of a hormonal response that dampens the inflammation that is key for training adaptations. But you can use cool water immersion any time after a long, hard endurance activity to redistribute blood flow, flush out the metabolites, and get "fresh" blood to your muscles.

Nutritionally, athletes often consume antioxidant supplements such as vitamins C and E because they believe that by fighting the potentially cell-damaging free radicals that your body produces during hard exercise, they can accelerate recovery and enhance performance. While that sounds like a good idea on paper, we now know that in the long run (and maybe even short term), it does more harm than good.

How's that? Inside your cells are molecular furnaces called mitochondria. It's the place where your body takes the food you eat and converts it to the energy you use to power your muscles. This energy-production process is powered by oxygen and is aptly called oxidation. Endurance athletes rely on this process to produce a steady power output as they swim, run, bike, row, and so forth. As with any energy-generating method, some waste is produced in the process. In this case the waste byproducts are reactive oxygen species, commonly known as free radicals.

Free radicals do have the potential to damage your cells as they take oxygen molecules from your healthy cells to stabilize themselves. This sets off a harmful chain reaction like molecular musical chairs, known as oxidative stress, which is one of the major contributors to DNA damage and disease. This is where antioxidants come to the rescue. They step in and neutralize free radicals as they develop, preventing cell damage.

But here is the key concept that supplement users have missed. Your body is actually very good at defending itself, and it creates its own natural antioxidants to quell free radicals. As you train harder, your body gets better at this. This adaptation follows the same pattern as all training adaptations. You stress the body; the body gets a little damaged; you recover; the body comes back stronger. So when you do a very long or very high-intensity workout, you increase your free-radical production. To overcome this influx of free radicals, your body boosts its antioxidant capacity. When you add more antioxidants into this mix by taking supplements, your body doesn't fully adapt, and the backlash is more harmful than neutral.

During the acute recovery period right after a hard workout, antioxidant supplements actually seem to work against the beneficial effects of exercise. Because the free radicals are dimmed before the body can react and adapt to them, your muscles aren't able to do their recovery job as well. In fact, when researchers examined key blood markers of muscle damage and cell rupture, people taking antioxidant supplements had the same level of damage as nonsupplementers, and sometimes the supplementers even appeared to have more muscle injury and slower recovery. Several studies have found that taking vitamins E and C (two very popular antioxidants) blunts the usual insulin-sensitizing effects of exercise, so the muscles aren't able to pull in the glycogen and nutrients they need to restock and repair. Antioxidant supplements like vitamins E and C have also been found to block anabolic signaling pathways and therefore impair adaptations to resistance training, which is the last thing women want.

We aren't as smart as nature. Our bodies need the chance to understand and overcome stress, which is the whole concept behind training and adaptation. Eat real food for functional recovery, and leave the bottle of supplements on the shelf (see Chapter 15 for more information on antioxidants and supplements).

WORK OUT THE KNOTS

Repetitive activity can cause inflammation in your muscles, which in turn leads to tension and adhesions or muscle knots that decrease your mobility and cause discomfort. A foam roller or a pair of lacrosse or tennis balls stuffed in a sock are excellent tools and can help compress and massage stuck spots. Breaking up the adhesions and scar tissue within the muscle and fascia that covers the muscle allows for greater mobility.

"Normal healthy muscles shouldn't hurt during compression," says Dr. Kelly Starrett, a coach, physiotherapist, and author. "If you lie on a lacrosse ball or foam roller and find pain, those are tissues that aren't gliding correctly." By rolling your muscles, you can smooth out any tight spots with compression. If you press so hard that you have to hold your breath, you're going too deep and triggering your fight-or-flight response, which will only further exacerbate the problem.

Here are a few excellent foam roller and lacrosse ball moves that hit the hips, lower back, Achilles, and foot regions that tend to get tight and knotted in women. Roll until you feel relief in your tight or tender spots or about a minute or so.

PLANTAR ROLL

Place your foot on top of a lacrosse ball and press down to apply pressure as you roll along the length of your foot and back to relieve tightness in the plantar fascia. You can also use a golf ball for better precision.

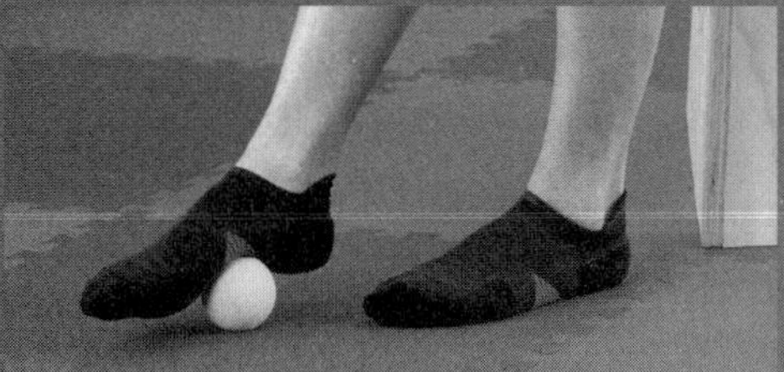

LOWER-BACK SMASH

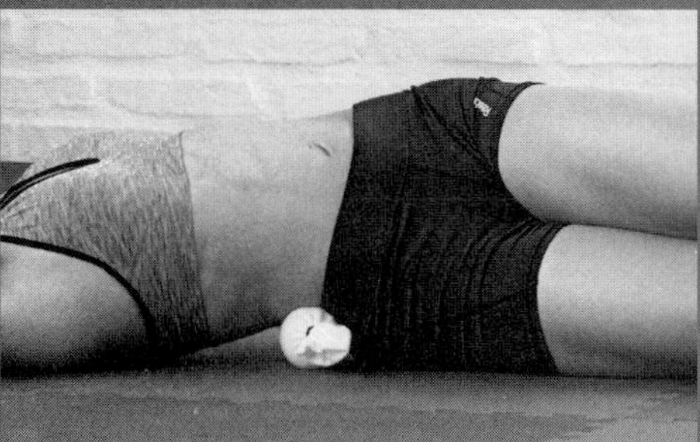

Place two lacrosse balls in a sock and twist the sock between the balls to create space between them. Lie on the floor with your knees bent, feet flat on the floor. Lift your hips and place the balls on your lower back at the base of your lumbar spine so each ball is on either side of your spine. Lower your back but keep your hips off the floor. Drop your left knee toward your right side and rotate your hips slightly to the right, making sure your shoulders stay in contact with the floor. Then rotate your hips to the opposite side. Rotate from side to side until you feel the tension release. Then move up to the next vertebra and repeat, continuing this sequence to the top of the lumbar spine (where your lower-back curve ends).

GLUTE SMASH

Sit on the floor with your knees bent and position a lacrosse ball on the side of your left hip. Press into the ball with your hip (slightly under your butt) and drop your left knee out toward the floor. Slowly roll from side to side across your glute. If you come across a particularly painful area, contract and relax, and keep applying gentle pressure to release the tissue. Return to center and repeat on the opposite side.

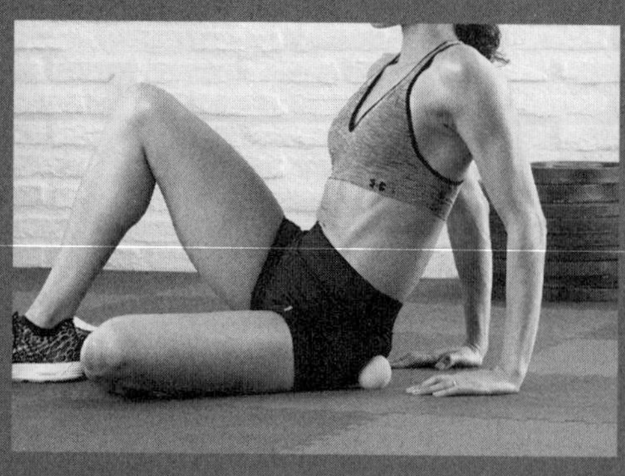

IT BAND ROLL

Lie on your right side with a foam roller under your right hip. Bracing your abs and glutes for balance and using your arms for support, slowly roll down from your hip to your knee. Switch to the other side and repeat.

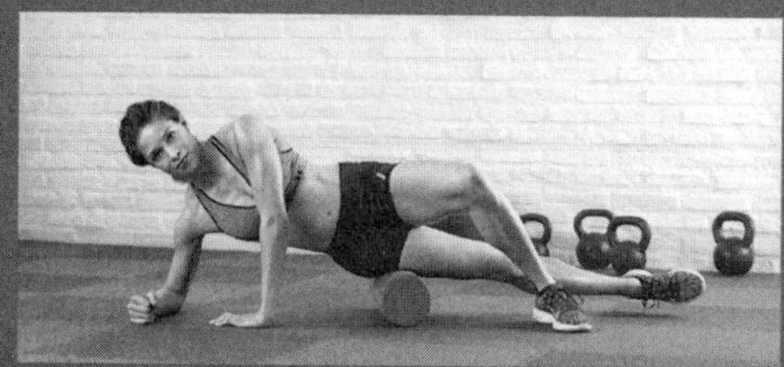

QUAD ROLL

Lie facedown on the floor and place a foam roller under your hips. Lean on your right leg and roll up and down the front of your thigh from your hip to your knee. Switch legs.

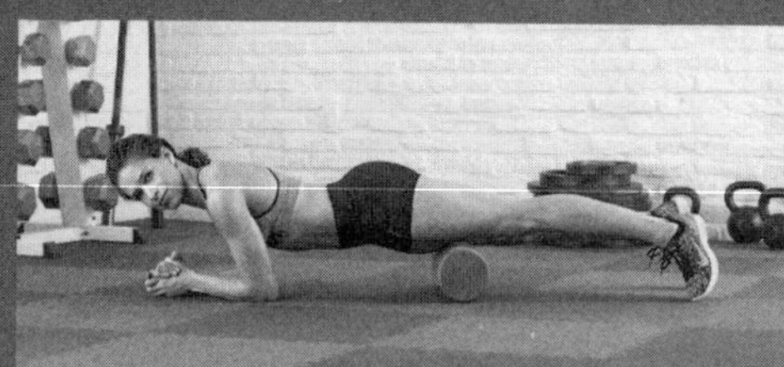

HAMSTRING ROLL

Sit with your left hamstring on the roller; bend your right knee and place your right foot on the floor. Place your hands on the floor behind you and roll up and down from your knee to just under your left butt cheek. Switch legs and repeat.

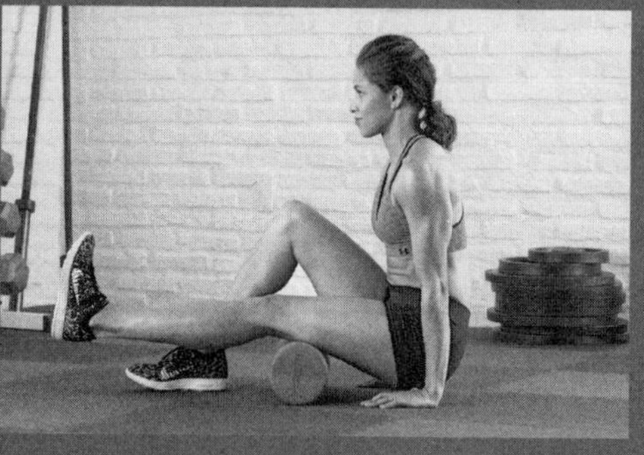

ARE YOU UNDER-RECOVERED?

When I talk about overtraining (which is a commonly used term that really means being under-recovered) with amateur athletes, they often act surprised, as if it's just a problem for the pros. Nothing could be further from the truth! Everyday active people can be more prone to staleness and neglecting recovery, which are marked by persistent fatigue and poor performance, because they don't have the luxury of putting their feet up and getting proper rest after their hard training sessions. Instead they're staying up late finishing work, shuttling kids to doctor appointments, cleaning the house, mowing the lawn, walking the dogs—you know, life!

It's fine to train hard, and often it's appropriate to train hard. But remember, those killer CrossFit workouts of the day and marathon training sessions take a toll on pretty much every system in your body. The point is to push the body to its limits, but then you have to back off and let it rebuild. If you don't, you'll find yourself sliding away from your goal; feeling tired, blue, and slow; and battling weight gain and sickness instead of feeling invigorated, fresh, fast, and healthy. The recovery techniques outlined in this chapter can help, but you also need pure rest: good-quality sleep and at least 1 day of no exercise (extremely light activity is okay) each week.

Remember that proper nutrition is essential for recovery. I see many active women limiting their sugar and carb intake, and the veggies they eat freely have tons of fiber, so they're getting full without getting the nutrients they need to recover. This leads to constantly elevated stress hormones, low growth hormones, and systemic inflammation. In combination with regular exercise, they're overtrained before they even know it. I talked to a neuroscientist recently who told me there's an upward trend of young, fit women on antidepressants (depression can be a symptom of overtraining) for this very reason. Some of these ladies may not actually need the medication; they just need to eat more, particularly carbs!

Which leads to my next point. One surprisingly easy way to stay fresh is to monitor your moods, which can help you detect creeping staleness before it becomes full-blown overtraining. Staleness is the end result of biological disruptions such as rising stress hormones, dips in feel-good neurochemicals such as serotonin, and muscle breakdown. Your emotions are an early indication of when these biological factors are heading south. So while it's natural to feel a little tired and agitated after a hard training block or a few really tough workouts, your mood should rebound with rest, and you should feel ready to go for the next hard session. If you're still cranky, irritable, and down, dial back your efforts until you feel recharged. Are you getting enough sleep? You should feel refreshed from a good night's sleep or two. If you're consistently waking up after a full 8 or 9 hours of sleep and still feeling bone tired (this happens easily with the combination of life stress and hard training), you need to really dial down your workouts, take a day or two off, and improve your diet.

As a good rule to follow, you shouldn't have more than three high-stress exercise sessions each week, and those should be punctuated with easy or off days in between.

RECOVERY BETWEEN INTERVALS: IT'S DIFFERENT FOR WOMEN

Most of this chapter focuses on postexercise recovery, the recovery you do after a workout and from day to day to make the most of your training. If you're doing high-intensity interval training (and as we mentioned in Chapter 7, you should definitely be doing high-intensity interval training), you also need to consider the acute recovery that happens between intervals, which is generally prescribed as RBI, or rest between intervals. As mentioned in Chapter 7, the RBI is designed to allow your body to recover so you can hit the next interval just as hard. It may surprise you to learn that those times are different between women and men.

When it comes to repeated high-intensity bouts of exercise, research finds that females, compared to males, have more fatigue resistance and improved recovery despite having a higher cardiovascular strain and perceived exertion. This might be because females appear to have faster ATP (an energy-carrying molecule used to produce energy) recovery. A 2020 study on female and male runners performing a 4-week HIIT plan that had women and men doing either 4 × 30-second sprints with 180 seconds recovery or 4 × 30 sprints with 30 seconds recovery twice a week found that the females performing the shorter-rest HIIT sessions increased their speed per bout and average speed per session at the end of the trial, compared to no effect in their female peers performing the longer-rest HIIT sessions.

What does that mean from a practical standpoint? If you're looking to improve your repeated running ability, which is key for sports like soccer and basketball, consider implementing shorter (i.e., 30 seconds) recovery periods in your interval workouts.

COMING BACK FROM INJURY

Whether you ride mountain bikes, schuss down alpine slopes, play point guard, or push your limits in power lifting competitions, injuries are a common part of the game. Find yourself with a broken collarbone, blown ACL, or a torn muscle and you could be looking at an arduous recovery process. You can't magically heal yourself overnight, but you can take measures to help your body every step of the way.

The initial concern is hanging on to your muscle tissue when you can't move it. Injuries and surgery create hormonal and inflammatory stress that triggers rapid muscle loss. You can lose 150 to 400 grams of muscle mass during the first 2 weeks of having a single immobilized limb, which is worsened by metabolic changes that reduce your ability to build muscle. You also experience strength loss that isn't related to muscle loss but rather disuse. Finally, you lose skeletal calcium and magnesium stores that are necessary for muscle contractions. In general, you lose strength three times as fast as you lose muscle following an injury that leaves you immobilized.

While it's natural that you won't be eating as much when you're not as active, it's essential to manipulate your diet to minimize this muscle loss. That means maintaining adequate daily protein intake (about 0.9 to 1.1 grams per pound/2 to 2.4 grams per kilogram of body weight, or about 122 to 148 grams for a 135-pound/61.5 kilogram woman). This will slow the rate of muscle loss but not alleviate it completely, because of anabolic resistance, or the hormonal changes that decrease your body's ability to build muscle.

How can you overcome anabolic resistance? It's more than just eating more protein. The amount of protein you eat is important, but the type of protein plays an even larger role.

This is where the specific anabolic (muscle growth and protein synthesis) properties of protein come into play. For protein to wield maximum muscle-building ability, it must be easily absorbed, and it must contain the right amino acids to stimulate muscle growth. For example, whey protein, which is more rapidly digested and absorbed than soy or casein, has been shown to be more anabolic. However, even when soy or casein protein is treated to have similar digestion and absorption rates to whey, it still doesn't provoke the same anabolic response. This is where the amino acid profile plays an important role. Your muscles need leucine. Leucine is the key amino acid that needs to saturate the muscle to create a "trigger" for optimal muscle protein synthesis. The leucine threshold is said to be 2.5 to 3 grams for pre-menopausal women, and 3 to 3.7 grams for peri- and postmenopausal women.

Why leucine? High-stress exercise, injury, and postexercise recovery all change amino acid and protein metabolism in your muscles and increase the metabolism of leucine. The damage in the muscle tissue stimulates muscle-cell breakdown, releasing amino acids. In recovery, tissue levels of leucine must be increased in order to slow this breakdown to a halt. The more rapidly you get your blood levels of leucine up, the faster it can saturate the muscle, triggering signals for muscle protein synthesis (i.e., the more quickly your body begins to send out signals to make muscle). For the best results, aim to take in at least 30 grams of protein that contain about 3 grams of leucine three times a day. Good injury-recovery foods include lean meat, low-fat Greek yogurt, nut butter on sprouted grain bread, and BCAAs found in green tea.

Keep in mind that this isn't the time to pull out the traditional recovery drinks formulated with carbohydrates, which stimulate insulin release and generally work with leucine to improve muscle building. When you're in a state of anabolic resistance, such as after an injury, adding carbs slows the rate at which the protein is digested and absorbed and *does not improve* the rate of muscle synthesis. What you need now is primarily protein.

Instead, omega-3 fatty acids like the kind found in fish oil can make protein work a little better. Take about 4 grams a day to make your muscles more reactive to the muscle-building effects of amino acids found in protein.

For example, let's use a hypothetical 130-pound/59-kilogram woman who has a major crash and ends up with a broken collarbone and a significant quadriceps crush injury. To reduce muscle-mass loss and preserve strength during her recovery, the ideal recommended daily protein intake is 116 to 140 grams of protein, ideally spread across four main meals (30 to 32 grams per meal with 2 to 3 grams of leucine) eaten every 3 to 5 hours. This amount counteracts the anabolic resistance caused by her injuries, and the equal timing keeps her muscle-synthesis rates elevated over a 24-hour period. A split supplementation of 4 grams of omega-3 fatty acids (2 grams in the morning, 2 grams before bed) will maintain the upturn of muscle-synthesis signaling.

Injuries, crashes, and high stress are unfortunately unavoidable in the world of sports, but knowing how to manipulate your body's responses to minimize muscle and strength loss will shorten the recovery time and get you back out there in no time!

PRIORITIZE YOUR SLEEP

We saved the biggest recovery tool for last here. Though all these techniques are helpful for repair and performance, sleep is number one when it comes to exercise recovery (and good health!). A 2021 study of 175 elite athletes from 12 sports including both team and individual sports published in the *International Journal of Sports Physiology and Performance* reported that elite female and male athletes need 8.3 hours of sleep to feel rested. Yet 71 percent of them failed to hit that mark most nights. Unfortunately, females represented only 17 percent of the athletes studied in this paper, but in my experience plenty of active women are not getting sufficient sleep.

How Sleep Helps You Recover

It may not look like you're doing anything when you're all tucked in, fast asleep, but your brain and body are as active as they are during the day as they get to work removing metabolic waste and making tissue repairs. As you dip into deep sleep, your body produces the majority of one of your body's greatest performance enhancers, human growth hormone (HGH), which helps you burn fat and stimulates tissue growth to build muscle and allow you to recover faster. When you shortchange your sleep—getting fewer than 7 to 9 hours of slumber a night—your HGH production stalls. That slump is particularly pronounced when you go to bed late, says renowned sleep specialist Christopher Winter, MD, author of *The Sleep Solution: Why Your Sleep Is Broken and How to Fix It.*

"The majority of your body's HGH secretion happens between 11 p.m. and 1 a.m. and then it starts shutting down," says Winter. As you get older, it's particularly important to heed the early-to-bed advice because your production of HGH naturally declines with age, and by age 55, your HGH levels are about one-third lower than they are in people ages 18 to 35. So it's particularly important to try to get to bed earlier and take advantage of that HGH-production window as we approach midlife and menopausal years.

Shortchanging your sleep is also stressful on your body. That means levels of stress hormones like cortisol remain elevated deep into the evening hours when they would naturally begin to decline. Research shows that cortisol declines six times more slowly in people who are short on sleep than in those who are properly rested. That not only disrupts your moods but also hinders your recovery by impairing tissue repair and growth. It also paves the way for insulin resistance, increased abdominal fat storage (which is linked to metabolic disease), injury, and overtraining.

Insufficient sleep also disrupts your appetite regulation. Research shows that sleep deprivation is linked to higher levels of the appetite stimulator ghrelin and lower levels of the appetite suppressor leptin. That's why you might find yourself constantly grazing or on the hunt for sugary snacks after a night (or more) of short sleep.

SLEEP STAGES

There are four primary stages of sleep that impact your health and performance:

Awake: As the name suggests, this is the time you're not asleep. It includes sleep latency, or the time it takes to fall asleep and sleep disturbances, which are the times you wake in the night to turn over, use the bathroom, or just wake up and look at the clock. Ideally, this accounts for about 5 percent of your sleep time.

Light: About half of your sleep time is spent in light sleep. As the name suggests, this is a transitory stage where your heart rate is lowering and your breathing is slowing, but you're easier to wake.

Deep (slow wave): This is where your tissue regeneration happens, where you're building bone and muscles and your immune system is getting a boost. Ideally, you should spend about 25 to 30 percent of your total night's sleep in slow wave sleep. Anything that accelerates your sympathetic nervous system, like alcohol or caffeine, will disturb this slow wave sleep, as will eating a big meal before bed.

REM: This is your rapid eye movement sleep, which you know as your dream sleep. This is where memory consolidation happens. In the early part of the night, your REM sleep phases are short, and they get longer as the night goes on. Healthy sleep includes about 20 percent REM sleep. If you don't have enough melatonin, you may find you're not getting that much REM sleep. This is important during perimenopause and beyond because your levels of melatonin decrease. (This is where using tart cherry juice, as we've already talked about, can be very helpful!)

Your body doesn't restock its glycogen supply as well when you don't get enough sleep. Prolonged sleep deprivation blunts insulin response. Some research finds even one night of sleep deprivation can reduce insulin sensitivity by a third. That makes it harder for you to restock your glycogen supply, which you need to feel fresh and fully recovered.

And it's not just your muscles that aren't fully restocked. Hard training like sprint workouts and Olympic lifting sessions demand lots of ATP (adenosine triphosphate) to power you through. The by-product of burning through ATP is adenosine, which builds up in your brain (and makes you drowsy) as well as your body. "The only way to clear it out is sleep," says Winter. As you slumber, your brain fires up the clean-up crews and clears the adenosine, which makes room for your brain to restock its own glycogen supply. Without sleep, the waste products remain, and your brain doesn't get all the energy it needs.

It's hard to perform your best when you're not properly rested. Your reaction time slows down and your endurance performance suffers when you don't get enough sleep. Exercise also feels harder. How rested you are impacts your perceived exertion during exercise. So when you're fully rested, those hard sessions feel relatively easy, and when you're not, they feel harder than they should.

Note: Do not let all this freak you out even further the night before a marathon or big event, when you're bound to be tossing and turning all night with nervous energy. Multiple studies have shown that one night of disrupted sleep, especially before an event, doesn't hurt endurance or power. Your race day energy will be fine. It's chronically poor sleep we're concerned about. Concentrate on getting a solid night's sleep two nights out and rest as well as you can the night before.

As mentioned in Chapter 3, sleep issues can arise for many women as they enter the menopause transition and postmenopause. Follow the advice on pages 49 and 55–56 if you're in the menopause transition and need help with sleep.

SLEEP & RECOVERY TRACKING

Long before trackers and apps, women were left to listen to their bodies to tell if they were rested and recovered. And that still works pretty well! If you have a spring in your step and you can bound up the stairs without feeling like you're scaling a mountainside, you're likely well recovered.

If you prefer data, you can tap into modern technology. Devices like the Whoop Strap and the Ōura Ring monitor your activity during the day and track your heart rate, respiration rate, body temperature, and sleep stages, as well as many other sleep metrics like restfulness, latency (how long it took you to fall asleep), and sleep efficiency, at night to deliver sleep and readiness scores. They also give you activity recommendations based on those scores.

They work well and allow you to clearly see the consequences of your behavior (both good and bad). Too much wine before bed? You can see your recovery and readiness drop as your heart rate stays elevated later into the night and you fail to drift into the deeper, restorative sleep stages you need. Early to bed with a book? You can see your recovery rise.

However, it's important to remember those scores won't always reflect how you actually *feel.* You may get a "high readiness" score because your heart rate and heart rate variability and sleep are good, but your legs are still pretty tender from a strength session. And sometimes you might get a low readiness score, but then go out and nail a workout.

The real benefit of these devices is that they allow you to peer into the overall trends of your physiology so as you're trying new training techniques, dietary shifts, and lifestyle interventions, you can see what is (and isn't) working and adjust accordingly. They also help you stay on track. No one likes getting a low score, so knowing that staying up to watch just one more episode of your favorite Netflix binger or topping off that glass of wine before bed will dock you some rest and readiness points (not to mention actually harm your health and performance in real life), you're more likely to do what you know you should do. (For more on sleep tracking pros, cons, and potential shortcomings regarding female physiology see page 322.)

Make Good Sleep Hygiene a Habit

There is no shortage of sleep supplements. And sometimes, especially in menopause, you can use a little extra help. Before you reach for assistance, make sure you're following the fundamentals for a good night's sleep:

Go easy on alcohol. Alcohol makes you feel drowsy, but it wrecks your sleep. Drinking, especially close to bedtime, lengthens your non-REM sleep and shortens your REM sleep during the first half of the night, so you don't get into that deep restorative sleep for very long. As your liver clears out the ethanol from your bloodstream, your body can go into a bit of withdrawal during the second half of the night, making you restless and more likely to toss and turn. Not drinking is best. But if you do, have that glass with dinner, but switch over to tart cherry juice (which is a natural sleep aid) before bedtime.

Eat dinner earlier. Making your body work on digestion can interfere with your parasympathetic needs of sleep. This is especially true if you have a larger meal that can cause bits of indigestion you may not even register but that wake you up enough to be disruptive and prevent you from falling into those deep, restorative sleep stages. Give yourself at least 2, preferably 3, hours before your last meal and bedtime. If you have evening workouts that make that impossible, have a light dinner early, before your workout. Do your session. Then have a protein-rich snack directly afterward, and wind down to be in bed without a bellyful of food. Or, if your regular schedule is evening exercise and you get home late every night, you can consider making your main meal in the early afternoon, a really large lunch, and then have a mini meal before and after training. If you're hungry before bed, try a casein-rich snack to stabilize blood sugar and promote muscle protein synthesis.

Pick up a book. You've heard it before, we'll say it again: being on your phone or laptop right up till bedtime can be bad news for your sleep. The best way to wind down is with some soft reading light and a book.

Turn down the temps. Cooler is better for sound sleep. The ideal temp for your bedroom is about 65°F (18°C), give or take, depending on your preference. You also can find cooling sheets, mattress toppers, and even mattresses to help keep you in the comfortable sleep temperature zone if you're a warm sleeper or a woman in menopause who has hot flashes at night. I also recommend taking a cool shower to help bring down your core temperature and lull you to sleep as well. Start with the water on warm (so you don't shock your system) and gradually turn the hot water down until the temperature is cool and you feel chilled. Then get in your PJs, curl up in your sheets, and feel the pleasant tiredness wash over you.

Block out light and noise. Ambient light and noise can keep you from drifting into that deep restorative state of sleep. Hang some blackout curtains and turn on a white noise machine to block out the sleep-disturbing light and sound. Or simply try wearing a sleep mask and earplugs.

Keep a bedside journal. If you have a busy mind at bedtime, keep a journal at your bedside and write down what's occupying your mind and the steps you'll take the next day to address it before you go to bed, so the problem solver in you is satisfied. If you wake up with more thoughts that won't let you rest, jot them down rather than lying there letting them race around inside your head. It will help you get back to sleep.

Try a later exercise time. Despite what you may have heard, exercising in the evening is not an automatic sleep wrecker. In fact, it can be better than dragging yourself out of bed at 5 a.m. after a restless night and then sleepwalking through the day. A 2019 meta-analysis of 23 studies found that not only did evening exercise not have a negative effect on sleep, but also, in some cases, improved it, as long as the session wrapped up at least an hour before bedtime. For an even better sleep-inducer, top off your sweat session with a cool shower to bring your body temperature down and set the stage for quality shuteye.

Keep caffeine in check. Caffeine is a wildly popular drug because it works. Remember that chemical called adenosine that clears during sleep? Even without hard exercise, it builds during the day and binds to specific nerve receptors to make you feel drowsy. Caffeine is an adenosine decoy that floats through your bloodstream and binds to those receptors. So now instead of slowing down, those nerves hit the gas and your pituitary gland gives you a shot of adrenaline. That's fine early in the day. But the half-life of caffeine is about 6 hours. So if you have a 200-milligram mug of coffee at 3 p.m., you still have a shot's worth of espresso kicking around at 9 p.m. That's not conducive to sleep. Try to avoid caffeine after 2 p.m., or at least make it a small cup.

Manage stress. Nothing keeps you awake like stress. Deep breathing exercises practiced periodically throughout the day and before bed can activate the vagus nerve and help you move out of a sympathetic (fight-or-flight) state and trigger parasympathetic (rest-and-digest) activity. Meditation also helps. Apps like Headspace offer structured meditation sessions to talk you through the process. Or wind down at night with a relaxing sleep story. There are audiobooks and apps that offer bedtime stories for adults that work just as well as they did when you were a kid.

GET A DOSE OF YOGA NIDRA (AKA NONSLEEP DEEP REST)

Naps are a well-established way to help boost recovery, especially after hard training or a night of short sleep. But they're not always practical and can sometimes interfere with sleep. Instead, you can try an ancient practice called yoga nidra, which is picking up steam in the United States as nonsleep deep rest (NSDR). The goal of these practices is to drift into a state of deep relaxation where you're hovering in a dreamy state between consciousness and sleep.

These "shallow naps" not only improve your cognitive function and rejuvenate your energy during the day, but they also set you up for a better night's sleep and may help manage chronic insomnia because they train your brain to go into rest mode. You can find 10- to 20-minute yoga nidra and/or NSDR guided meditations on YouTube or numerous apps on your smart phone.

ROAR ▸▸▸ SOUND BITES

▸ Postexercise blood flow is different between men and women. Women tend to shunt blood away from their muscles, where it's needed to deliver nutrients and oxygen and take away waste, while men tend to have an enhanced blood flow to their muscles.

▸ By using recovery techniques such as an easy cooldown combined with cooling and/or compression, women can push more blood back into central circulation and enhance blood flow to the muscles to flush out waste and encourage muscle repair.

▸ Key tools for recovery include massage, cooling and/or compression devices such as Game Ready, and small electrical muscle-stimulation devices such as the Marc Pro.

▸ Soft-tissue recovery includes using a lacrosse or tennis ball to target specific areas that are prone to tightness and inflammation.

▸ Delay the intake of antioxidants for 4 to 5 hours postexercise in order to allow a key adaptation to occur at the level of the mitochondria (cells' energy-producing furnaces).

▸ Sleep is queen for recovery. Aim for 7 to 9 hours a night. Also work in periods of nonsleep deep rest (yoga nidra) to recharge during the day.

15

HIGH PERFORMANCE IN A PILL?

SOME SUPPLEMENTS CAN BE HELPFUL, WHILE OTHERS CAN DERAIL YOUR PERFORMANCE

The sheer number of supplements people take constantly amazes me. You open their medicine cabinet and it looks like the backroom of a pharmacy, packed with pills and powders and magic potions. Active, healthy people are the biggest consumers of these products because we work hard to get fit and strong, so we are particularly susceptible to products that promise to boost performance, hasten recovery, and otherwise make us bulletproof.

Don't believe the hype. Depending on your situation, a few supplements may improve your performance and general health, but many are a waste of money, and some may actually be detrimental. On top of that, the FDA really doesn't do much in the way of regulating what you're buying. We have seen in the herbal supplement industry that tested products sometimes contain mere traces of what's promised on the label.

With that in mind, here's a review of which supplements you might want to look into as an active woman and which ones to leave on the health food store shelves. (Note: The supplements addressed here are daily dietary supplements, not the occasional-use supplements such as valerian that I have mentioned in other chapters, which may be beneficial in special circumstances such as sleep disturbances during menopause.)

SUPPORT FOR YOUR SYSTEM

My overriding philosophy is that you should work with your physiology to be the best you can be. So any supplement you take should serve that purpose. There are a few supplements that women commonly need for a boost, at least during certain periods of their lives.

Iron: Iron is essential for energy. It helps your body deliver oxygen to your working muscles and participates in the energy-making process in your mitochondria. It's also a key player in cognitive function and keeping your immune system strong. Active women need more iron, and maintaining healthy iron levels is important to avoid iron deficiency, which is low iron, as well as iron-deficiency anemia, where you have both low iron and a lack of hemoglobin, the iron-rich protein in your blood cells that carry oxygen. Iron-deficiency anemia can leave you chronically tired, hamper your workouts, and cause more random symptoms, such as irritability and frequently feeling cold.

Iron deficiency is more common in women in general, especially premenopausal women, because monthly blood loss depletes iron stores and increases demand. The heavier your periods, the higher your risk. Perimenopausal women are at higher risk because estrogen helps downregulate an iron-regulating hormone called hepcidin. When estrogen declines and hepcidin rises, iron is harder to absorb. In female athletes, iron deficiency is an even more common diagnosis because of the even greater iron loss through red cell breakdown, losses in sweat, gastrointestinal bleeding (from running impact, gut distress, and NSAID use), and an increase in cytokine expression (inflammation by-products that interfere with the absorption of iron) from the constant acute inflammation response to exercise. Other factors that lead to a negative iron balance include the hormone hepcidin (more on that in a bit), environmental stressors like altitude, and genetics.

It is also common for women to suffer from low energy availability (so many nutrients, like iron, may be insufficient) and/or follow a meatless diet—the RDAs for vegetarians are 1.8 times higher than for people who eat meat because heme iron from meat is more bioavailable than nonheme iron from plant-based foods.

Research shows that 1 in 10 women will have anemia at any point in time and about a third of women suffer with anemia at some point in their lifetime. While about 5 to 11 percent of male athletes have iron deficiency, that number jumps to 15 to 35 percent among females. Worse, a recent study in *The Lancet Haematology* reports that current test thresholds for detecting iron deficiency in women (as well as children) may be too low because physiological changes like fatigue, impaired physical performance, and decreased work productivity can occur well before iron levels reach the stage of deficiency as currently defined by blood tests.

Anemia is such a concern among exercising women that a study published in the journal *Medicine* concluded that active women should get screened for anemia as part of their general care. (I suggest, and research supports, that women get screened biannually or quarterly, depending on their previous history of iron deficiency.)

In the study, researchers surveyed 300 active premenopausal women, average age 31, for risk factors and signs of iron deficiency and anemia. Nearly 80 percent of women had risk factors for anemia. More than 43 percent had a previous history of iron deficiency; 26 percent were vegetarian or vegan; and more than 43 percent had heavy menstrual bleeding.

More than 80 percent of women also had at least one symptom relating to iron deficiency. The most common symptom was brain fog, with half the women reporting fuzzy cognition. More than a quarter reported shortness of breath. And 35 percent reported heart palpitations. It's important to note that many women don't even realize that these can be symptoms of iron deficiency, making the case for testing even stronger. If a woman isn't unusually fatigued, she might not think, "Oh, my iron might be low."

Other symptoms that the survey didn't include that are relevant to athletes are poor recovery and a reduction in performance, particularly when you wouldn't expect it, like when your training load is constant or not particularly strenuous or during a recovery, deload week.

According to the Recommended Daily Allowance, women younger than 50 should aim for 18 milligrams of iron a day. Women 51 years and older should aim for 8 milligrams of iron a day. I have to say, this longstanding recommendation has never sat well with me because the recommendation is grounded in menopausal status, *not* age. Sure, the average age of menopause is 51, but some women go through menopause considerably earlier or later. The better recommendation is aiming for 18 milligrams when you're pre- and perimenopausal and 8 milligrams postmenopause. The richest sources of heme iron include animal-based foods like beef, poultry, and seafood. Plant foods rich in non-heme iron include nuts, beans, leafy green vegetables, and fortified grain products like cereals and breads.

You can optimize your iron absorption by consuming your iron-rich foods with vitamin C–rich foods like oranges and peppers and avoiding taking them with foods that impair iron absorption like calcium-containing foods such as dairy, as well as caffeine (e.g., coffee and tea).

If you go the supplement route, be aware that oversupplementing can cause iron-overload (e.g., too much iron), which can cause symptoms similar to anemia, like fatigue, poor recovery, and shortness of breath. So, you should get your iron tested with a blood test to determine your iron stores before you start supplementing.

For premenopausal women: If you're on the low end of normal, supplementing with your cycle will help you increase your iron stores. Take an iron supplement every other day, in the morning, during the low-hormone phase (about days 3 to 16) of your cycle before training or at least 3 hours after training. This will help you work with your natural hepcidin responses and absorb the iron you take.

For peri- and postmenopausal women: If you're on the low end of normal, supplementing with your hepcidin circadian rhythm will help you increase your iron stores. In a perfect world, you would take your iron supplement first thing along with vitamin D3 (which helps lower hepcidin and improve absorption) before training, because hepcidin can be elevated after training for up to 24 hours in late perimenopausal and postmenopausal women. If you're a coffee or tea drinker, take your supplement at night; just be sure to take your vitamin D3 supplement (more on that in a bit) after your day's training to help bring those naturally higher hepcidin levels down.

As for what iron compound to take, it is best to discuss with your doctor to determine how much elemental iron you need; but if you are buying over the counter, look for iron bisglycinate or carbonyl iron, both of which are easy to absorb.

If you tend to run low on iron, you may find that supplementation improves your performance on nearly every level. A meta-analysis of iron supplements and female exercise performance done by Australian researchers found that female athletes (particularly those low in iron) who took iron supplements improved their maximum power as well as their exercise efficiency, meaning they put out more power at a lower heart rate.

Vitamin D: Vitamin D can be tricky to get from food unless you eat a lot of fatty fish, such as salmon, tuna, and mackerel. Fortified milk, cheese, and egg yolks also contain vitamin D, but the primary source for most humans is the sun, which reacts with your skin to synthesize the essential nutrient.

Turns out many of us aren't getting enough from any source. In fact, some researchers have gone so far as to call vitamin D deficiency a pandemic! Some experts believe it's because we spend so much of our modern lives indoors, and when we do go out, we cover ourselves in clothes and sunblock. The sunblock part is iffy. Some studies have found that sunblock can indeed hinder vitamin D synthesis from sunshine. Others have found the effect negligible. Ultimately, you don't need to go out and deliberately bake yourself, but we can't ignore the problem either, because vitamin D is a key player in many essential metabolic functions.

For one, vitamin D aids in the absorption of calcium and phosphorus, so it is paramount for bone health, which although not just a women's issue, it tends to be a more urgent issue for women. (See Chapter 9 for more information on bone health.) Vitamin D is also important for downregulating hepcidin, which as mentioned above, is essential for maintaining positive iron balance.

As science probes further, we're also discovering that vitamin D may be a major muscle maker (and maintainer) and may help with physical performance on nearly every level. In fact, research shows that increasing your vitamin D to 75 to 100 nanomoles per liter (nmol/L) could boost your aerobic capacity, muscle growth, and muscle power while shortening your recovery time from hard exercise bouts and improving bone density. The Recommended Dietary Allowance for adults 19 and older is 600 IU daily, and for adults over 70 it is 800 IU daily. More than that is not better. Even in the dark months of winter, 800 to 1,000 IUs is adequate. Very high levels (more than 125 nanomoles per liter) can have negative side effects and have even been linked to increased mortality. You can stay safe by not exceeding the tolerable upper intake level of 4,000 IU of vitamin D3 (the most effective type for increasing vitamin D plasma levels) per day.

Magnesium: Magnesium is an essential mineral that your body uses for maintaining healthy blood pressure, regulating blood sugar, muscle and nerve function, bone development, and more. It also helps with muscle relaxation and helps regulate neurotransmitters that are related to sleep.

It's easy to get through a healthy diet, as it is widely distributed in a variety of plant and animal foods including green leafy vegetables, legumes, nuts, seeds, and whole grains, as well as fish, poultry, and beef.

If you're highly active, however, consider taking a 400-milligram magnesium supplement to keep your levels in the optimum zone. When you exercise strenuously, you pee and sweat out enough magnesium to increase your requirements by up to 20 percent, according to research. That means if you routinely get the 320 milligrams recommended each day for adult women, you could easily be deficient if you're very active.

This is a concern, since research shows that maintaining healthy magnesium levels is especially important for maintaining muscle and preventing muscle loss in women as they age. Perimenopausal and postmenopausal women also often find that magnesium supplementation can improve sleep efficiency, sleep latency, early morning awakening, and insomnia.

SUPPLEMENTS FOR PERFORMANCE ENHANCEMENT

Research on female college athletes shows that more than 65 percent of them use some type of supplement at least once a month. I don't know what the percentage is among performance-minded women outside of the collegiate ranks, but based on my experience, I'll say it's as high if not higher.

I am obviously not antisupplement, since I use a few ergogenic aids like essential amino acids, caffeine, and adaptogens myself. But I think it's important for women to recognize that just as women have been traditionally understudied in sports science in general, we have been very understudied in the realm of ergogenic aids. Based on what we know about how women respond differently to strategies like intermittent fasting and ketogenic diets, we should also take a closer look at how we might respond (or not) to sports supplements.

A 2016 study published in the *Strength and Conditioning Journal* titled "The Ergogenic Effects of Supplemental Nutritional Aids on Anaerobic Performance in Female Athletes" did just that and provided a good springboard into some of the most recent research to paint a picture of what you can expect from some of the most popular sports supplements. Just remember: Supplements are exactly that—*supplements.* They are designed to enhance (and sometimes only truly marginally so) the work you are doing. Before you jump on the newest supplement trends, make sure you have the basics—recovery, sleep, nutrition, training, etc.—covered first.

Creatine Monohydrate

If you're going to supplement with any performance-enhancing supplements, I recommend starting with creatine. Creatine is a naturally occurring substance found in your muscle cells that helps them produce energy during high-intensity exercise and heavy lifting. Ninety-five percent of all creatine is stored in your skeletal muscles, and you can bump up those creatine reserves by about 20 percent with supplementation.

Women naturally have 70 to 80 percent lower creatine stores than men, and we typically consume significantly lower amounts of dietary creatine, which comes primarily from animal foods like beef, compared to men. So, it's little surprise that research finds that women may benefit more from supplementing this ergogenic aid.

The 2016 study found that females had greater relative performance improvements over males, with males experiencing about a 6 percent increase in performance and females enjoying a 15 percent increase in performance—more than double the benefit.

More recently, a 2021 review of the literature published in *Nutrients* reported that "creatine supplementation may be of particular importance during menses, pregnancy, post-partum, during and post-menopause" and that "females with varying levels of training and fitness may experience improvements in both anaerobic and aerobic exercise performance from both short-term and long-term creatine supplementation."

Creatine is traditionally viewed as an ergogenic compound known to promote cell survival and influence the production and usage of energy for fast and high-demanding energetics of the body, in particular the brain. It may also help with mood disorders.

The review included interesting research on brain health in women; identifying research that women with a major depressive disorder who augmented their daily antidepressant with 5 grams of creatine responded twice as fast and experienced remission of depression at twice the rate of women who took just the antidepressant. The researchers recommend a traditional loading dose (0.3 gram per kilogram of body weight a day for 5 to 7 days) or a routine daily dose (3 to 5 grams) for 4 weeks as effective for women, regardless of age. The traditional side effect of weight gain (due to water retention) does not occur with this low dose, yet the health and performance outcomes increase significantly.

Beta-Alanine

Beta-alanine is an amino acid found in poultry, meat, and fish. Your body uses it to produce carnosine, which serves as an acid buffer and helps improve exercise performance. Beta-alanine also improves muscle fiber firing rates and recovery.

Carnosine levels are naturally lower in females than males, according to the 2016 study, but females experience greater relative increases in carnosine after beta-alanine supplementation. Studies on female masters athletes show performance gains with beta-alanine supplementation, including improving lower-body exercise performance and improving cycling time trial performance. A study on premenopausal soccer players found that beta-alanine supplementation during plyometric training appeared to add further adaptive changes in endurance and repeated sprinting and jumping ability.

If you are in the menopausal transition and suffer hot flashes during exercises, a dose of beta-alanine, which helps open your blood vessels, before you head out can help ward them off.

Research has shown exercise improvements with consumption of 3.2 to 6.4 grams a day. Some people get pins-and-needles sensations at the higher end of that recommended dosage. You can avoid that by taking it in two separate doses over the course of the day.

SUPPLEMENTS THAT MAY HELP AND HURT IN THE HEAT

The same supplements that work in cool to moderate temperatures may not be as effective—or worse, may be counterproductive—when you use them in high temperatures, when the body is already challenged by the heat. Two of the most widely used ergogenic aids—caffeine and nitrates—top this list.

Though most of us don't think of caffeine as a "supplement" per se, and I'm not suggesting you go cold turkey without your morning coffee or tea before a big event in a hot climate, it's a good idea to go easy on how much caffeine you put in your system before and during a hot-weather event. Caffeine can increase your core temperature, which you obviously don't want. One study found that when regular caffeine users had the equivalent of 4 to 5 cups of coffee (the equivalent of 350 milligrams of caffeine for a 154-pound/70-kilogram person) before a steady-state exercise test in a hot lab, they experienced increased core temperature and decreased blood flow to the skin on the arms and back. Go easy on caffeinated sports products during events in the heat, and try drinking cold brew/iced coffee (sticking to about 2 cups) ahead of the event to avoid the heating effect of drinking a hot beverage.

Nitrates are a vasodilator, so they open your blood vessels to increase blood flow. But their effectiveness dissipates when the body is under heat stress because your body is already doing all it can to vasodilate the vessels to off-load heat. So, there are no additional benefits to taking supplemental nitrates.

Beta-alanine is still effective in the heat for reducing muscle fatigue, both through its buffering capabilities and its ability to improve calcium release for muscle contraction.

Two supplements that might be helpful in the heat: curcumin and glutamine. Curcumin can be especially beneficial if you struggle with gut issues in the heat. Recent research has demonstrated that taking 500 milligrams a day for 3 days before an exercise heat stress test improved gut function and physiological strain responses. Supplementing with glutamine (0.9 gram/kilogram) 2 hours before exercise can help decrease intestinal permeability and improve the integrity of the mucosal lining (protective lining of the gut).

FILE UNDER QUESTIONABLE

I'd like to also call out a few supplements that many women—especially active women—believe they should be taking (sometimes in very high doses), and they probably don't need to (and maybe shouldn't), unless they've been directed to by a health care provider.

Calcium: Surprised to see this one on the list? You're not alone. Women have been pushed and prompted to take calcium as a preventive measure against osteoporosis for decades. And you know what? It might be a wash. In 2013, the US Preventive Services Task Force recommended that postmenopausal women refrain from taking calcium (as well as vitamin D, as they are often taken in tandem). After reviewing more than 135 studies, the task force concluded that calcium supplementation didn't prevent fractures. Worse, a few studies suggested that calcium supplements seemed to increase the risk of heart attack and death from heart disease.

On the flip side, a few large studies such as the Women's Health Initiative have reported benefits, specifically a reduction in hip fracture (with no increase in heart attacks) among postmenopausal women on hormone therapy (which is likely the key player here; hormone therapy is FDA approved for preventing osteoporosis in at-risk women) taking 1,000 milligrams of calcium and 400 IU of vitamin D a day. And the National Osteoporosis Foundation stands by supplement use for women with osteoporosis or significant risk factors for a fracture. It's important to note, however, that this is the recommendation for women who are low in calcium to begin with. Too much calcium supplementation, especially when you're getting what you need from food, is what appears to be problematic.

In the end, it is wise to err on the side of common sense and get the calcium you need through your diet, not a pill. Some scientists speculate that it's the pills—not the nutrient itself—that may cause the heart problems in some people. When you take a huge bolus of calcium, it just gets dumped into your bloodstream all at once rather than in the smaller doses you'd get throughout the day with your diet, and this can result in calcium deposits in your arteries.

If you're younger than 50, you need 1,000 milligrams a day. Women over 50 need 1,200 milligrams a day. Getting the 1,000 to 1,200 milligrams you need daily is pretty easy. Three servings of plain yogurt (415 milligrams per 8 ounces) can help you get there quickly. One and a half ounces of part-skim mozzarella and 3 ounces of sardines both deliver about 330 milligrams (33 percent of your daily recommendation) of calcium. For those who don't eat dairy, fortified cereal and greens such as kale are also good sources. No supplementation necessary.

Antioxidants—all of 'em: Listen up, active-antioxidant-loving gals. I repeat, put down the vitamin C, E, and beta-carotene and walk away. While you're at it, check the sports nutrition you're using for hefty doses of these nutrients. If they're fortified with them, cease and desist using them. You're doing yourself a disservice. As mentioned in Chapter 14, antioxidants can actually impair your training adaptations and recovery. And in case you're not convinced, there's more. High-dose supplements also seem to be detrimental to your overall health.

Once again, we got sucked into overly simplistic thinking. Just because a little is a good thing, then a lot (most supplements give you a lot of one nutrient) must be even better! This thinking is dangerous (more in a second), but first and foremost it comes down once again to getting the nutrients you need through the food you eat. Natural foods not only contain proper amounts of specific nutrients, but they also naturally pair those nutrients with others that work synergistically to provide the health benefit. Nowhere is that more true than with antioxidants.

To recap, antioxidants are molecules that step in and neutralize potentially cell-damaging by-products called free radicals. Free radicals have been blamed for everything from cancer to skin wrinkles, even aging itself! So looking back, it's not hard to see where our infatuation with antioxidants came from. Boatloads of epidemiological data (large population studies) found that folks who ate a diet filled with antioxidant-rich fruits, vegetables, and drinks had lower rates of disease and lived longer and healthier lives. But when people started taking high-dose supplements of these antioxidants, it didn't work. They actually got sicker. Two large studies on more than 47,000 smokers taking beta-carotene had to be halted because the groups taking the antioxidants were actually getting cancer, as well as heart disease, at higher rates than those taking dummy pills. The researchers discovered that though foods rich in beta-carotene seemed protective for smokers, one whopping dose of the antioxidant seemed to fortify the free radicals and cause great harm.

THE TRACK STACK*

For those who are seeking ways to supplement their training that actually work and are not harmful (or illegal), I present the track stack—a blend of compounds that work together to prime your pump and get you fully ready for action. Take it 20 minutes before go time. *(Note: This is for specific use only and should not be taken every day. Do not take this if you have any history of heart problems or blood pressure issues, as this creates a very strong vasodilation response.)*

1 × 100 milligrams of caffeine (stimulant)

1 × 81 milligrams of baby aspirin if no contraindications to aspirin (dilates blood vessels)

1,500 milligrams of beta-alanine (improves muscle fiber firing rate)

* This dose is for smaller individuals. If you weigh more than 155 pounds, increase the dose to 150 milligrams of caffeine, 1 × 81 milligrams of baby aspirin if no contraindications to aspirin, and 2,000 milligrams of beta-alanine.

As an athlete, you don't need any antioxidant supplements—that includes fortified bars, drinks, or gels—because they could in fact be harmful to getting fitter and faster. We can't outsmart nature. We need to let our bodies naturally overcome exercise-induced stress and make the appropriate adaptations. Look to real food to get everything your body needs to work its magic, and limit supplementation to very specific and medically necessary situations.

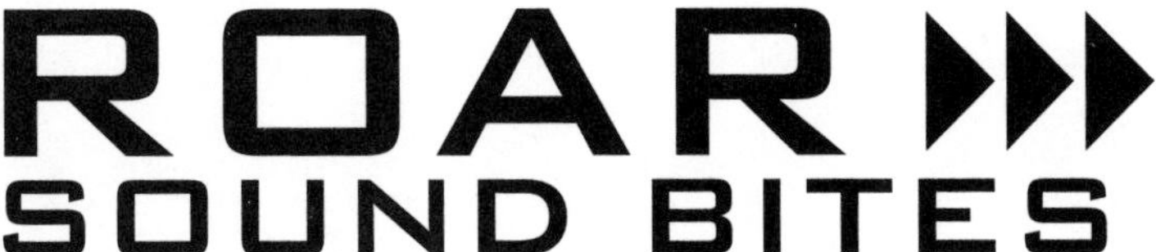

▸ Be sparing with supplements. Most vitamin pill lovers take far more than they need—or than is good for them.

▸ Calcium supplements may do more harm than good. Get your recommended daily dose from food sources.

▸ Megadoses of antioxidants may be dangerous.

▸ If you're racing, competing, or aiming for peak performance, a few well-studied supplements such as beta-alanine are worth a look.

▸ For most nutrients, food is still your best source.

16

BRAIN TRAINING

IT'S NOT ALL IN YOUR HEAD; WOMEN AND MEN DO THINK DIFFERENTLY

Girls are good at reading. Boys are good at math. Men never ask for directions. Women are intuitive and good multitaskers. You've heard all the gender stereotypes (and probably then some). Of course, they are just that, stereotypes, and they do not define us. Women's and men's brains are more similar than they are different. That said, there are some key unique elements to the female brain that can impact the way we train and perform, especially in team situations. It also influences how we perceive ourselves and the self-talk that follows.

"A lot of these are broad-brush generalizations, and of course there are exceptions, but female athletes generally do bring a perspective to training and sport that is unique from their male counterparts'," says sports psychologist Kristin E. Keim of Keim Performance Consulting. "It's useful for women to know and appreciate those differences, especially when they're working with a male coach or male teammates, who may literally think differently than they do."

IT'S ALL IN OUR CONNECTIONS

When neuroscientists wanted to understand the fundamental differences between the minds of men and women, they did what scientists do best—they lined up a few hundred volunteers and studied them. In a study published in the *Proceedings of the National Academy of Sciences*, researchers analyzed nearly 1,000 brain scans of men and women (428 males and 521 females). Though more research is needed and the "presence, magnitude, and significance of sex differences" between female and male brains is a topic of debate in the scientific community, the key differences they found are compelling.

For one, as you might expect, women's brains are smaller—by about 8 percent—than men's by virtue of our bodies being smaller overall. That doesn't limit our intelligence, however (average IQ scores are the same across gender lines). Research also shows there are sex differences in the volume of various parts of the brain with women having greater volumes in the prefrontal cortex, orbitofrontal cortex, superior temporal cortex, lateral parietal cortex, and insula and males on average having greater volume in the ventral temporal and occipital regions.

As one study put it, the larger amounts of gray matter volume in the prefrontal areas in women are "functionally important for executive functioning, such as planning, working memory, inhibition, mental flexibility as well as the initiation and monitoring of action, but also for emotional control, moral considerations and processing of language." Men, by contrast, had larger gray matter volume in areas involved in motor function.

There may also be important differences in the way our brain circuitry is wired and activated. In women, our brain circuitry is heavily connected between our left and right hemispheres. By contrast, men's connections are strongest between the front and back regions of their brains. Generally speaking, that means that male brains "may be optimized for motor skills, and female brains may be optimized for combining analytical and intuitive thinking," as noted in *Scientific American*. Again, these findings apply to the population as a whole and are not an absolute for individuals; they may also change over the lifespan and with development, but they provide valuable insights into other ways we are not small men.

Perhaps the most important sex difference is chemical. It's well known that women are diagnosed with depression and anxiety far more often than men. That may be because there are significant differences in our serotonin systems, with one study finding that women have a greater number of the most common serotonin receptors than men, but they also have lower levels of the protein that transports serotonin back into the nerve cells that secrete it. It is this protein that the most common antidepressants (SSRIs) block. This is yet another reason why women need to be very careful about extremely low-carb diets, because restricting this macronutrient causes your brain to produce even less serotonin, setting you up for mood disorders, especially if you're already prone to them.

Women's brains also physically change during the menopause transition, according to the vital work being done by Dr. Lisa Mosconi, director of the Women's Brain Initiative at Weill Cornell Medicine in New York. Her research shows there is a dip in gray and white matter volume and glucose metabolism in the brain during the menopause transition (aka perimenopause). When estrogen declines during this time, the brain goes through some structural and metabolic changes. But, as those follow-up scans showed, it also adapts and for most women returns to structure and function levels similar to premenopause once they enter postmenopause. Not everyone's brain recovers fully, however, which may explain why women are at greater risk for Alzheimer's disease. Research on this is ongoing. (I'll note that in another vote for doing more strength training, resistance training is good for your brain and helps lower the risk.)

Finally, there's a reason you don't see as many women in daredevil, high-risk sports such as base jumping (aka parachuting off a cliff face). That's not to say some women don't participate or women cannot participate; we're just not wired to seek and engage in risk-taking behaviors in the same way men are.

ARE CONCUSSIONS DIFFERENT FOR FEMALES?

When it comes to brain injury during sport, women may be more susceptible. Some research finds that women are 50 percent more likely to have a concussion than men. That may set them up for trouble down the road because the same study found that athletes who suffered a previous concussion were three times as likely to have another compared to their peers who had never had one. Other research has found that women have greater rates of concussion in baseball/softball, basketball, ice hockey, and soccer than men. Females also seem to be more vulnerable to developing post concussion migraine.

When it comes to recovery from concussion, some studies find that females are at a higher risk for prolonged recovery, while other research finds that female and male athletes take approximately the same amount of time to recover. That discrepancy may be related to the impact of the menstrual cycle. Importantly, research has found that women injured during the luteal phase of their menstrual cycle, when progesterone concentration is high, had significantly lower scores on quality of life assessments 1 month after their injury than women injured during the follicular phase of their cycle or women taking oral contraceptives. Research I'm overseeing is finding longer time to recovery and greater lingering post concussion fatigue if the concussion occurred in the luteal phase. Also, menstrual cycle dysfunction/irregularity appears to happen for 4 to 5 months post concussion. Recent research shows that some of this discrepancy may be because females tend to get delayed concussion care compared to males (if you hit your head, get care ASAP!).

More research is essential here, but we do know that, regardless of sex, brain injury is to be taken seriously, and athletes of both sexes have better outcomes when they seek care as soon as they sustain the injury. If you hit your head, get checked out.

MINDFULNESS IN MOTION

What does all this mean for you as you train, compete, and recover? Just as you dial in your nutrition, hydration, and training to complement your unique female physiology, you can work with rather than fight against your unique brain structure and circuitry to gain physical and competitive advantages.

Know the why. If you've ever felt unmotivated to do a particular workout or follow a certain plan, ask yourself why you were planning to do it in the first place. If you can't answer the question, it could explain your lack of motivation. As a woman, you may be wired for intuitive and analytical thinking, so it's important that you know why you're doing what you're doing. "Women want and do better when they have the whole perspective," says Dr. Keim, "whereas a guy will often just want you to tell him what to do and then go do it. Women want to know why."

If you work with a coach, make exercise explanations part of your plan. If you're out doing your own thing, do a little background research to learn exactly how the workouts you're doing benefit you. If you understand why hill sprints are so important for marathon training, you'll be more motivated to do them.

Find your flock. Because of our social nature, there is no shortage of women-specific clubs and groups for just about any sport or activity. "Women are deeply rooted in their relationships and connections," says Dr. Keim. "So it's not surprising that they may find it more satisfying to be part of a community when they're working out."

By becoming part of a women's running or cycling club, soccer team, or gym class, you can work out in the camaraderie of like-minded women while creating bonds that continue beyond the gym walls or playing field. Your group doesn't necessarily have to be gender specific: Decades of research confirm that you're far more likely to consistently stick to your exercise plans when you have someone (or a group) to whom you feel accountable.

Understand your inner conflict. Women may be more likely to be conflicted with competition because they're more hardwired to be empathetic and sympathetic, according to Dr. Keim. "That can have a negative impact on you in a competitive environment." It's natural to feel bad for a competitor who is having trouble; just save your sympathy for after the competition is done.

Monitor your moods. Are you feeling happy about lacing up your shoes and heading out the door? Or are you miserable, searching for the energy to get changed for your next exercise bout? Women are more prone to overtraining, which is marked by high-stress hormones such as cortisol, low feel-good neurochemicals such as serotonin, and fatigue. Persistent low mood is an early indication that you're heading toward overtraining and the first sign that you should pull back your intensity and let yourself get adequate rest and recovery. "Women take longer to recover from overtraining," says Dr. Keim. "So it's important to see the signs before you have full-blown symptoms."

Be objective with yourself. When a man has a performance in his event, he will likely come in blaming the conditions, the equipment, his nutrition, and any litany of outside factors that contributed to his downfall. A woman will be tempted to blame herself. That's a sweeping generalization, of course, but women are more likely to put poor performance on their own ability or lack thereof, says Dr. Keim. "Women are prone to personalizing a bad performance." There are times when it pays to "think like a dude." This is one. Take an objective look at what happened. Was it inordinately hot or cold? Did your nutrition go as planned (assuming there was a plan)? In the end, you (both men and women) need to take some level of personal responsibility for the outcome of any given competition. But identifying the factors that contributed to your performance, whether positive or negative, helps you develop a concrete plan going forward. Feeling like you failed does not.

Set the scene. Because as a woman your brain is wired to take in the whole picture, visualization can be a particularly potent training tool, says Dr. Keim. "I find women really gravitate to and do well with this exercise." Whether you're gunning for that tenth pullup or lining up for a 10-K, play it out in your head. Imagine your lats, biceps, and deltoids lighting up and firing in a beautifully synchronized feat of strength. Picture yourself skimming over the asphalt, your feet turning over lightly and quickly as you run through the streets. It not only calms your mind, it actually helps you perform better. Research shows that when you visualize an action, your brain maps it out in your body, so your muscles are primed to perform. In one study, scientists found that volunteers who just imagined exercising their biceps 5 days a week for 12 weeks improved their strength by more than 13 percent, though they never actually moved a muscle, while those who did no imaginary exercise reaped no strength gains. That's powerful stuff.

Talk nice. The words you say to yourself have a powerful impact on your performance. Unfortunately, women can be prone to negative self-talk. If you keep saying, "I'll never qualify for the Boston Marathon," or "I'll never pull off a muscle-up," you'll probably prove yourself right. So change the script in your head to a more positive one. Even if it's not particularly how you're feeling at the time, you can actually trick yourself into a better performance. One study from 2014 found that cyclists undergoing endurance tests felt like the task was less taxing and actually pedaled nearly 2 minutes longer when they gave themselves a little positive reinforcement. So tell yourself, "I've got this." Then go get it.

Practice mindfulness. Because we're such good multitaskers, it can actually be challenging for us to completely focus and immerse ourselves in the task at hand. You're doing yourself a disservice by not focusing. By thinking past what you're doing, you're not allowing yourself to get the most out of what you're currently doing. As such, you're also setting yourself up for mistakes, such as being slack on your nutrition and hydration during a marathon, because your mind is on a million different things (you'd be surprised how often people will admit that they forgot to eat and drink).

Practice being engaged in the moment. How do your muscles feel? What's going on around you? What do you need to be doing right now to maintain or improve your performance? That's not to say your thoughts will never drift to your cousin's wedding this weekend or your son's algebra grades. But with practice, you can let those thoughts drift through your mind while you pull your focus back to the task at hand.

HEAR HER ROAR

THE PRO CYCLIST WHO NEEDED SELF-CONFIDENCE

Success should breed confidence. But sadly for women, that is often not the case. Not only do women tend to have lower self-confidence than their male peers, but far too often belittling coaches and envious peers knock them down even further. When they do win, they have a tendency to downplay it instead of using the victory to build themselves up. They're also more prone to depression, which they often battle alone, thinking they need to be tough. Now in the era of social media where everyone shows you only the rosiest side of their lives, successful athletes can feel very alone.

Despite this, it is still a surprise when an accomplished athlete such as Amber Pierce, pro cyclist and member of the US national team, whose race résumé is jam-packed with wins, comes to your door because she's having trouble staying above water. It's something sport psychologist Kristin Keim sees all too often. "There are still too many coaches who will be critical instead of nurturing, when women tend to respond better to nurturing."

So Dr. Keim gave Amber, who had been through her share of confidence-crushing situations, just what she needed most: a sympathetic, nonjudgmental ear. "Even when things were going well, my main struggle was not having confidence that matched my ability or achievements. There's a lot of negative self-talk that goes with that," says Amber.

Making matters worse, Amber struggled with society's view of women in general. She says, "Confidence and competitiveness in women is often socially equated to bitchiness. Speaking in broad terms, men are rewarded for those traits, while women are put down. The considerable and negative social feedback for feeling confident and embracing it can be really, really difficult. In the first place, we struggle with confidence more than men and have difficulty reconciling our competitiveness. On top of that, we're not rewarded when we actually do embrace those characteristics."

All this added up to a whole lot of wasted energy. "I was spending a great deal of mental and emotional energy managing stress," recalls Amber. "I realized that while I had shown a great deal of resiliency, I was barely keeping my head above water. I was effectively staving off depression and managing pretty well. But really, when you're competing on an elite level—or any level—you don't want to be 'managing pretty well.' You want to optimize. Stagnating at 'pretty well' robs you of motivation and vigor, so you can't perform your best."

Through a lot of talking and reflection, Amber was able to reframe the issues that were troubling her. "I came to the conclusion that women are praised for being selfless and punished for being selfish, which I can't really change," says Amber. However, she was able to look at the situation from a different perspective and successfully boost her self-confidence. "We have to invest in our capacity to give and to motivate others. I can look at my time cycling, training, and racing as selfish, or I can look at it as building my capacity to give back to others. Cycling makes me come alive and empowers me to give."

Amber also changed her view on what it means to be competitive. "I've come to view competition as a form of cooperation," she says. "None of us can do as well solo as we do in a race when we compete with others. Your competitor is helping you to discover your limits and potential and how you have more in yourself than you thought possible. She is your greatest ally in that self-discovery, and you are the same for her," says Amber. "Regardless of whether you win or lose, you are creating an arena in which you can reach peak performance. You are competing together because you bring out the best performance from each of you. In that regard, training hard and being as prepared as possible to give your best effort during competition is the best gift you can give your competitor, because she has to reach that much higher to find her own personal excellence."

Try these philosophies for yourself. They may help inspire some newfound confidence in simply being true to yourself.

Embrace your identity. Many women are reluctant to identify themselves as athletes even when they are, which has some downsides but also some upsides, says Dr. Keim. "She'll say whatever her occupation is, that she's a mom, all these other things before she says athlete, if she even says athlete at all." That sounds like it could be a negative thing for someone who is indeed primarily an athlete, but it's well-roundedness that Dr. Keim also believes plays to a woman's advantage. "Male athletes are more likely to get their self-worth and identity very closely tied to their athletic selves and performance, and it can be troublesome for them," she says. "Women, on the other hand, have all these other identities that they can lean on when the athletic one isn't going as well as they'd like." Embrace your well-roundedness. Just remember that it's okay to include your athletic self as part of your identity.

ROAR SOUND BITES

- Women's brains are wired differently from men's. We have stronger connections side to side, which may make us better at combining analytical and intuitive thinking.
- As a woman, you are more prone to depression and anxiety and Alzheimer's disease later in life. (Resistance training helps attenuate this risk!)
- Women like to know why they're doing what they're doing. Ask yourself why you are training.
- Women are more susceptible to overtraining, so keep track of those moods.
- Self-confidence can be a struggle. Find a supportive cheerleader and believe in yourself.

17

BE YOUR OWN BIOHACKER

TAKE A PEEK INSIDE YOUR PHYSIOLOGY TO OPTIMIZE HOW YOU EAT, DRINK, TRAIN, AND PERFORM

As active, maybe even competitive women, we monitor our exercise and training progress by our output. We have watches and bike computers that can tell us if we're getting faster. Power meters can tell us to a watt how much stronger we are. We can track how much weight we rack up in the gym. That's all great. But there's more. You can tap into your physiology to see how your diet, training, and lifestyle are affecting your physical being. This can empower you to make adjustments to your input—what you eat, how you train, and your daily habits—to improve how you feel and perform!

BIOHACKING 101

This process of looking inside your physiology is what some call biohacking. Just like a computer hacker unlocks previously secret codes to get sensitive information, you're hacking into your unique physiology. By learning what makes you tick, you can effectively optimize your physiology for peak performance.

Biohacking is a rapidly growing field that includes everything from basic over-the-counter urinalysis strips (pee sticks) to full-on genetic DNA analysis. If you want to monitor it, there's a sensor for it. You can buy optical sensors, which literally peer beneath your skin and into your muscles and veins to inform you of your muscle oxygen saturation (how much oxygen is in your muscles and when you're approaching your lactate threshold). You can wear a continuous glucose monitor (CGM) to see your blood sugar levels rise and drop in (virtually) real time. Want to know how the heat's affecting you? Swallow a core body temperature capsule and wear a dermal patch to learn how hot you are inside and out. You can monitor your heart rate and respiration along with your watts. You can wear a Whoop Strap or Ōura Ring to track how much you toss and turn in your sleep and how ready and recovered your central nervous system is when you wake in the morning. You can even ship off some blood and saliva samples for a full panel of your hormones, vitamins, minerals, and other key biomarkers, as well as your overall health and athletic genetic makeup.

The big question is, should you be monitoring all these metrics? And if so, what do you do with all this data? The answer, of course, is it depends. How serious are you about your training and/or racing? Are you making progress? How much progress do you want to make? Are there specific situations, such as the heat, that tend to be particularly difficult for you? Biohacking is a great way to see what's going on inside and how it affects your output as well as solve training problems. So while I'm not sure everyone needs to undergo intensive chromosomal scrutiny to improve their 5-K performance, I do see the benefit in a number of these measures and have seen clients integrate them into their training with great success. I'll start with the basics before painting a head-to-toe biohacking scenario.

BIOHACKING, TRACKING, AND DATA-DRIVEN PERFORMANCE

Though we tend to think of biohacking as this new field, we've really been doing it for decades. The following are common biohacking techniques, tracking devices, and, most important, what that data does or does not mean for you.

Heart Rate Monitoring

One of the most basic biohacking devices is the heart rate monitor. A heart rate monitor is a two-part device. The first part is a transmitter that sits on your breastbone right over your heart, fixed in place with a strap that wraps around your torso (there are now also some wristwatch-style models). The second part is a computer readout that you wear as a watch or mount on your handlebars if you're cycling. It acts as a cardiovascular dashboard and tells you how many beats per minute your heart is thumping.

A heart rate monitor will tell you just how hard you're working, but only to a point. Heart rate can be somewhat fickle and is often influenced by dehydration, caffeine, menstruation, rest (or lack thereof), hormones, mood, and weather. There's also a great deal of variation from one rider to the next. You might start huffing and puffing and going into the red at 85 percent of your maximum heart rate, while someone just getting started on an exercise plan may hit hers at 75 percent.

If you invest in a heart rate monitor, you'll find instructions for setting your training zones based on your maximum heart rate (MHR), the highest number of beats your heart can pump out in 1 minute. Those instructions might include an MHR formula: 220 minus your age. Don't use it. It's antiquated and inaccurate. A better formula is 211 minus 64 percent of your age. So a 45-year-old woman would have a max heart rate of 182. As with all formulas, however, there is a margin of error, so the most accurate way to determine your MHR is an old-school field test.

First, warm up thoroughly. Then run, ride, row (or whatever you do) as hard as possible for 10 minutes, leaving it all out there for the final 30 seconds. Then actively cool down and check your monitor for your MHR. Repeat this test one or two more times (with rest days in between) and use the average result to find your true MHR. For the best results, prepare for the field test as you would a race. You should be well rested, well hydrated, well fed, and feeling good going into the tests. It also helps to do it with a faster friend who can motivate your competitive side and really push you to your limit.

Once you've determined your max, break your heart rate down into training zones to accomplish goals including endurance training, lactate threshold training, and recovery. Calculate your zones based on your MHR (see page 309). There are many different ways to divvy up your training zones. Below is an extremely basic example of what those zones can look like. For example, a rider with a 180 beats per minute (bpm) max would have a recovery heart rate around 115 bpm. The equation is MHR (180) × % of MHR (0.64) = 115. Keep in mind that monitoring your heart rate during training can be tricky because there's a lag between when you start pushing yourself and your heart rate response. It's meant to be used as a guide, not gospel.

HEART RATE ZONES

TRAINING ZONE	PERCENT OF MAXIMUM HEART RATE (MHR)
Zone 1 (recovery, easy day)	60–64
Zone 2 (aerobic endurance)	65–74
Zone 3 (high-level aerobic—tempo)	75–84
Zone 4 (lactate threshold—race pace)	85–94
Zone 5 (max effort)	95–100

With training, your resting heart rate drops, so if you're new to training, you'll find that your resting heart rate may be lower than is considered "normal" as you get fitter. A normal resting heart rate for a woman is often cited as 60 to 100 beats per minute. A well-trained woman may have a resting heart rate between 40 to 60 bpm.

Like your quads and calves, your heart gets stronger and more efficient with training. It can squeeze out more blood with every beat, so it doesn't have to work as hard to circulate oxygen and nutrient-rich blood through your system. Your cardiovascular system also becomes more adept at using that oxygen. So efforts that used to send your heart rate into Zone 3 or 4 will feel easier and you can complete them at a lower heart rate.

Heart rate also is a good indicator of your training/recovery status. If you're not fully recovered, your heart rate will not increase to where it needs to be to supply the necessary blood flow during exercise. This contributes to the sluggishness or staleness athletes often experience at the onset of overtraining. Even if you try to work harder, you will still feel like someone has put a lid on your performance because your heart rate cannot elevate to give you the blood supply you need. The result is a frustrating and psychologically damaging workout. The best thing you can do is go home, eat, and sleep.

Heart Rate Variability

Many women tell me that they use heart rate variability (HRV)—the variance in time between beats of your heart—for tracking recovery. HRV is the metric that Whoop Strap, Ōura Ring, and other recovery tracking devices use to tell you how rested or ready you are. It's a good indicator, but, like many physiological factors, female hormones affect it, so that number is not telling you the whole story—and sometimes it's telling a false story. If you're tracking HRV, here's what you need to know.

Your HRV is the result of the interplay between the parasympathetic (rest-and-digest) and sympathetic (fight-or-flight) branches of your autonomic nervous system. It describes the variability in the time between your heartbeats. When your HRV increases, that means your body is resilient to stress. When it decreases, you have less stress resilience.

Sounds straightforward—until you factor in sex hormones. Estrogen tends to increase vagal tone (i.e., the ability of your ventral vagal nerve to regulate your heartbeat), which is what devices measure to give you HRV. Progesterone, though "calming" in the brain, has the opposite effect on the vagal nerve and overrides estrogen's effect on increasing vagal tone. In naturally cycling women, when progesterone goes up, estrogen is still there, but progesterone is the dominant hormone, decreasing vagal tone. When progesterone drops, estrogen becomes the dominant hormone, which increases vagal tone.

In premenopausal women, HRV is influenced by the menstrual cycle. In the low-hormone (follicular) phase, HRV is highest. After ovulation, as progesterone rises, it stimulates the sympathetic nervous system, which in turn increases resting heart rate and respiratory rate while reducing HRV.

What does all this mean? For one, your recovery metrics in the late luteal phase will always be lower as compared to the follicular phase because of those changes in the autonomic nervous system and how they affect HRV. So, you may be recovered, but because the devices are not based on an algorithm that understands hormone fluctuations, you may get a false low-recovery score telling you that you are not fully recovered when you are. (You'll note that what your device tells you and how you feel do not always match up.)

Of course, many women do experience lower recovery during the late luteal phase because of these and other physiologic changes. You can work with your physiology during this time to help counter these effects by addressing the systemic inflammation (which also impacts your recovery scores) that comes with the peak and drop of sex hormones right before your period starts.

I recommend using 1 gram of omega-3 fatty acids (DHA and EPA), which helps counter the inflammatory cytokine prostaglandin E2, which is increased by estrogen. Make sure you're getting enough magnesium and zinc. And if you tolerate aspirin, take one 80-milligram baby aspirin to counter the inflammatory receptor sites COX-1 and COX-2 and keep those receptor sites muted.

Oral contraceptives also impact HRV. A paper I recently published looked at recovery responses across the natural and hormonal contraception (HC) driven menstrual cycles. We know that HRV is higher in the low-hormone phase and decreases as estrogen and progesterone increase across the natural cycle. But what is interesting are the patterns of recovery for women using HC. In the first few days of starting HC, HRV was elevated, but it significantly decreased across the active pill weeks, finding its lowest point in the first 2 days of the placebo pill, before increasing again.

Why? Because when we are taking exogenous hormones, it takes a few days for the hormone levels to build up, and subsequent ingestion influences the vagal nerve; when the active pill and withdrawal bleed start, those exogenous hormones drop, reducing their influence over the vagal nerve. How does this fit into training when you are using HC? The body is most resilient to stress and high loads in the first 5 days of pill use, then gradually becomes less resilient (needs more recovery between hard sessions) until the last five placebo pills, when the body is primed to take on stress again.

Finally, in perimenopausal women, the hormone ratios are completely different, and in postmenopausal women, they are flatlined, so the hormonal influences on the vagal nerve are altered. In both cases, you end up with more fight-or-flight activity and less rest-and-digest activity, especially after menopause.

There is minimal research on active women in the peri- and postmenopausal phases of their lives; however, it is known that HRV decreases in the menopause transition and a new baseline is established in postmenopause. When we look at how this physiological decrease can affect recovery and recovery scores, we know that the current algorithms of wearables do not detect this change and cannot accurately predict true recovery. What we can do is monitor our trends in HRV, respiratory rate, and sleep quality. When you see lower HRV and higher respiratory rate (especially along with lower-quality sleep), it's time to back off.

To increase your HRV, you need to step in and activate those parasympathetic responses with changes to your lifestyle and behavior. Practice good sleep hygiene. Getting enough essential amino acids (EAAs) can help reduce central fatigue. Reduce your consumption of alcohol (which can reduce your HRV). Mindfulness and breathwork, exercising in nature, and a bit of cold-water exposure are also strong vagus nerve stimulants.

Urinalysis (Pee Sticks)

I'm all about the pee sticks and what you can learn from them. "Everyone knows that if your pee is dark yellow, you're not well hydrated," says CrossFit and yoga enthusiast Lisa Hunt, whom I've worked with for years. "But there's so much more to it. Pee sticks are just about the coolest thing. They're kind of like power meters: They don't

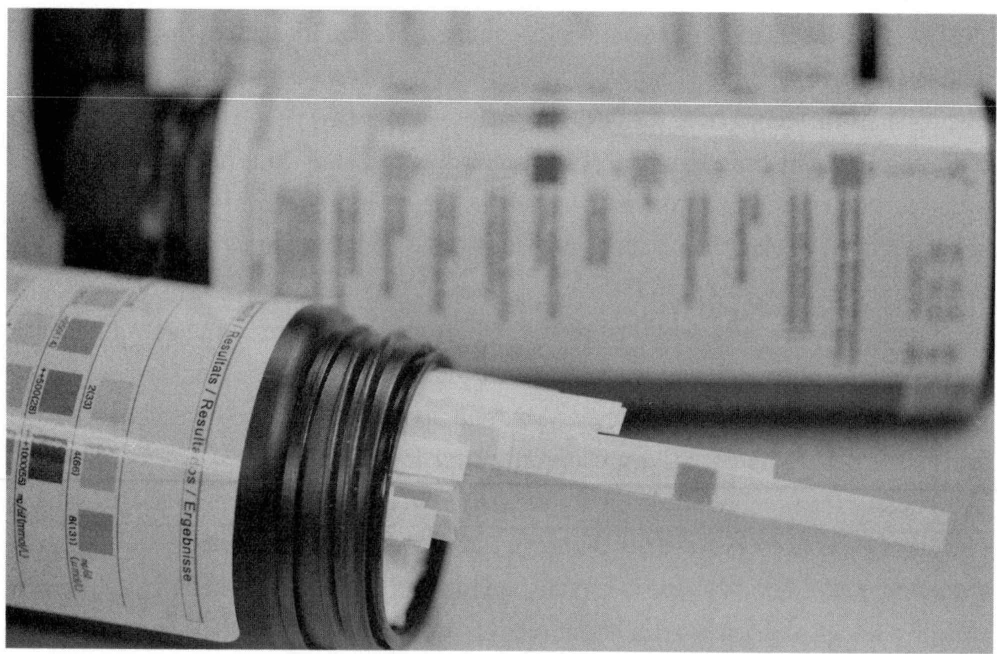

lie. Every morning I pee on a stick. I can tell if I'm recovered, if I'm getting sick, if I'm hydrated. Eek, too much protein in my pee? Back off! You've got to love data."

Lisa just about sums up the benefits, but let me add some science. Your urine is a waste product that shows you very clearly what your body is getting rid of. It can change dramatically depending on your diet and the stress of training. Urinalysis is a useful tool for monitoring these changes as well as for monitoring your recovery.

You use them just as you would imagine. Pee on the strip. Then hold it horizontally (so the chemicals from the pads don't bleed into one another). Compare the color change of the reagent pads to the corresponding color chart on the bottle's label. Here's what the colors mean (in the order of the reagent pad).

Leukocytes (LEU): These test for disease-fighting white blood cells in your urine. No change in color means there is no indication of leukocyte presence. A positive test will yield a purple color, and the severity of leukocyte presence is indicated by the shade of purple. The day after a hard training session, any positive results indicate inadequate recovery. Take an easy day! If you haven't done anything particularly hard and still get a positive test, it suggests the onset of illness (viral, bacterial). Get some quality sleep, hydrate, eat a clean, nutrient-rich diet, and keep track of your heart rate (high resting heart rate means your body is stressed).

Nitrites (NIT): This is not a training indicator but rather a bacterium that causes urinary tract infections (UTIs), which are very common in women. If you get a positive test result, consult with your doctor; you likely have a UTI.

Urobilinogen (URO): This is an indicator of liver function. We don't typically look at this one for training purposes. But again, good to know since high values warrant a trip to your doctor.

Protein (PRO): Protein isn't normally found in urine, so yellow indicates a normal test result (no protein). Any green is a positive marker for protein presence. This test should be normal in the few hours after exercise. If you still get a positive result the morning after training, you're not adequately recovered. Hydrate and increase your protein intake across the day. Take an easy aerobic or active recovery day to improve blood flow and facilitate recovery.

pH: This marker indicates how acidic your urine is. This isn't a number to worry too much over. Normal urine pH is slightly acid in the morning (pH = 6.5 to 7.0), generally becoming more alkaline (pH = 7.5 to 8.0) by the evening. You may find that your pH increases for up to 2 hours postexercise, but this rise is directly related to the amount of lactate produced during exercise (expect to see a greater rise after anaerobic exercise). If you read incredibly low or incredibly high consistently, it can be a medical issue, which is something to see a doctor about.

Blood (BLO): Any green spots or color development within 60 seconds indicates the presence of hemoglobin—blood in your urine. From a training standpoint, that means you have muscle and cellular damage, so you need to significantly back off!

Women may see green color development in the 2 to 3 days before menstruation, as blood traces will show up in urine prior to it being visible by the naked eye. This test can be useful for keeping track of your menstrual cycle.

Specific gravity (SG): This is the key for hydration status. Distilled water sits at 1.000. Normal body water in humans is 1.005 to 1.020. When you approach 1.025, this indicates hypohydration or low body water (down 1 percent body water). Greater than 1.028 indicates dehydration. You know what to do (if not, see Chapter 12).

Ketones (KET): These are the end product of excessive fatty-acid breakdown, and they're usually not present in urine. A positive test result suggests that you're either not eating enough carbs (low-carb and keto followers are notorious for this) or you rely too much on fat for resting fuel. Ketones will be steady during training, as you are using fat for fuel. However, a dark purple result means you need to add a bit more carbohydrates to your training fuel; otherwise you run the risk of hitting the wall and not recovering well.

Bilirubin (BIL): This is not a training indicator, but it is another important window of liver function. It's not usually found in urine, but a positive test result can indicate liver or gallbladder problems.

Glucose (GLU): A marker of sugar in your urine, which shouldn't be there. We don't look at this for training, but if your reading is high, it could indicate diabetes or pregnancy.

PEE STICKS PUT TO THE TEST

The beauty of pee sticks is that you can use them not just to monitor your recovery status, but also to see how your body is reacting to training and fueling so you can make appropriate adjustments in real time. During a visit to my office in California, my coauthor, Selene Yeager, used them during a series of training rides to evaluate her ride nutrition and hydration. In her words:

"It was eye-opening. I rolled out with a few other bike racers and triathletes on a 40-mile ride that included four 12-minute threshold efforts up Route 1 from Muir Beach—between 6 and 8 percent climb. After each effort, we rolled back down the hill and ducked behind some roadside construction to pee on our sticks. Among the things we were checking: specific gravity (are we staying hydrated?); pH (blood acid buffering, so your muscles keep contracting without burning and shutting down) to be able to ride with intensity and recover without compromising the effort; protein (are we becoming catabolic and eating into our own muscles?); and ketones (are we taking in enough food for fuel?).

"Up the hill. Down the hill. Duck and pee. Analyze. What did I learn? Well, that I do a pretty good job of hydrating, but not such a good job of eating, as evident by my rising protein levels. The next day we rolled out for more efforts and analyzing, this time banging out eight 1-minute full-throttle efforts punctuated by 2 minutes of recovery up Mount Tam from Stinson Beach. This time I drank a sports drink with sodium bicarbonate, sodium citrate, and amino acids before we rolled out. I also made sure to eat half a bar about an hour into the ride. It worked. Despite all the eye-popping efforts on this second day, my protein levels didn't budge. I never became ketonic, and I remained respectably hydrated. I also felt great. It's not like I'm going to stop and pee on sticks on every training ride. But it was empowering to see my hydration and nutrition strategies really work."

I challenge you to do the same. At the very minimum, use pee sticks and monitor your hydration. On days where you actually stay within a urine specific gravity (SG) of 1.015 to 1.020, you will notice less of a decline in power and a stronger recovery.

Muscle Oxygen Saturation

One of the biggest benchmarks of endurance training is max VO_2, a measurement of how much oxygen your body can use. Some of it is determined by genetics, but it's also very trainable. A high max VO_2 means you can use a lot of oxygen to produce energy, which in turn means you can do a lot of aerobic work before fatiguing. You can't really monitor your max VO_2 outside of a lab, but there are optical sensors that claim to peek inside your muscles to see how much oxygen is in your capillaries and where that oxygen is being consumed.

Watching the sensor findings in real time tells you a few things, such as when your muscles are literally warmed up from vessel dilation and blood flow as well as when muscle saturation plummets during high-intensity work. It can also tell you when your muscles are recovered and ready to exert again. You also can use these devices to track training progress, since as your fitness level improves, so does your ability to use oxygen and increase your lactate threshold.

These sensors can teach you how to breathe better (a lesser-appreciated use). One study conducted by the Australian Sports Commission found that up to 50 percent of elite athletes experienced significant declines in oxygen saturation during their sports performance. Practicing deep, rhythmic breathing can help limit the decline.

This is all interesting from a scientific standpoint, and when *ROAR* first came out, there was a push to bring this technology into the mainstream with devices like BSX Insight and Humon, which were relatively affordable sensors athletes could wear, such as in a neoprene sleeve over the calf. But it never caught on in the mainstream, and both BSX and Humon stopped selling their sensors. The devices would give athletes muscle oxygenation levels, but it was mostly up to them to figure out what to do with it. It wasn't practical.

There is still one major player in this market, Moxy, but they're quite expensive (about $800 US) and geared toward coaching and training professionals to use on their athletes. In the context of a coaching relationship, this type of biohacking may make more sense. And on the highest competitive levels, they yield some interesting data. Nike scientists used them during their Breaking2 project (the attempt to break the 2-hour marathon), and they saw that the balance of muscle oxygen supply and demand was a "critical metabolic rate" that separated a sustainable effort from one that was not.

For everyday athletes, however, the technology just isn't there for ease of use and translating the numbers you're getting into meaningful training adaptations. You can certainly achieve elite-level performance without it.

Blood Testing

That red fluid coursing through your veins contains a gold mine of information. Think about it: Everything your muscles and organs need to function is delivered through your blood. That's why your doctor performs routine blood work during checkups—to make sure you have all the stuff you need in the right amounts. It's also why companies such as InsideTracker offer blood-screening services aimed at improving athletic performance.

These services analyze your own lab-performed blood screening or one provided from a home finger-prick kit. Results are sent via e-mail in about 10 days and include raw data on up to 43 biomarkers for energy and metabolism, muscle and bone health, inflammation, strength and endurance, and general health, as well as interpretations as they relate to sports performance and recommendations for improving your metrics.

My coauthor, Selene Yeager, has had extensive experience with such screening on and off over the course of her racing career. Here is an adaptation of the story she shared with readers at Bicycling.com.

My initial readings were okay, but nothing worth crowing about. To be honest, there was considerable room for improvement. Between trying to finish up a huge writing project on top of my regular writing gigs, training 15 hours a week, and managing daily life, I was burning through precious resources without replacing them. So my body was going into emergency mode, eating into its own tissues to get what it needed, and my blood was becoming a bit of a mess. The first round of readings looked like this:

Glucose: Borderline high. This has been the case for the past few years. Routine blood work reveals that my fasting glucose hovers above 100, when it should be below, especially for my exercise level and body composition.

Total cholesterol: High. Like glucose, this one is always a little higher than I'd like, sitting between 213 and 240 (239 is the cutoff for high). My HDL is generally between 110 and 120.

Vitamin D: On the low side at 36 ng/mL, when it should be between 40 and 50 ng/mL.

Vitamin B_{12}: A little low at 322 pg/mL. Should be closer to the 500 to 800 range. This is an important one for cyclists, because [Vitamin B_{12}] helps make red blood cells and turn the protein you eat into pedal-pushing muscles.

Iron: My iron levels were good—for now—but unless I got my [B_{12}] in line, I learned that I could be on my way to anemia, not good for an endurance athlete.

Cortisol: My stress hormone levels were borderline high and just a few ticks from being fully in the red. Since cortisol is responsible for providing energy, maintaining blood glucose, and helping with carbohydrate, protein, and fat metabolism, when this number is high, it can mess up the other biomarkers. Judging from those numbers above, this appears to be the case.

So what was going on? Two main things: One was my diet, which is an endless work in progress. I'm always tinkering and tweaking it to find the sweet spot where my energy is high, weight is stable, and performance and recovery are solid. The other factors were lifestyle related. All the work and training I was trying to juggle led to that extra espresso midmorning to rev up and that extra glass of wine to wind down. My outlet was my training, but it was also adding to the layers of stress, especially since I wasn't fueling properly. (See "Hear Her Roar: The Endurance Athlete's Deficient Daily Diet" on page 193 for a detailed analysis of Selene's diet and how her blood results were used in combination with dietary changes to improve her overall health and performance.)

Selene continues, "I would have never guessed any of these markers were out of whack. I felt great in training and was getting good results in my races. That's just how I am, though. I feel pretty good even when on paper I should feel lousy, which sounds like a good problem to have, but it's still a problem, because I could be silently and slowly doing damage to my overall health without seeing the signs.

"It was empowering to have this data along with some concrete recommendations of how to alter my diet and lifestyle to bring those markers into a range that not only helps with my performance and recovery but also general health and well-being.

"After just 3 weeks of following my plan, I had another blood draw and got my results. Improvements across the board. Most notably, my glucose fell below 100, which is where it should be. My LDL cholesterol went down. My vitamin D and [B_{12}] went up, and most importantly my cortisol dropped into the optimal zone."

As this example shows, general blood screening can be a great tool. It can provide specific, detailed information about your overall health, empowering you to tweak your diet or lifestyle to get enough of all the nutrients you need and reach your performance goals.

DNA Screening

Companies such as 23andMe, DNAFit, and InsideTracker (who also offer DNA screening) promise that you can use your DNA to maximize what Mother Nature gave you. These companies use saliva samples to read your DNA. In return, you receive information on everything from your muscle fiber types (so you can tell if you're built more for power or endurance) to your risk of common diseases and conditions that can affect athletes, such as atrial fibrillation, an abnormal heart rhythm.

These home kits are relatively affordable and super easy to perform. I had mine done and found out that I carry the gene for hemochromatosis (iron overload), which may help explain why I've never had issues with anemia. Is it necessary? Of course not. But it's another tool you can use to tailor your training and nutrition to your unique physiology. You may discover that you are a slow caffeine metabolizer, which means that afternoon cup of joe will definitely interfere with your sleep; or you may find that you are genetically predisposed to putting on belly fat from a carbohydrate sensitivity. With this knowledge, you can tailor your carbohydrate intake to meet just your training demands and improve your overall body composition.

Just bear in mind that this is a constantly evolving science. If you're interested in following it in real time, you can go to genome.gov/human-genome-project for up-to-date interpretation of genes and their relationship to disease. I'll note that this is also where genetic information is strongest, in my opinion. The data are not robust enough to say that people with one genotype should always be sprinters and people with another should always be endurance athletes. But there are some genes that are well established for increasing your risk for certain diseases, and that knowledge can help you make lifestyle changes accordingly to help mitigate your risk.

Menstrual Cycle Tracking

Menstrual cycle tracking isn't "biohacking" per se, but it's definitely a way to get valuable insights into your physiology so you can make adjustments to get the most out of each training session and feel and perform your best.

Unless you're postmenopausal, you should be tracking your menstrual cycle. Tracking can be as simple as using a pen and paper and marking the day of your cycle and how you feel. If you use an online training tool like TrainingPeaks, you can put little notes in the comment box. It doesn't have to be fancy. The goal is just to make you aware of where you are within your cycle and how you feel during each phase. For example, you might go back into your logs and see that on day 14 you had a fabulous workout or on day 26 you felt tired and lethargic before your period started 3 days later. Too often women will push through off days, thinking they're just stressed or, worse, unfit, without making the connection that there is an underlying physiological aspect related to their cycle that's making them feel that way. It's not their fitness; it's their physiology.

Another benefit of tracking your menstrual cycle is that you can see if you're starting to creep into overtraining/underrecovery/underfueling territory, because the first indicator is often a glitch in your menstrual cycle. You'll have a bit of endocrine dysfunction, and your cycle might get shorter or longer. When I'm evaluating team data from athletes I work with, I can tell by their tracking if they've traveled, if it was a high period of competition, or when they're back in town recovering because of the length of their cycles. Stress has a very big impact on your cycle, but if you don't track it, you don't know.

If you want to be more high tech, you can use an app. There's a lot of Femtech out there to help with tracking. WILD.AI uses artificial intelligence to take the information you provide on the days of your cycle and how you're feeling to help you see patterns as well as make training and nutrition recommendations. Apps like FitrWoman are designed for the active woman to track her cycle and give generalized information on phase recovery and nutrition. Other apps like HelloClue and FLO are geared more toward fertility, without any insights into recovery and nutrition for active women. The thing to remember when using an app is that you want to maintain your agency here. You might have an app telling you that you're in a certain part of your cycle, so you "should or shouldn't" do something, but that is based on a generalization of physiology that may not be applicable to *you*, the individual. The goal is to learn your own body, understand how your physiology may be impacting how you feel, and train accordingly to maximize that session. It's not to be completely tied to an algorithm. These apps really shine when you can use them with a coach. The US soccer team uses FitrWoman, for example. The athletes themselves aren't looking at the data day to day; their coach is and uses that as another piece of information about each athlete to help maximize training and performance.

If you want to add some actual biohacking into your tracking (and you are naturally cycling as opposed to on hormonal contraceptives), you can track the length of your cycle and the phases using an over-the-counter ovulation predictor kit and couple it with a basal body thermometer you can get from the pharmacy. (The caveat is that most women have one to three anovulatory cycles per year. An anovulatory cycle often comes across as a shortened cycle due to an earlier signal/feedback to shed the lining.)

The estrogen surge right before ovulation lowers your internal temperature 1°F/0.5°C. After ovulation, your internal temperature goes up by 1°F/0.5°C because progesterone is thermogenic. Once you see that upsurge in temperature, you know you're in the luteal phase. When you see a dip and then a rise, you know you're around ovulation. If you're using an IUD (both copper and progestin-only, more on these below), you can use this strategy as well. The benefit of this is knowing the length of your low-hormone (follicular) phase, because the high-hormone phase stays constant, but the follicular phase changes from 12 days to longer or shorter.

If you're on oral contraceptives, it's still worthwhile to track where you are in the pack and how you're feeling. Generally, we see that there is better stress resilience in the first 5 days of active pills and progressively less stress resilience and the need for more recovery as the active pills continue until about day 2 of the placebo/sugar pill, when the hormones have been flushed out and you're primed to take on higher stress again. Tracking can help you see your own rhythms.

If you're on an IUD, your experience will be similar to a natural cycle. With the copper IUD, ovulation does not stop. With progestin-only (e.g., Mirena), ovulation usually resumes about 8 months after insertion. So at that point you can track using your basal body temperature. (Up until that point, you are akin to being in the low-hormone/follicular phase.)

Once you reach the menopause transition, you can expect to have more anovulatory cycles and your cycles become irregular, so the actual cycle length can vary significantly. It is beneficial to track to understand how your cycles are changing and symptoms that may become more frequent the week before your period starts.

Tracking can also help you realize when you're in perimenopause, so you can start implementing the advice from Chapter 3.

Sleep Tracking

I'll say it again: Sleep is queen for recovery. We covered sleep, sleep stages, and how it's essential for recovery and general health in Chapter 3. Now let's talk about sleep tracking. Many factors impact your sleep quality and quantity, including environment, diet, exercise, and the myriad factors we talked about previously. Your hormones also impact your sleep.

Women will sometimes tell me that their sleep is worse during their high-hormone phase. That's because our core body temperature rises with progesterone, which makes it harder to dip into that colder core body temperature ideal for sleep. Estrogen mitigates melatonin production, so when estrogen rises, you aren't producing as much melatonin, which also makes it more difficult to fall asleep. It's also common to have less REM sleep in the high-hormone phase, so you end up with more light sleep, which is easier to wake up from. Women who experience premenstrual dysphoric disorder (PMDD) and premenstrual syndrome (PMS) generally have more erratic sleep architecture in the week leading up to their periods as compared to those who don't. The hormonal swings that happen during perimenopause can wreak havoc on sleep by disrupting body temperature, melatonin levels, neurotransmitter activity, and much more. By tracking your sleep overtime, you can see your own natural rhythms, what impacts your sleep, and then test various sleep strategies and interventions to see what works best.

The best way to track your sleep is with a designated sleep-tracking device. I know many women use their Garmin watches for convenience. They're okay but not really the best tool for the job because Garmin uses actigraphy—a movement-based analysis—to record sleep. You move a little more in certain sleep stages than others, so Garmin uses how much you move (or not) during the night to approximate your sleep stages. When compared to more scientific sleep analysis, Garmin is about 65 to 70 percent accurate, which leaves a large margin of error. Devices like the Whoop Strap and Ōura Ring use special red and green lights to monitor superficial blood flow, heart rate, respiratory rate, body temperature, and other variables to monitor the quantity and quality of your sleep. They are both highly correlated with polysomnography, the gold standard laboratory sleep study. Note that like HRV and "readiness scores," sleep score algorithms are based on male data and don't take into account sex or menstrual cycle differences in sleep architecture. So don't get too hung up on the scores, and use the devices to watch global trends in your sleep as you implement various sleep strategies.

The best way to improve your sleep using a sleep tracker is to implement one sleep regimen per week and record how it impacts your sleep. Here is an example of how that works.

Step 1:

Pick a regimen that you have not tried before or an area that needs improvement (e.g., reducing screentime before bed).

1. Limit food intake 2 hours before bed except for 4 oz/115 ml cold tart cherry juice 30 minutes before bed.
2. Limit food intake 2 hours before bed except for 1 serving (15 g) of a casein-rich snack 30 minutes before bed (e.g., slow-release protein, yogurt, or milk).
3. Reduce screentime 2 hours before bed or use yellow glasses/blue light filter on devices.
4. If exercising within 4 hours of bedtime, use cooling strategies—e.g., cold shower; eating or drinking something ice cold within 30 minutes of finishing exercise.

Step 2:

For 2 days, record your current sleeping metrics for 2 nights, then implement your sleeping experiment for the next 4 days and record your sleeping metrics. Make note of your training stress and any other stressors (work deadline/child interrupting sleep, illness, etc.) that are greater than normal. See how well it works. Then, if you still want improvement, try another the following week, and so forth.

BIOHACKING SLEEP RECORDING SHEET

	DAY 1	DAY 2	DAY 3	DAY 4	DAY 5	DAY 6
Training session(s)						
Intensity						
Duration						
Mode						
Notes						

	DAY 1	DAY 2	DAY 3	DAY 4	DAY 5	DAY 6
Date						
Perceived sleep metrics						
What time did you go to bed?						
How long did it take you to get to sleep?						
How many times did you get up during your sleep?						
How many hours did you sleep for (h)?						
How was the quality of your sleep? 0 = poor, 3 = average, 5 = amazing						
How tired were you upon waking? 0 = exhausted, 3 = average, 5 = energetic						
How hungry are you upon waking? 0 = no appetite, 3 = average, 5 = very hungry						

	DAY 1	DAY 2	DAY 3	DAY 4	DAY 5	DAY 6
Date						
Gadget sleep metrics						
Total hours of sleep						
Time in deep sleep/slow wave sleep (h:min)						
Time in light sleep (h:min)						
Time in REM (h:min)						
Awake time (h:min)						
Resting heart rate (bpm)						
Heart rate variability (ms)						
Other notes						

Continuous Glucose Monitoring

One of the more recent trends in biohacking has been the use of continuous glucose monitors (CGMs) in sport. People with diabetes (especially type 1) have used CGMs to manage their blood sugar for years. Now companies like Supersapiens, Levels, and NutriSense are marketing CGMs to a nondiabetic population with promises of improving health and, in some cases, athletic performance. From what we've seen thus far, you may be able to improve some general health metrics with a CGM plan, but the jury is out (and it's looking less promising) on using them during exercise for performance benefits.

CGMs are circular sensors about the size of a quarter that have a fine wire filament that goes into your skin and is attached to a transmitter that pairs via Bluetooth with a companion app. Using a special applicator, you press the sensor (which is layered with adhesive) onto the back of your arm. The needle goes into the fat layer under your skin, where it registers the concentration of glucose in milligrams per deciliter (mg/dL) that is circulating in your interstitial fluid—the fluid that surrounds every cell of the human body. The transmitter beams that information to your phone so you can read your glucose levels on a companion app. Supersapiens also integrates with certain exercise devices like bike computers and some sports watches.

For general health purposes, spending some time with a CGM can be instructive. You can see how your blood sugar spikes in response to stress, how it's elevated after a poor night's sleep, how various foods cause spikes and drops, and how it responds to exercise. In that way it helps reinforce healthy behaviors like stress management, daily walks, avoiding superprocessed foods, and the like.

What a CGM is not is a fuel gauge during activity. You can't just look down at your cycling computer and know when and what to eat based off the number you see, and even if you keep your blood sugar in a predetermined "ideal" range, that doesn't guarantee you're going to perform a certain way.

A recent analysis published in the *International Journal of Sport Nutrition and Exercise Metabolism* put it best, concluding: "Due to the complexities of the interactions between carbohydrate ingestion and exercise, carbohydrate availability, energy availability, and systemic glucose, further research is required to determine the utility of CGM technology as a tool to assess fueling strategies and energy availability among athletes."

That was my coauthor's experience during her several months of CGM testing. "I was able to get some useful insights into my physiology. My blood sugar is more balanced when I eat more complex carbs. I'm mindful of pairing more simple carbs with some protein and/or fat to prevent big spikes. I've come to appreciate the health value of an evening walk. But during training sessions, the data was less useful. Sometimes I would feel a bit draggy and see my glucose levels were low. But other times, the levels were spot on and my energy was not."

One of my PhD students collected data using CGM in ultraendurance runners between menstrual cycle phases and also found that the outcomes still do not provide data that lets us make concrete training and fueling decisions during exercise in real time. For one, there's a lag time of about 15 minutes between the blood and interstitial fluid, so the CGM results are not exactly real time. Athletes without diabetes have better metabolic control to deal with wide fluctuations than those with diabetes (who very much do benefit from these devices), and the variations in blood glucose cannot be tracked to indicate what kind of fueling should be used during exercise.

In short, if you're interested in learning more about how your blood sugar responds to your diet and lifestyle, especially if you know you have prediabetes or other metabolic concerns, a CGM program can be a useful tool. If you're trying to hack into some unseen fuel tank to know exactly what to eat and when to maximize performance, you can take a pass.

Sweat Testing

As mentioned in the hydration chapter, sweat testing involves taking a small amount of sweat and seeing how much sodium is in it. You can do this in a lab or, more simply, by wearing a special patch on your skin that captures your sweat as you exercise. As I mentioned previously, in the majority of cases, this is unnecessary and not useful.

The premise of doing a sweat test is that by knowing how much sodium is in your sweat, you know how much sodium you need while training and/or racing. But it doesn't work that way. What you are sweating out is so variable that you can't say what you need based on one—or many—sweat tests.

For example, women have a higher amount of sodium in their sweat during the high-hormone phase. The more fit you are, the more dilute your sweat is. There's variability with the change of seasons. There is variability with temperature fluctuations; if you haven't acclimated to the heat and you run on a hot day, you'll have more salt in your sweat. How much salt you've been eating in your diet can cause variability. The whole idea of sweat patches and sweat testing is a marketing myth. Take a pass.

Metabolic Testing

Metabolic testing is generally done in the lab. It's generally used in research to determine max VO_2 and onset of blood lactate accumulation. It also measures your respiratory exchange ratio (RER), which is the ratio between the amount of carbon dioxide produced in metabolism and the oxygen used. This measurement shows the contribution of fat and carbohydrates to energy expenditure during exercise. As with sweat testing, this one is being misused in the mainstream.

There are people who want that data so they can manipulate their diet and training to become more metabolically efficient at burning fat. But that happens naturally through training. As you train, you improve your cardiovascular fitness and become "metabolically efficient." You'll be able to stay aerobic at higher exercise thresholds. In the end, what really drives metabolic flexibility is exercise and fitness. It's the outcome of what you're doing. It's not something you're trying to artificially manipulate to get fit.

• • • • •

Finally, when all is said and done, don't forget the most important piece of biohacking: Ask yourself, "How do I feel?" Even the most sophisticated sports laboratories in the world always ask you to rate your perceived exertion during exercise performance tests. All the data in the world doesn't matter if it doesn't match how you actually feel.

ROAR ▶▶▶ SOUND BITES

▶ Heart rate monitoring was an early form of biohacking—and it's still a very relevant one!

▶ You can learn an awful lot from monitoring your urine.

▶ Sorry, trend followers, you really don't want to see a lot of ketones in your pee.

▶ A little blood work goes a long way in telling you how well (or not) your training and nutrition are working.

▶ The most important measurement of all is the answer to the question "How do I feel?"

APPENDIX

RECIPES

CHAPTER 3

QUINOA BOWL

- 1 cup organic unsweetened almond milk
- 1 cup water
- 1 cup organic quinoa
- 2 cups organic blackberries
- ½ teaspoon ground cinnamon
- ⅓ cup chopped toasted pecans
- 4 teaspoons maple syrup

In a medium saucepan, combine the almond milk, water, and quinoa. Bring to a boil over high heat. Reduce the heat to medium-low. Cover and simmer for 15 minutes, or until most of the liquid is absorbed. Turn off the heat and let stand, covered, for 5 minutes. Stir in the blackberries and cinnamon. Transfer to a bowl and top with the pecans and maple syrup.

MAKES 4 SERVINGS

GREEN GODDESS SMOOTHIE

- 1 cup cold almond milk
- ⅔ cup frozen mango pieces
- 1 medium fresh or frozen ripe banana
- 3 leaves stemmed kale (about ½ cup packed)
- 2 tablespoons unsweetened flaked coconut
- 1 teaspoon raw flaxseeds

Place the milk, mango, banana, kale, coconut, and flaxseeds in a blender and process until smooth.

MAKES 1 LARGE OR 2 SMALL SERVINGS

QUINOA, BROCCOLI, APPLE, AND POMEGRANATE SALAD WITH LIME VINAIGRETTE

1 head broccoli
2 tablespoons olive oil
½ teaspoon salt
2 apples
Juice and zest of 1 organic lime
1 pomegranate
3 cups white quinoa, cooked and left to cool
⅓ cup Lime Vinaigrette

Separate the broccoli into small florets. Peel the stalk and chop into bite-size pieces. In a frying pan, pan-roast the broccoli in olive oil until it is nicely browned but still has bite and vibrant green color. Season with salt.

Quarter the apples, remove the cores, cut into small cubes, and toss with the lime juice and zest. Halve the pomegranate. Line the bottom of a large bowl with a paper towel. Hold half the pomegranate over the bowl (cut surface down) and tap the pomegranate with a wooden spoon so the seeds drop out. Continue with the other half and remove any remnants of the white membrane from the bowl.

Toss the quinoa with the broccoli, apples, and lime vinaigrette. Arrange the salad in a bowl and sprinkle with the pomegranate seeds.

MAKES 4 SERVINGS

Recipe courtesy of Hannah Grant and The Grand Tour Cookbook

LIME VINAIGRETTE

3 tablespoons lime juice
Zest of 2 organic limes
3 tablespoons honey
1 teaspoon wasabi
½ teaspoon tamari (Japanese gluten-free soy sauce)
⅔ cup cold-pressed olive oil

In a bowl, whisk together the lime juice, lime zest, honey, wasabi, and tamari until the honey is dissolved. While whisking, slowly add the olive oil. Continue whisking until the mixture is nice and emulsified. Season with additional tamari and lime juice.

MAKES 12 SERVINGS

TOASTED ALMOND SPREAD WITH CINNAMON

- **3½ cups raw almonds**
- **½ tablespoon coconut oil**
- **1 teaspoon ground cinnamon**
- **1 tablespoon creamed honey**
- **½ teaspoon salt flakes**

Preheat the oven to 350°F. Place the almonds on a baking sheet and toast them in the oven until golden, about 8 to 10 minutes. Blend in a food processor while they are still warm. Initially, the almonds will turn to flour and then to liquid (about 10 minutes). Add the coconut oil, cinnamon, honey, and salt and blend thoroughly into a complete homogeneous mixture. Transfer the almond spread to a jar with a lid or a resealable container. Keeps in the refrigerator for up to 2 weeks.

MAKES 16 SERVINGS (1 TABLESPOON EACH)

Recipe courtesy of Hannah Grant and The Grand Tour Cookbook

OATMEAL WITH BLUEBERRIES AND CHIA SEEDS

- **2 cups water**
- **½ teaspoon ground cinnamon**
- **¼ teaspoon dried ginger**
- **3 tablespoons sunflower seeds**
- **3 tablespoons chia seeds**
- **2⅓ cups gluten-free oatmeal**
- **¼ teaspoon salt**
- **20 grams protein powder (vanilla or unsweetened)**
- **1 cup fresh blueberries**
- **Honey (to taste)**

Bring the water to a boil with the cinnamon, ginger, sunflower seeds, and chia seeds. Add the oatmeal and cook, stirring constantly. Turn down the heat and let the oatmeal simmer until it has the desired consistency, adding more water if needed. Remove from the heat and stir in the salt and protein powder. Serve with blueberries and honey. Note: The result is best with a mixture of fine-rolled oats and coarse/steel-cut oats.

MAKES 4 SERVINGS

Recipe courtesy of Hannah Grant and The Grand Tour Cookbook

CARAMELIZED CAULIFLOWER AND ALMOND SALAD WITH CIDER VINEGAR VINAIGRETTE

1 head cauliflower
3 tablespoons olive oil
⅔ cup raw almonds
3 cups mixed baby lettuce
3 tablespoons goji berries
4 tablespoons Cider Vinegar Vinaigrette

Preheat the oven to 350°F. Separate the cauliflower into bite-size florets and chop the stalk into chunks of the same size. In a frying pan, pan-roast the cauliflower in the olive oil until nicely caramelized, sweet, and tender with a bit of bite, about 20 minutes. Cool to room temperature.

Meanwhile, place the almonds on a baking sheet and toast in the oven for 7 to 8 minutes, or until golden. Let them cool. Rinse the lettuce and drain.

Toss the cauliflower with the almonds, lettuce, goji berries, and vinaigrette.

MAKES 4 SERVINGS

Recipe courtesy of Hannah Grant and The Grand Tour Cookbook

CIDER VINEGAR VINAIGRETTE

¼ cup cider vinegar
1 tablespoon Dijon mustard
1 tablespoon honey
½ teaspoon salt
⅔ cup cold-pressed olive oil

In a bowl, whisk together the vinegar, mustard, honey, and salt until the honey and salt are dissolved. While whisking, slowly add the olive oil, whisking until it is nice and emulsified. Season with additional salt and vinegar.

MAKES 12 SERVINGS

DATE BROWNIE

5 Medjool dates, pitted
⅔ cup toasted hazelnuts
Juice and zest of 1 organic orange
½ cup dark, unsweetened cocoa powder
Pinch of salt

In a food processor, blend the dates to a puree. Add the hazelnuts, orange juice, orange zest, cocoa powder, and salt. If the mixture is too dry, add a bit more orange juice. Press the brownie mixture into an 8" × 8" pan and refrigerate for at least 1 hour before cutting.

MAKES 12 BROWNIES

Recipe courtesy of Hannah Grant and The Grand Tour Cookbook

CHAPTER 5

VEGAN NUT BUTTER BALLS

- ½ cup natural nut butter or Toasted Almond Spread with Cinnamon (page 331)
- ¼ cup quick-cooking oats
- ⅓ cup vanilla protein powder
- ¼ cup unsweetened flaked coconut
- ½ teaspoon ground cinnamon
- ¼ cup apple cider
- 1 tablespoon maple syrup
- ⅓ cup rice cereal (optional)

In a bowl, add all the ingredients except the rice cereal, and mix until thoroughly combined.

Gently mix in the rice cereal, if using. Shape the mixture into 16 balls, each 1" in diameter. Store the balls in the refrigerator for up to 3 weeks.

MAKES 16 SERVINGS

Recipe courtesy of Hannah Grant and The Grand Tour Cookbook

WARM POTATO SALAD WITH BROCCOLI AND CRANBERRIES AND ORANGE VINAIGRETTE

- 1 pound new potatoes
- 2 tablespoons coconut oil
- Pinch of salt
- 1 head broccoli
- 3 tablespoons dried cranberries
- Zest of 1 organic lemon
- ¼ cup Orange Vinaigrette (page 334)

Scrub the potatoes and cut them into bite-size pieces. In a frying pan, pan-roast them over medium heat in the coconut oil and season with salt. Remove the potatoes from the pan. Separate the broccoli into small florets. Rinse, drain, and pan-roast it with coconut oil until the florets are nicely browned but still have a bite and a vibrant green color. Season with salt. In a bowl, combine the potatoes, broccoli, and cranberries. Rinse the lemon and zest it onto the salad. Toss with the dressing.

MAKES 4 SERVINGS

Recipe courtesy of Hannah Grant and The Grand Tour Cookbook

ORANGE VINAIGRETTE

- ¼ cup orange juice
- Zest of 2 organic lemons
- 3 tablespoons Dijon mustard
- 2 tablespoons cider vinegar
- 1 tablespoon honey
- ½ teaspoon salt
- ⅔ cup cold-pressed olive oil
- Pinch of freshly ground black pepper

In a bowl, whisk the orange juice with the lemon zest, mustard, vinegar, honey, and salt until the salt and honey are dissolved. While whisking, slowly add the olive oil, whisking until it's nice and emulsified. Season with additional salt, vinegar, and the pepper.

MAKES 12 SERVINGS

RESOURCES

Introduction

Charkoudian, N., E. C. J. Hart, J. N. Barnes, M. J. Joyner. "Autonomic Control of Body Temperature and Blood Pressure: Influences of Female Sex Hormones." *Clinical Autonomic Research* 27, no. 3 (May 2017): 149–155. https://pubmed.ncbi.nlm.nih.gov/28488202.

"European Championships Munich 2022: Dina Asher-Smith Calls for More Period Sports Science." BBC, August 19, 2022. https://www.bbc.com/sport/athletics/62598938.

"Menstrual Cycle 'Last Taboo' for Women in Sport—Annabel Croft." BBC, January 20, 2015. https://www.bbc.com/sport/tennis/30908551.

Morse, Ben. "Lydia Ko Praised for Talking about Period after Surprising Reporter with Honest Answer." CNN, May 3, 2022. https://edition.cnn.com/2022/05/03/golf/lydia-ko-period-pain-lpga-spt-intl/index.html.

Phillips, Tom. "'It's Because I Had My Period': Swimmer Fu Yuanhui Praised for Breaking Taboo." *The Guardian*, August 15, 2016. https://www.theguardian.com/sport/2016/aug/16/hinese-swimmer-fu-yuanhui-praised-for-breaking-periods-taboo.

Chapter 1

Almonroeder, T. G., and L. C. Benson. "Sex Differences in Lower Extremity Kinematics and Patellofemoral Kinetics during Running." *Journal of Sports Sciences* 35, no. 16 (August 2017): 1575–81, https://www.tandfonline.com/doi/abs/10.1080/02640414.2016.1225972?journalCode=rjsp20.

Anderson, Owen. "Science of Sport: The Gender Gap." *Running Research News*, April 22, 2005. http://www.runnersweb.com/running/news/rw_news_20050422_RRN_Gender_Gap.html.

Anderson, Owen. "Female and Male Performance Times." *Sports Performance Bulletin*, Green Star Media Ltd., 2014. http://www.pponline.co.uk/encyc/0240.htm.

Bartolomei, S., G. Grillone, R. Di Michele, and M. Cortesi. "A Comparison between Male and Female Athletes in Relative Strength and Power Performances." *Journal of Functional Morphology and Kinesiology* 6, no. 1 (February 2021): 17. https://www.ncbi.nlm.nih.gov/pmc/articles/PMC7930971.

Bellemare F., A. Jeanneret, and J. Couture. "Sex Differences in Thoracic Dimensions and Configuration." *American Journal of Respiratory and Critical Care Medicine* 168, no. 3 (August 2003): 305–12. https://pubmed.ncbi.nlm.nih.gov/12773331.

Bruening, D., A. R. Baird, K. J. Weaver, A. T. Rasmussen. "Whole Body Kinematic Sex Differences Persist across Non-Dimensional Gait Speeds." *PloS One.* (August 2020). https://journals.plos.org/plosone/article?id=10.1371/journal.pone.0237449.

Chumanov, E. S., C. Wall-Scheffler, and B. C. Heiderscheit. "Gender Differences in Walking and Running on Level and Inclined Surfaces." *Clinical Biometrics* 23, no. 10 (December 2008). https://www.clinbiomech.com/article/S0268-0033(08)00229-5/fulltext.

Ferreira, L. F. "Mitochondrial Basis for Sex-Differences in Metabolism and Exercise Performance." *American Journal of Physiology. Regulatory, Integrative and Comparative Physiology* 314, no. 6 (June 2018): R848–R849. https://www.ncbi.nlm.nih.gov/pmc/articles/PMC6032305/.

Ganru, M., J. M. Cremer, S. Schmeichel, M. Kunkel, and W. Bloch. "Comparisons of Blood Parameters, Red Blood Cell Deformability and Circulating Nitric Oxide Between Males and Females Considering Hormonal Contraception: A Longitudinal Gender Study." *Frontiers of Physiology* 9 (December 2018). https://www.frontiersin.org/articles/10.3389/fphys.2018.01835/full.

Henderson, G. C., J. A. Fattor, M. A. Horning, N. Faghihnia, M. L. Johnson, M. Luke-Zeitoun, G. A. Brooks. "Glucoregulation Is More Precise in Women Than in Men during Postexercise Recovery." *The American Journal of Clinical Nutrition* 87, no. 6 (June 2008): 1686–94.

Horton, M. G., and T. L. Hall. "Quadriceps Femoris Muscle Angle: Normal Values and Relationships with Gender and Selected Skeletal Measures." *Physical Therapy* 69, no. 11 (November 1989): 897–901.

Ichinose-Kuwahara, T., Y. Inoue, Y. Iseki, S. Hara, Y. Ogura, and N. Kondo. "Sex Differences in the Effects of Physical Training on Sweat Gland Responses during a Graded Exercise." *Experimental Physiology* 95, no. 10 (2010): 1026. doi:10.1113/expphysiol.2010.053710.

Kim, Han, Clark Richardson, Jeanette Roberts, Lisa Gren, and Joseph L. Lyon. "Cold Hands, Warm Heart." *Lancet* 351, no. 9114 (May 16, 1998): 1492.

Knechtle, B., T. Rosemann, and C. A. Rüst. "Women Cross the 'Catalina Channel' Faster than Men." *SpringerPlus* 4, no. 8 (July 2015): 332. https://www.ncbi.nlm.nih.gov/pmc/articles/PMC4495100/.

Lee, Chang Woock, Mark E. Newman, and Steven E. Riechman. "Oral Contraceptive Use Impairs Muscle Gains in Young Women." Presented at Experimental Biology 09 FASEB 2009; Abstract 4197.

Maud, P. J., and B. B. Shultz. "Gender Comparisons in Anaerobic Power and Anaerobic Capacity Tests." *British Journal of Sports Medicine* 20, no. 2 (June 1986): 51–54.

McClelland, E. L., and P. G. Weyand. "Sex Differences in Human Running Performance: Smaller Gaps at Shorter Distances?" *Journal of Applied Physiology* 133, no. 4 (October 2022): 876–85. https://journals.physiology.org/doi/abs/10.1152/japplphysiol.00359.2022.

Meyer, Robinson. "We Thought Female Athletes Were Catching Up to Men, but They're Not." *Atlantic*, August 9, 2012. http://www.theatlantic.com/technology/archive/2012/08/we-thought-female-athletes-were-catching-up-to-men-but-theyre-not/260927/.

Miller, A. E., J. D. MacDougall, M. A. Tarnopolsky, and D. G. Sale. "Gender Differences in Strength and Muscle Fiber Characteristics." *European Journal of Applied Physiology and Occupational Physiology* 66, no. 3 (1993): 254–62.

Miotto, P.M., C. McGlory, T. M. Holloway, S. M. Phillips, and G. P. Holloway. "Sex Differences in Mitochondrial Respiratory Function in Human Skeletal Muscle." *American Journal of Physiology.*

Regulatory, Integrative and Comparative Physiology 314, no. 6 (June 2018): R909–R915. https://www.ncbi.nlm.nih.gov/pmc/articles/PMC6032304.

Munatones, Steven. "Men vs. Women in Endurance Sports." Active.com. n.d. http://www.active.com/swimming/articles/men-vs-women-in-endurance-sports.

Murphy, W. G. "The Sex Differences in Haemoglobin Levels in Adults—Mechanisms, Causes, and Consequences." *Blood Reviews* (2014): http://www.sah.org.ar/pdf/eritropatias/CADAE1408C.pdf.

Pierre, S. R., M. Peirlinck, and E. Kuhl. "Sex Matters: A Comprehensive Comparison of Female and Male Hearts." *Frontiers of Physiology* 13 (March 2022). https://www.frontiersin.org/articles/10.3389/fphys.2022.831179/full.

Sharma H. B., and J. Kailashiya. "Gender Difference in Aerobic Capacity and the Contribution by Body Composition and Haemoglobin Concentration: A Study in Young Indian National Hockey Players." *Journal of Clinical and Diagnostic Research* 10, no. 11 (November 2016): CC09–CC13. https://www.ncbi.nlm.nih.gov/pmc/articles/PMC5198313.

Staron, Robert S., Fredrick C. Hagerman, Robert S. Hikida, Thomas F. Murray, D. P. Hostler, M. T. Krill, K. E. Ragg, and Kumika Toma. "Fiber Type Composition of the Vastus Lateralis Muscle of Young Men and Women." *Journal of Histochemistry and Cytochemistry* 48, no. 5 (2000): 623–29.

Chapter 2

Alfaro-Magallanes, V. M., L. Barba-Moreno, N. Romero-Parra, et al. "Menstrual Cycle Affects Iron Homeostasis and Hepcidin Following Interval Running Exercise in Endurance-trained Women." *European Journal of Applied Physiology* 122 (2022): 2683–2694.

Badenhorst, Claire E., Kazushige Goto, Wendy J. O'Brien, and Stacy Sims. "Iron Status in Athletic Females, A Shift in Perspective on an Old Paradigm." *Journal of Sports Sciences* 39, no. 14 (February 2021): 1565–75. https://www.tandfonline.com/doi/full/10.1080/02640414.2021.1885782.

Bankhead, Charles. "FASEB: Oral Contraceptives Blunt Women's Muscle Gain." *MedPage Today*, April 17, 2009. http://www.medpagetoday.com/PrimaryCare/ExerciseFitness/13797.

Berbic, M. "Immunology of Normal and Abnormal Menstruation." *Women's Health* 9, no. 4 (2013): 387–95. https://journals.sagepub.com/doi/pdf/10.2217/WHE.13.32.

Bruinvels G, R. Burden, N. Brown, T. Richards, and C. Pedlar. "The Prevalence and Impact of Heavy Menstrual Bleeding (Menorrhagia) in Elite and Non-Elite Athletes." *PloS One* 11, no. (February 2016); e0149881. https://pubmed.ncbi.nlm.nih.gov/26901873/.

Clancy, K. B., Baerwald, A. R., and Pierson, R. A. "Systemic Inflammation Is Associated with Ovarian Follicular Dynamics during the Human Menstrual Cycle." *PloS One* (May 2013). https://journals.plos.org/plosone/article?id=10.1371/journal.pone.0064807.

Constantini, Naama W., Gal Dubnov, and Constance M. Lebrun. "The Menstrual Cycle and Sport Performance." *Clinics in Sports Medicine* 24, no. 2 (April 2005): e51–e82.

Curtis, Vickie, C. J. K. Henry, E. Birch, and A. Ghusain-Choueiri. "Intraindividual Variation in the Basal Metabolic Rate of Women: Effect of the Menstrual Cycle." *American Journal of Human Biology* 8, no. 5. Article first published online, December 7, 1998.

Dalgaard, Line B., et al. "Influence of Oral Contraceptive Use on Adaptations to Resistance Training." *Frontiers of Physiology* 10 (July 2018). https://www.frontiersin.org/articles/10.3389/fphys.2019.00824/full.

Dean, M. "Glycogen in the Uterus and Fallopian Tubes Is an Important Source of Glucose during Early Pregnancy." *Biology of Reproduction* 101, no. 2 (August 2019): 297–305. https://pubmed.ncbi.nlm.nih.gov/31201425.

ESPN The Magazine, Body Issue Confidential, July 18, 2014. http://espn.go.com/espnw/athletes-life/article/11199365/espn-magazine-body-issue-confidential.

Folscher, Lindy-Lee, Catharina C. Grant, Lizelle Fletcher, and Dina Christina Janse van Rensberg. "Ultra-Marathon Athletes at Risk for the Female Athlete Triad." *Sports Medicine Open* 1, no. 1 (2015): 29. doi:10.1186/s40798-015-0027-7.

Fridén, Cecilia. "Neuromuscular Performance and Balance during the Menstrual Cycle and the Influence of Premenstrual Symptoms." Departments of Surgical Sciences and Woman and Child Health, Karolinska Institutet, and the University College of Physical Education and Sports, Stockholm, Sweden. https://openarchive.ki.se/xmlui/bitstream/handle/10616/38957/thesis.pdf?sequence=1.

Garcia, A. M. C., M. G. Lacerda, I. A. T. Fonseca, F. M. Reis, L. O. C. Rodrigues, and E. Silami-Garcia. "Luteal Phase of the Menstrual Cycle Increases Sweating Rate during Exercise." *Brazilian Journal of Medical and Biological Research* [online] 39, no. 9 (2006): 1255–61.

Gold, E. B., C. Wells, and M. O. Rasor. "The Association of Inflammation with Premenstrual Symptoms." *Journal of Women's Health* 25, no. 9 (September 2016): 865–74. https://www.ncbi.nlm.nih.gov/pmc/articles/PMC5311461.

Groeger, A., C. Cipollina, M. Cole et al. "Cyclooxygenase-2 Generates Anti-inflammatory Mediators from Omega-3 Fatty Acids." *Nature Chemical Biology* 6 (May 2010): 433–41. https://www.nature.com/articles/nchembio.367#:~:text=Omega%2D3%20fatty%20acids%20are,adduct%20to%20protein%20and%20glutathione.

Hervé, M. A. J., G. Meduri, F. G. Petit, T. S. Domet, G. Lazennec, S. Mourah, and M. Perrot-Applanat. "Regulation of the Vascular Endothelial Growth Factor (VEGF) Receptor Flk-1/KDR by Estradiol through VEGF in Uterus." *Journal of Endocrinology* 188, no. 1 (November 2005): 91–99. https://joe.bioscientifica.com/view/journals/joe/188/1/1880091.xml.

Hughes, S.M., C. N. Levy, R. Katz, et al. "Changes in Concentrations of Cervicovaginal Immune Mediators across the Menstrual Cycle: A Systematic Review and Meta-Analysis of Individual Patient Data." *BMC Medicine* 20, 353 (2022). https://bmcmedicine.biomedcentral.com/articles/10.1186/s12916-022-02532-9.

Hutchinson, Alex. "The 'Last Taboo' in Sports: The Menstrual Cycle." *Globe and Mail*. February 15, 2015. http://www.theglobeandmail.com/life/health-and-fitness/fitness/how-the-menstrual-cycle-influences-athletic-performance/article22989539/.

Janse, Jonge. "Effects of the Menstrual Cycle on Exercise Performance." *Sports Medicine* 33, no. 11 (2003): 833–51.

Janse, Jonge, M. W. Thompson, V. H. Chuter, L. N. Silk, and J. M. Thom. "Exercise Performance over the Menstrual Cycle in Temperate and Hot, Humid Conditions." *Medicine and Science in Sports and Exercise* 44, no. 11 (2012): 2190–98.

Kruse T., H. Reiber, and V. Neuhoff. "Amino Acid Transport across the Human Blood-CSF Barrier: An Evaluation Graph for Amino Acid Concentrations in Cerebrospinal Fluid." *Journal of Neurological Sciences* 70, no. 2 (September 1985): 129–38. https://www.sciencedirect.com/science/article/abs/pii/0022510X85900826.

Lee, Chang Woock, Mark E. Newman, and Steven E. Riechman. "Oral Contraceptive Use Impairs Muscle Gains in Young Women." Presented at Experimental Biology 09 FASEB 2009; Abstract 4197.

Li, Yuyuan, Yuanyi Wei, Feng Zheng, Youfei Guan, and Xiaoyan Zhang. "Prostaglandin E2 in the Regulation of Water Transport in Renal Collecting Ducts." *International Journal of Molecular Sciences* 18, no. 12 (2017): 2539. https://www.ncbi.nlm.nih.gov/pmc/articles/PMC5751142/.

Lowe D. A., K. A. Baltgalvis, and S. M. Greising. "Mechanisms behind Estrogen's Beneficial Effect on Muscle Strength in Females." *Exercise and Sport Sciences Reviews* 38, no. 2 (2010): 61–67. https://www.ncbi.nlm.nih.gov/pmc/articles/PMC2873087/.

Meek, I. L., M. A. van de Laar, H. E. Vonkeman. "Non-Steroidal Anti-Inflammatory Drugs: An Overview of Cardiovascular Risks." *Pharmaceuticals (Basel)* 3, no. 7 (July 2010): 2146–62. https://www.ncbi.nlm.nih.gov/pmc/articles/PMC4036661.

Menkes, D. B., D. C. Coates, and J. P. Fawcett. "Acute Tryptophan Depletion Aggravates Premenstrual Syndrome." *Journal of Affective Disorders* 32, no. 1 (September 1994): 37–44. https://www.sciencedirect.com/science/article/pii/0165032794900590.

Moran, V. H., H. L. Leathard, and J. Coley. "Cardiovascular Functioning during the Menstrual Cycle." *Clinical Physiology* 20, no. 6 (2000): 496–504.

Mountjoy, Margo, et al. "The IOC Consensus on Relative Energy Deficiency in Sport (RED-S): 2018 Update." *British Journal of Sports Medicine* 52 (2018): 687–97.

Nasiadek, M., J. Stragierowicz, M. Klimczak, and A. Kilanowicz. "The Role of Zinc in Selected Female Reproductive System Disorders." *Nutrients* 12, no. 8: (August 2020). https://www.ncbi.nlm.nih.gov/pmc/articles/PMC7468694.

Nørregaard, Rikke, Tae-Hwan Kwon, and Jørgen Frøkiær. "Physiology and Ppathophysiology of Cyclooxygenase-2 and Prostaglandin E2 in the Kidney." *Kidney Resesarch and Clinical Practice* 34, no. 4 (December 2015): 194–200.

Pivarnik, J. M., C. J. Marichal, T. Spillman, and J. R. Morrow Jr. "Menstrual Cycle Phase Affects Temperature Regulation during Endurance Exercise." *Journal of Applied Physiology* 72, no. 2 (1992): 543–48.

Solomon, S. J., M. S. Kurzer, D. H. Calloway. "Menstrual Cycle and Basal Metabolic Rate in Women." *The American Journal of Clinical Nutrition* 36, no. 4 (October 1982): 611–16. https://pubmed.ncbi.nlm.nih.gov/7124662/.

Sung, Eunsook, Ahreum Han, Timo Hinrichs, Matthias Vorgerd, Carmen Manchado, and Petra Platen. "Effects of Follicular versus Luteal Phase-Based Strength Training in Young Women." *SpringerPlus* 3, no. 668 (2014). doi:10.1186/2193-1801-3-668.

Tomarchio, Cameron. "Sport's Most Uncomfortable Questions Answered." July 30, 2014. news.com.au. http://www.news.com.au/sport/more-sports/sports-most-uncomfortable-questions-answered/news-story/8e0d396f75350739b2fb298ced3941eb.

"Vaginal Immune System Ebbs and Flows Depending on Menstrual-Cycle Stage." News Medical Life Sciences. October 7, 2022. https://www.news-medical.net/news/20221007/Vaginal-immune-system-ebbs-and-flows-depending-on-menstrual-cycle-stage.aspx.

Vannuccini, S, F. Fondelli, S. Clemenza, G. Galanti, and F. Petraglia. "Dysmenorrhea and Heavy Menstrual Bleeding in Elite Female Athletes: Quality of Life and Perceived Stress." *Reproductive Sciences* 27, no. 3 (2020): 888–94. https://pubmed.ncbi.nlm.nih.gov/32046446.

Verhoef, S. J., M. C. Wielink, E. A. Achterberg, M. Y. Bongers, and S. M. T. A. Goossens. "Absence of Menstruation in Female Athletes: Why They Do Not Seek Help." *BMC Sports Science, Medicine and Rehabilitation* 13, no. 1: (November 201): 146. https://www.ncbi.nlm.nih.gov/pmc/articles/PMC8609260.

Chapter 3

Abildgaard, J., A. T. Pedersen, C. J. Green, N. M. Harder-Lauridsen, T. P. Solomon, C. Thomsen, A. Juul, M. Pedersen, J. T. Pedersen, O. H. Mortensen, H. Pilegaard, B. K. Pedersen, and B. Lindegaard. "Menopause Is Associated with Decreased Whole Body Fat Oxidation during Exercise." *American Journal of Physiology: Endocrinology and Metabolism* 304 (2013): E1227—E1236.

Amabebe, Emmanuel, Sonia I. Omorodion, Janet O. Ozoene, Andrew C. Ugwu, and Leonard F. Obika. "Sweating and Thirst Perception in Premenopausal, Perimenopausal and Postmenopausal Women during Moderate Exercise." *Journal of Experimental and Integrative Medicine* 3, no. 4 (2013): 279–84.

American Physiological Society. "Water Retention Linked to Changes in Sex Hormone Levels." June 22, 2015. news-medical.net. http://www.news-medical.net/news/20150622/Water-retention-linked-to-changes-in-sex-hormone-levels.aspx.

Beddhu, Srinivasan. "2-Minute Walk Every Hour May Help Offset Effects of Sitting." *Clinical Journal of the American Society of Nephrology* (April 30, 2015).

Biswas, Aviroop, Paul I. Oh, Guy E. Faulkner, Ravi R. Bajaj, Michael A. Silver, Marc S. Mitchell, and David A. Alter. "Sedentary Time and Its Association with Risk for Disease Incidence, Mortality, and Hospitalization in Adult." *Annals of Internal Medicine* 162, no. 2 (January 2015): 123–32. https://www.acpjournals.org/doi/10.7326/m14-1651.

Burd, Nicholas A., Jason E. Tang, Daniel R. Moore, and Stuart M. Phillips. "Exercise Training and Protein Metabolism: Influences of Contraction, Protein Intake, and Sex-Based Differences." *Journal of Applied Physiology* 106, no. 5 (May 1, 2009): 1692–701.

Collins, B. C., E. K. Laakkonen, and D. A. Lowe. "Aging of the Musculoskeletal System: How the Loss of Estrogen Impacts Muscle Strength." *Bone* 123 (June 2019): 137–144. https://www.sciencedirect.com/science/article/pii/S8756328219301206.

Day, Anna. "Hormone Replacement Therapy Lessons from the Women's Health Initiative: Primary Prevention and Gender Health." *Canadian Medical Association Journal* 167, no. 4 (August 20, 2002): 361–62.

Dillon, E. L., M. Sheffield-Moore, D. Paddon-Jones, C. Gilkison, A. P. Sanford, S. L. Casperson, J. Jiang, D. L. Chinkes, and R. J. Urban. "Amino Acid Supplementation Increases Lean Body Mass, Basal Muscle Protein Synthesis, and Insulin-Like Growth Factor-I Expression in Older Women." *The Journal of Clinical Endocrinology and Metabolism* 94, no. 5 (May 2009): 1630–1637. https://www.ncbi.nlm.nih.gov/pmc/articles/PMC2684480/.

Fonseca, Helder, Daniel Moreira-Gonçalves, Rita Ferreira, Francisco Amado, Mário Vaz, and José Duarte. "AR1 Estrogen Loss Leads to Reduced Motor Activity: Neural versus Muscular Role?" *Medicine and Science in Sports and Exercise* 42, no. 10 (October 2010): 64–65.

Gould, L. M., A. N. Gordon, H. E. Cabre, A. T. Hoyle, E. D. Ryan, A. C. Hackney, and A. E. Smith-Ryan. "Metabolic Effects of Menopause: A Cross-sectional Characterization of Body Composition and Exercise Metabolism." *Menopause* 29, no. 4 (February 2022): 377–389. https://pubmed.ncbi.nlm.nih.gov/35231009.

Greendale, Gail A., Carol A. Derby, and Pauline M. Maki. "Perimenopause and Cognition." *Obstetrics and Gynecology Clinics of North America* 38, no. 3 (September 2011): 519–35.

Hadley, Susan, and Judith J. Petry. "Valerian." *American Family Physician* 67, no. 8 (April 15, 2003): 1755–58. Hormone Replacement Therapy Also Called: ERT, Estrogen Replacement Therapy, HRT, Menopausal Hormone Therapy. U.S. National Library of Medicine, NIH: National Heart, Lung, and Blood Institute, August 4, 2014.

Johnson, Jodee. "Dietary Bioactive Components: Antioxidant and Anti-Inflammatory Effects of Dietary Bioactive Components" section of the annual meeting of the American Society of Nutrition, held in conjunction with the Experimental Biology 2014 meeting in San Diego.

Katzmarzyk, P. T., T. S. Church, C. L. Craig, and C. Bouchard. "Sitting Time and Mortality from All Causes, Cardiovascular Disease, and Cancer." *Medicine and Science in Sports and Exercise* 41, no. 5 (May 2009): 998–1005.

Landau, Meryl Davis. "Is It Possible to Cure Hot Flashes?" *National Geographic*. December 8, 2017. https://www.nationalgeographic.co.uk/science-and-technology/2022/12/is-it-possible-to-cure-hot-flushes-we-may-be-getting-closer.

Lebrun, Constance M. "Effect of the Different Phases of the Menstrual Cycle and Oral Contraceptives on Athletic Performance." *Sports Medicine* 16, no. 6 (December 1993): 400–430.

Macdonald, I. "Influence of Fructose and Glucose on Serum Lipid Levels in Men and Pre- and Postmenopausal Women." *American Journal of Clinical Nutrition* 18, no. 5 (May 1966): 369–72.

Manson, J. E., R. T. Cheblowski, M. L. Stefanick, A. K. Aragaki, J. E. Rossouw, R. L. Prentice, G. Anderson, B. V. Howard, C. A. Thomson, A. Z. LaCroix, J. Wactawski-Wende, R. D. Jackson, M. Limacher, K. L. Margolis, S. Wassertheil-Smoller, S. A. Beresford, J. A. Cauley, C. B. Eaton, M. Gass, J. Hsia, K. C. Johnson, C. Kooperberg, L. H. Kuller, C. E. Lewis, S. Liu, L. W. Martin, J. K. Ockene, M. J. O'Sullivan, L. H. Powell, M. S. Simon, L. Van Horn, M. Z. Vitolins, and R. B. Wallace. "Menopausal Hormone Therapy and Health Outcomes During the Intervention and Extended Poststopping Phases of the Women's Health Initiative Randomized Trials." *JAMA* 310, no. 13 (October 2, 2013): 1353–68. doi:10.1001/jama.2013.278040. PMID: 24084921.

Moore, Anne. "Hormone Replacement Therapy: Dilemmas in 2002." *Transactions of the American Clinical and Climatological Association* 114 (2003): 233–40.

Moore, Daniel R., Eric P. Williamson, Nathan Hodson, Stephanie Estafanos, Michael Mazzulia, Dinesh Kumbhare, and Jenna B. Gillen. "Walking or Body Weight Squat 'Activity Snacks' Increase Dietary Amino Acid Utilization for Myofibrillar Protein Synthesis During Prolonged Sitting." *Journal of Applied Physiology* 133, no. 3 (September 2022): 777–85.

National Heart, Lung, and Blood Institute. "More Guidance for Hormone Replacement Therapy." October 28, 2013. http://www.nih.gov/news-events/nih-research-matters/more-guidance-hormone-replacement-therapy.

National Osteoporosis Foundation. "What Women Need to Know." http://nof.org/articles/235 National Sleep Foundation. "Menopause and Sleep." September 16, 2010. https://sleepfoundation.org/sleep-topics/menopause-and-sleep.

Pigeon, W. R., M. Carr, C. Gorman, and M. L. Perlis. "Effects of a Tart Cherry Juice Beverage on the Sleep of Older Adults with Insomnia: A Pilot Study." *Journal of Medicinal Food* 13, no. 3 (June 2010): 579–83. doi:10.1089/jmf.2009.0096.

Poehlman, E. T. "Menopause, Energy Expenditure, and Body Composition." *Acta Obstetrica Gynecologica Scandinavica* 81, no. 7 (July 2002): 603–11.

Shanks, Lori J. "60 Minutes of Exercise per Day Needed for Middle-Aged Women to Maintain Weight." *Harvard Gazette*, March 23, 2010.

Smith, G. I., D. T. Villareal, D. R. Sinacore, K. Shah, and B. Mittendorfer. "Muscle Protein Synthesis Response to Exercise Training in Obese, Older Men and Women." *Medicine and Science in Sports and Exercise* 44, no. 7 (July 2012): 1259–66. doi:10.1249/MSS.0b013e3182496a41.

Tappy, Luc. "Markedly Blunted Metabolic Effects of Fructose in Healthy Young Female Subjects Compared with Male Subjects." *Diabetes Care* 31, no. 6 (June 2008): 1254–56. "The 2022 Hormone Therapy Position Statement of The North American Menopause Society." *Menopause* 29, no. 7 (2022): 767–794.

Chapter 4

Alajmi, N., K. Deighton, J. A. King, A. Reischak-Oliveira, L. K. Wasse, J. Jones, R. L. Batterham, and D. J. Stensel. "Appetite and Energy Intake Responses to Acute Energy Deficits in Females versus Males." *Medicine and Science in Sports and Exercise*, October 12, 2015 [epub ahead of print].

Clapp, J. F., and E. Capeless. "The VO_2max of Recreational Athletes before and after Pregnancy." *Medicine and Science in Sports and Exercise* 23, no. 10 (October 1991): 1128–33.

Darroch, Francine, Amy Schneeberg, Ryan Brodie, Zachary M. Ferraro, Dylan Wykes, Sarita Hira, Audrey R. Giles, Kristi B. Adamo, and Trent Stellingwerff. "Effect of Pregnancy in 42 Elite to World-Class Runners on Training and Performance Outcomes." *Medicine and Science in Sports and Exercise* 55, no. 1 (January 2023): 93–100. https://journals.lww.com/acsm-msse/Abstract/2023/01000/Effect_of_Pregnancy_in_42_Elite_to_World_Class.10.aspx.

O'Connor, P. J., M. S. Poudevigne, M. E. Cress, R. W. Motl, and J. F. Clapp 3rd. "Safety and Efficacy of Supervised Strength Training Adopted in Pregnancy." *Journal of Physical Activity and Health* 8, no. 3 (March 2011): 309–20.

Teerapornpuntakit, J., A. Klanchui, N. Karoonuthaisiri, K. Wongdee, and N. Charoenphandhu. "Expression of Transcripts Related to Intestinal Ion and Nutrient Absorption in Pregnant and Lactating Rats as Determined by Custom-Designed CDNA Microarray." *Molecular and Cellular Biochemistry* 391, no. 1, 2 (June 2014): 103–16. doi:10.1007/s11010-014-1992-8. Epub February 12, 2014.

U.S. Department of Health and Human Services. ODPHP Publication. UO036. Washington, DC, USA: U.S. Department of Health and Human Services. 2008 Physical Activity Guidelines for Americans. http://www.health.gov/PAGuidelines/.

Zavorsky, G. S., and L. D. Longo. "Adding Strength Training, Exercise Intensity, and Caloric Expenditure to Exercise Guidelines in Pregnancy." *Obstetrics and Gynecology* 117, no. 6 (June 2011): 1399–402. doi:10.1097/AOG.0b013e31821b1f5a.

Chapter 5

Arciero Paul J., Stephen J. Ives, Alex E. Mohr, Nathaniel Robinson, Daniela Escudero, Jake Robinson, Kayla Rose, Olivia Minicucci, Gabriel O'Brien, Kathryn Curran, Vincent J. Miller, Feng He, Chelsea Norton, Maia Paul, Caitlin Sheridan, Sheriden Beard, Jessica Centore, Monique Dudar, Katy Ehnstrom, Dakembay Hoyte, Heather Mak, Aaliyah Yarde. "Morning Exercise Reduces Abdominal Fat and Blood Pressure in Women; Evening Exercise Increases Muscular Performance in Women and Lowers Blood Pressure in Men." *Frontiers in Physiology* 13 (2022). https://www.frontiersin.org/articles/10.3389/fphys.2022.893783.

Chang, Chin-Sun, I-Ting Liu, Fu-Wen Liang, Chia-Chun Li, Zih-Jie Sun, Yin-Fan Chang, Ting-Hsing Chao, and Chih-Hsing Wu. "Effects of Age and Gender on Body Composition Indices as Predictors of Mortality in Middle-Aged and Old People." *Scientific Reports* 12 (May 2022). https://www.nature.com/articles/s41598-022-12048-0.

Redman, L. M., L. K. Heilbronn, C. K. Martin, L. de Jonge, D. A. Williamson, J. P. Delany, E. Ravussin, and Pennington CALERIE Team. "Metabolic and Behavioral Compensations in Response to Caloric Restriction: Implications for the Maintenance of Weight Loss." *PLoS One* 4, no. 2 (2009): e4377.

Richards, Evie. "Mountain Bike World Championships 2022: 'Young female athletes need to know what's normal and what's not'—Evie Richards." BBC, August 24, 2022. https://www.bbc.com/sport/cycling/62600029.

"Survey Finds Disordered Eating Behaviors among Three out of Four American Women." UNC Health Care and UNC School of Medicine, May 17 at the Academy for Eating Disorders' 2008 International Conference on Eating Disorders in Seattle.

Tomiyama, A. J., T. Mann, D. Vinas, J. M. Hunger, J. Dejager, and S. E. Taylor. "Low Calorie Dieting Increases Cortisol." *Psychosomatic Medicine*, April 5, 2010 [epub ahead of print].

Weyer, C., R. L. Walford, I. T. Harper, M. Milner, T. MacCallum, P. A. Tataranni, and E. Ravussin. "Energy Metabolism after Two Years of Energy Restriction: The Biosphere 2 Experiment." *American Journal of Clinical Nutrition* 72, no. 4 (2000): 946–53.

Wilke, Joy. "In U.S., Majority 'Not Overweight,' Not Trying to Lose Weight." June 10, 2014. Gallup. http://www.gallup.com/poll/171287/majority-not-overweight-not-trying-lose-weight.aspx.

Chapter 6

Assaly, Shiren. "Effectiveness of Neuromuscular Conditioning to Prevent Anterior Cruciate Ligament Injuries in Female Athletes: A Critical Synthesis of Literature." *Orthopaedic Practice* 23, no. 3: 11.

Csapo, R., C. N. Maganaris, O. R. Seynnes, and M. V. Narici. "On Muscle, Tendon and High Heels." *Journal of Experimental Biology* 213 (2010): 2582–88. doi:10.1242/jeb.044271.

Gottschall, Jinger S., Jackie Mills, and Bryce Hastings. B-38 Free Communication/Poster—Resistance Exercise: June 1, 2011, 1:00 PM–6:00 PM: ROOM: Hall B, Core Exercises That Incorporate Distal Trunk Muscles Maximize Primary Trunk Muscle Activation: 1692: Board #225 June 1, 3:30 p.m.–5:00 p.m.

Huseynov, Alik, Christoph P. E. Zollikofer, Walter Coudyzer, and Marcia S. Ponce de León. "Developmental Evidence for Obstetric Adaptation of the Human Female Pelvis." *PNAS* 113, no. 19 (April 2016): 5227–32.

Orishimo, K. F., M. Liederbach, I. J. Kremenic, M. Hagins, and E. Pappas. "Comparison of Landing Biomechanics between Male and Female Dancers and Athletes, Part 1: Influence of Sex on Risk of Anterior Cruciate Ligament Injury." *American Journal of Sports Medicine* 42, no. 5 (May 2014): 1082–88. doi:10.1177/0363546514523928. Epub March 3, 2014.

Silvers-Granelli, Holly. "Why Female Athletes Injure Their ACL's More Frequently? What Can We Do to Mitigate Their Risk?" *International Journal of Sports Physical Therapy* 16, no. 4 (August 2021): 971–77. https://ijspt.scholasticahq.com/article/25467-why-female-athletes-injure-their-acl-s-more-frequently-what-can-we-do-to-mitigate-their-risk.

Chapter 7

Byerly, Rebecca. "The Woman Who Outruns the Men, 200 Miles at a Time." *New York Times*. December 5, 2018. https://www.nytimes.com/2018/12/05/sports/courtney-dauwalter-200-mile-race.html.

Chidi-Ogbolu, N., and K. Baar. "Effect of Estrogen on Musculoskeletal Performance and Injury Risk." *Frontiers in Physiology* 9 (2018): 1834. https://www.ncbi.nlm.nih.gov/pmc/articles/PMC6341375.

Human Kinetics. "Strength Training during Menopause Offers Multiple Benefits, Action Plan for Menopause 2005." http://www.humankinetics.com/excerpts/excerpts/strength-training-during-menopause-offers-multiple-benefits.

Reis, E., U. Frick, and D. Schmidtbleicher. "Frequency Variations of Strength Training Sessions Triggered by the Phases of the Menstrual Cycle." *International Journal of Sports Medicine* 16, no. 8 (1995): 545–50.

Schnettler, Chad, John Porcari, and Carl Foster, with Mark Anders. "Exclusive ACE Research Examines the Fitness Benefits of Kettlebells." (January/February 2010) ACE FitnessMatters. https://www.acefitness.org/getfit/studies/kettlebells0120.

Simons, R., and R. Andel. "The Effects of Resistance Training and Walking on Functional Fitness in Advanced Old Age." *Journal of Aging and Health* 18, no. 1 (February 2006): 91–105.

Temesi, John, Pierrick J. Arnal, Thomas Rupp, Léonard Féasson, Régine Cartier, Laurent Gergelé, S. Verges, V. Martin, and Guillaume Millet. "Are Females More Resistant to Extreme Neuromuscular Fatigue?" *Medicine and Science in Sports and Exercise* 47, no. 7 (July 2015): 1372–82.

Chapter 8

Cox, A. J., D. B. Pyne, P. U. Saunders, and P. A. Fricker. "Oral Administration of the Probiotic *Lactobacillus fermentum* VRI-003 and Mucosal Immunity in Endurance Athletes." *British Journal of Sports Medicine* 44, no. 4 (March 2010): 222–26. doi:10.1136/bjsm.2007.044628. Epub February 13, 2008.

Hilimire, Matthew R., Jordan E. DeVylder, and Catherine A. Forestell. "Fermented Foods, Neuroticism, and Social Anxiety: An Interaction Model." *Psychiatry Research* 228, no. 2 (August 15, 2015): 203–8.

Hua, Xinwei, Yueming Cao, David M. Morgan, Kaia Miller, Samantha M. Chin, Danielle Bellavance, and Hamed Khalili. "Longitudinal Analysis of the Impact of Oral Contraceptive Use on the Gut Microbiome." *Journal of Medical Microbiology* 71, no. 4 (April 2022). https://www.microbiologyresearch.org/content/journal/jmm/10.1099/jmm.0.001512?crawler=true.

Jiang, Irene, Paul J. Yong, Catherine Allaire, and Mohamed A. Bedaiwy. "Intricate Connections between the Microbiota and Endometriosis." *International Journal of Molecular Sciences* 22, no. 11 (May 2021): 5644. https://www.mdpi.com/1422-0067/22/11/5644.

Kim, Nayoung. "Sex Difference of Gut Microbiota." *Sex/Gender-Specific Medicine in the Gastrointestinal Diseases*. https://link.springer.com/chapter/10.1007/978-981-19-0120-1_22.

Liu, Rui, Chenhong Zhang, Yu Shi, Feng Zhang, Linxia Li, Xuejiao Wang, Yunxia Ling, Huaqing Fu, Weiping Dong, Jian Shen, Andrew Reeves, Andrew S. Greenberg, Liping Zhao, Yongde Peng, and Xiaoying Ding. "Dysbiosis of Gut Microbiota Associated with Clinical Parameters in Polycystic Ovary Syndrome." *Frontiers of Microbiology* 8 (February 2017). https://www.frontiersin.org/articles/10.3389/fmicb.2017.00324/full.

"The Microbiome." Harvard T. H. Chan School of Public Health. Last accessed August 3, 2023. https://www.hsph.harvard.edu/nutritionsource/microbiome.

Mihajlovic, Jovana, Michael Leutner, Bela Hausmann, Gudrun Kohl, Jasmin Schwarz, Hannah Röver, Nina Stimakovits, Peter Wolf, Katharina Maruszczak, Magdalena Bastian, Alexandra Kautzky-Willer, David Berry. "Combined Hormonal Contraceptives Are Associated with Minor Changes in Composition and Diversity in Gut Microbiota of Healthy Women." *Environmental Microbiology* 23, no. 6 (June 2021): 3037–47. https://ami-journals.onlinelibrary.wiley.com/doi/10.1111/1462-2920.15517.

Omara, Jaclyn M., Yen-Ming Chana, and Mitchell L. Jones. "*Lactobacillus fermentum* and *Lactobacillus amylovorus* as Probiotics Alter Body Adiposity and Gut Microflora in Healthy Persons." *Journal of Functional Foods* 5, no. 1 (January 2013): 116–23.

Pace, Fernanda, and Paula I. Watnik. "The Interplay of Sex Steroids, the Immune Response, and the Intestinal Microbiota." *Trends in Microbiology* 29, no. 9 (September 2021): P849–859. https://www.cell.com/trends/microbiology/fulltext/S0966-842X(20)30279-1?_returnURL=https%3A%2F%2Flinkinghub.elsevier.com%2Fretrieve%2Fpii%2FS0966842X20302791%3Fshowall%3Dtrue.

Pang, Michelle D., Gijs H. Goossens, and Ellen E. Blaak. "The Impact of Artificial Sweeteners on Body Weight Control and Glucose Homeostasis." *Frontiers in Nutrition* 7 (January 2021).

Rizk, Maryan G, and Varykina G Thackray. "Intersection of Polycystic Ovary Syndrome and the Gut Microbiome." *Journal of the Endocrine Society* 5, no. 2 (February 2021). https://academic.oup.com/jes/article/5/2/bvaa177/5983408?login=false%20Table%20or%20Box??.

Ruanpeng, D., C. Thongprayoon, W. Cheungpasitporn, and T. Harindhanavudhi. "Sugar and Artificially Sweetened Beverages Linked to Obesity: A Systematic Review and Meta-analysis." *QJM* 110, no. 8 (August 2017): 513–20. https://academic.oup.com/qjmed/article/110/8/513/3574201.

Salliss, Mary E., Leslie V. Farland, Nichole D. Mahnert, and Melissa M. Herbst-Kralovetz. "The Role of Gut and Genital Microbiota and the Estrobolome in Endometriosis, Infertility and Chronic Pelvic Pain." *Human Reproductive Update* 28, no. 1 (January–February 2022): 92–131. https://academic.oup.com/humupd/article/28/1/92/6412766?login=false.

Shin, Ji-Hee, Young-Hee Park, Minju Sim, Seong-Ah Kim, Hyojee Joung, and Dong-Mi Shin. "Serum Level of Sex Steroid Hormone Is Associated with Diversity and Profiles of Human Gut Microbiome." *Research in Microbiology* 170, no. 4–5 (2019): https://www.sciencedirect.com/science/article/pii/S092325081930035X.

Shing, Cecilia M., Jonathan M. Peake, Chin Leong Lim, David Briskey, Neil P. Walsh, Matthew B. Fortes, Kiran D. K. Ahuja, and Luis Vitetta. "Effects of Probiotics Supplementation on Gastrointestinal Permeability, Inflammation and Exercise Performance in the Heat." *European Journal of Applied Physiology* 114, no. 1 (January 2014): 93–103.

Turer, Emre, William McAlpine, Kuan-wen Wang, Tianshi Lu, Xiaohong Li, Miao Tang, Xiaoming Zhan, Tao Wang, Xiaowei Zhan, Chun-Hui Bu, Anne R. Murray, and Bruce Beutler. "Creatine Maintains Intestinal Homeostasis and Protects against Colitis." *PNAS* 114, no. 7 (January 2017): E1273–E1281. https://www.pnas.org/doi/10.1073/pnas.1621400114.

Valdes, A. M., J. Walter, E. Segal, and T. D. Spector. "Role of the Gut Microbiota in Nutrition and Health." *British Medical Journal* (2018): 361. https://www.bmj.com/content/361/bmj.k2179.

Williams, William V. "Hormonal Contraception and the Development of Autoimmunity: A Review of the Literature." *The Linacre Quarterly* 84, no. 3 (August 2017): 275–295. https://pubmed.ncbi.nlm.nih.gov/28912620.

Willingham, Emily. "Some Sugar Substitutes Affect Blood Glucose and Gut Bacteria." *Scientfic American*. August 19, 2022. https://www.scientificamerican.com/article/some-sugar-substitutes-affect-blood-glucose-and-gut-bacteria/.

Chapter 9

Bass, Martha A., Ankita Sharma, Vinayak K. Nahar, Stacy Chelf, Brittany Zeller, Linda Pham, and M. Allison Ford. "Bone Mineral Density Among Men and Women Aged 35 to 50 Years." *Journal of Osteopathic Medicine* 119, no. 6 (June 2019): 357–363. https://jom.osteopathic.org/abstract/bone-mineral-density-among-men-and-women-aged-35-to-50-years/.

Booth, Sarah L., Katherine L. Tucker, Honglei Chen, Marian T. Hannan, David R. Gagnon, L. Adrienne Cupples, P. W. Wilson, J. Ordovas, E. J. Schaefer, B. Dawson-Hughes, and Douglas P. Kiel. "Dietary Vitamin K Intakes Are Associated with Hip Fracture but Not with Bone Mineral Density in Elderly Men and Women." *American Journal of Clinical Nutrition* 71 (2000): 1201–8.

Booth, S. L., K. E. Broe, D. R. Gagnon, K. L. Tucker, M. T. Hannan, R. R. McLean, B. Dawson-Hughes, P. W. Wilson, L. A. Cupples, and D. P. Kiel. "Vitamin K Intake and Bone Mineral Density in Women and Men." *American Journal of Clinical Nutrition* 77, no. 2 (2003): 512–16.

Chen, Li, Ruiyi Liu, Yong Zhao, and Zumin Shi. "High Consumption of Soft Drinks Is Associated with an Increased Risk of Fracture: A 7-Year Follow-Up Study." *Nutrients* 12, no. 2 (February 19, 2020): 530. https://www.ncbi.nlm.nih.gov/pmc/articles/PMC7071508.

Feskanich, D., P. Weber, W. C. Willett, H. Rockett, S. L. Booth, and G. A. Colditz. "Vitamin K Intake and Hip Fractures in Women: A Prospective Study." *American Journal of Clinical Nutrition* 69 (1999): 74–79.

Feskanich, D., W. C. Willett, M. J. Stampfer, and G. A. Colditz. "Milk, Dietary Calcium, and Bone Fractures in Women: A 12-Year Prospective Study." *American Journal of Public Health* 87 (1997): 992–97.

Gosset, A, J. M. Pouilles, and Florence Tremollieres. "Menopausal Hormone Therapy for the Management of Osteoporosis." *Best Practice & Research Clinical Endocrinology & Metabolism* 35, no. 6 (December 2021): 101551. https://pubmed.ncbi.nlm.nih.gov/34119418.

Harvard School of Public Health. "Calcium and Milk: What's Best for Your Bones and Health?" *Nutrition Source*. http://www.hsph.harvard.edu/nutritionsource/calcium-full-story/.

Heinonen, Ari, Pekka Kannus, Harri Sievänen, Pekka Oja, Matti Pasanen, Marjo Rinne, Kirsti Uusi-Rasi, and Ilkka Vuori. "Randomised Controlled Trial of Effect of High-Impact Exercise on Selected Risk Factors for Osteoporotic Fractures." *The Lancet* 348, no. 9038 (November 1996): 1343–47. https://www.thelancet.com/journals/lancet/article/PIIS0140-6736(96)04214-6/fulltext.

Ilich, Jasminka Z., and Jane E. Kerstetter. "Nutrition in Bone Health Revisited: A Story Beyond Calcium." *Journal of the American College of Nutrition* 19, no. 6 (December 2000): 715–37. https://www.tandfonline.com/doi/abs/10.1080/07315724.2000.10718070.

Jang, Hae-Dong, Jae Young Hong, Kyungdo Han, Jae Chul Lee, Byung-Joon Shin, Seok Keun Choi, Seung Woo Suh, Jae Hyuk Yang, Si Young Park, and Chungwon Bang. "Relationship between Bone Mineral Density and Alcohol Intake: A Nationwide Health Survey Analysis of Postmenopausal Women." *PLoS One* 12, no. 6 (June 29, 2017): e0180132. https://journals.plos.org/plosone/article?id=10.1371/journal.pone.0180132.

Keay, Nicky. "Cumulative Endocrine Dysfunction in Relative Energy Deficiency in Sport (RED-S)." BJSM Blog. February 18, 2018. https://blogs.bmj.com/bjsm/2018/02/18/cumulative-endocrine-dysfunction-relative-energy-deficiency-sport-red-s.

Moore, D. R., J. Sygo, and J. P. Morton. "Fuelling the Female Athlete: Carbohydrate and Protein Recommendations." *European Journal of Sport Science* (2021): 1–13. doi:10.1080/17461391.2021.192250810.1080/17461391.2021.1922508.

National Institutes of Health. "New Recommended Daily Amounts of Calcium and Vitamin D." *NIH Medline Plus* 5, no. 4 (Winter 2011): 12.

Owusu, W., W. C. Willett, D. Feskanich, A. Ascherio, D. Spiegelman, and G. A. Colditz. "Calcium Intake and the Incidence of Forearm and Hip Fractures among Men." *Journal of Nutrition* 127 (1997): 1782–87.

Tai, Vicky, William Leung, Andrew Grey, Ian R. Reid, and Mark J Bolland. "Calcium Intake and Bone Mineral Density: Systematic Review and Meta-Analysis." *BMJ* (2015): 351. https://www.ncbi.nlm.nih.gov/pmc/articles/PMC4784773.

Tucker, K. L., K. Morita, N. Qiao, M. T. Hannan, L. A. Cupples, and D. P. Kiel. "Colas, but Not Other Carbonated Beverages, Are Associated with Low Bone Mineral Density in Older Women: The Framingham Osteoporosis Study." *American Journal of Clinical Nutrition* 84, no. 4 (October 2006): 936–42.

Watson, Steven L, Benjamin Kurt Weeks, Lisa J. Weis, Amy T. Harding, Sean Horan, and Belinda R. Beck. "High-Intensity Resistance and Impact Training Improves Bone Mineral Density and Physical Function in Postmenopausal Women with Osteopenia and Osteoporosis: The LIFTMOR Randomized Controlled Trial." *Journal of Bone and Mineral Research* 33, no. 2 (October 4, 2017): 211–20. https://pubmed.ncbi.nlm.nih.gov/28975661/.

"What Women Need to Know." Bone Health and Osteoporosis Foundation. Last accessed on August 3, 2023. https://www.bonehealthandosteoporosis.org/preventing-fractures/general-facts/what-women-need-to-know.

Zhao, Rongsheng, Meihua Zhao, and Liuji Zhang. "Efficiency of Jumping Exercise in Improving Bone Mineral Density among Premenopausal Women: A Meta-Analysis." *Sports Medicine* 44 (October 2014): 1393–1402. https://link.springer.com/article/10.1007/s40279-014-0220-8.

Chapter 10

Appel, L. J., F. M. Sacks, V. J. Carey, E. Obarzanek, J. F. Swain, E. R. Miller 3rd, P. R. Conlin, T. P. Erlinger, B. A. Rosner, N. M. Laranjo, J. Charleston, P. McCarron, L. M. Bishop, and OmniHeart Collaborative Research Group. "Effects of Protein, Monounsaturated Fat, and Carbohydrate Intake on Blood Pressure and Serum Lipids: Results of the Omniheart Randomized Trial." *JAMA* 294, no. 19 (November 16, 2005): 2455–64.

Berry, Jennifer. "What to Know about Omega-6 Fatty Acids," September 24, 2020. https://www.medicalnewstoday.com/articles/omega-6-fatty-acids#are-they-healthful.

Burke, Louise M., Avish P. Sharma, Ida A. Heikura, Sara F. Forbes, Melissa Holloway, Alannah K A McKay, Julia L. Bone, Jill J. Leckey, Marijke Welvaert, and Megan L. Ross. "Crisis of Confidence Averted: Impairment of Exercise Economy and Performance in Elite Race Walkers by Ketogenic Low Carbohydrate, High Fat (LCHF) Diet Is Reproducible." *PLoS ONE* 15, no. 6 (June 2020): e0234027. https://journals.plos.org/plosone/article?id=10.1371/journal.pone.0234027.

Burke, Louise M., Megan L. Ross, Laura A Garvican-Lewis, Marijke Welvaert, Ida A. Heikura, Sara F. Forbes, Joanne G. Mirtschin, et al. "Low Carbohydrate, High Fat Diet Impairs Exercise Economy and Negates the Performance Benefit from Intensified Training in Elite Race Walkers." *The Journal of Physiology* 595, no. 9 (February 2017): 2785–2807. https://physoc.onlinelibrary.wiley.com/doi/10.1113/JP273230.

Cadegiani, Flavio. "The Underappreciated Athlete: Overtraining Syndrome in Resistance Training, High-Intensity Functional Training (HIFT), and Female Athletes." In *Springer EBooks*, 131–54, 2020. https://link.springer.com/chapter/10.1007/978-3-030-52628-3_7.

Enríquez-Valencia, Salma A., Norma Julieta Salazar-López, Maribel Robles-Sánchez, Gustavo A. González-Aguilar, J. Fernando Ayala-Zavala, and Leticia Xochitl Lopez Martinez. "Propiedades Bioactivas de Frutas Tropicales Exóticas y Sus Beneficios a La Salud." *Archivos Latinoamericanos De Nutricion* 70, no. 3 (March 2021): 206–15. https://www.alanrevista.org/ediciones/2020/3/art-5/.

Fahrenholtz, Ida Lysdahl, Anna Melin, Paulina Wasserfurth, Andreas Stenling, Danielle M. Logue, Ina Garthe, Karsten Koehler, et al. "Risk of Low Energy Availability, Disordered Eating, Exercise Addiction, and Food Intolerances in Female Endurance Athletes." *Frontiers in Sports and Active Living* 4 (May 2022). https://www.frontiersin.org/articles/10.3389/fspor.2022.869594/full.

Glenn, Jordan M., Michelle Gray, Bruno Gualano, and Hamilton Roschel. "The Ergogenic Effects of Supplemental Nutritional AIDs on Anaerobic Performance in Female Athletes." *Strength and Conditioning Journal* 38, no. 2 (April 2016): 105–20. https://journals.lww.com/nsca-scj/pages/articleviewer.aspx?year=2016&issue=04000&article=00015&type=Fulltext&fbclid=IwAR3hhAHX6GycCIbI2FSgjOVC1yEZwCdIYkXGRPftp-1s8hexKx_YdiOcoec.

Guest, Nanci S., Trisha A. VanDusseldorp, Michael T. Nelson, Jozo Grgic, Brad J. Schoenfeld, Nathaniel D.M. Jenkins, Shawn M. Arent, et al. "International Society of Sports Nutrition Position Stand: Caffeine and Exercise Performance." *Journal of the International Society of Sports Nutrition* 18, no. 1 (January 2021). https://jissn.biomedcentral.com/articles/10.1186/s12970-020-00383-4.

Gregory, Rachel M, Hasan Hamdan, Danielle M. Torisky, and Jeremy D. Akers. "A Low-Carbohydrate Ketogenic Diet Combined with 6-Weeks of Crossfit Training Improves Body Composition and Performance." *International Journal of Sports and Exercise Medicine* 3, no. 2 (April 30, 2017). https://clinmedjournals.org/articles/ijsem/international-journal-of-sports-and-exercise-medicine-ijsem-3-054.php?jid=ijsem.

Hardy, Karen, Jennie Brand Miller, Katherine D. Brown, Mark G. Thomas, and Les Copeland. "The Importance of Dietary Carbohydrate in Human Evolution." *Quarterly Review of Biology* 90, no. 3 (September 2015): 251–68.

Holtzman, Bryan, and Kathryn E. Ackerman. "Recommendations and Nutritional Considerations for Female Athletes: Health and Performance." *Sports Medicine* 51, no. S1 (September 2021): 43–57. https://www.ncbi.nlm.nih.gov/pmc/articles/PMC8566643/.

Ihle, Rayan, and Anne B. Loucks. "Dose-Response Relationships Between Energy Availability and Bone Turnover in Young Exercising Women." *Journal of Bone and Mineral Research* 19, no. 8 (April 2004): 1231–40. https://asbmr.onlinelibrary.wiley.com/doi/full/10.1359/JBMR.040410.

Jesus, Filipe, Inês Castela, Analiza M. Silva, Pedro Branco, and Mónica Sousa. "Risk of Low Energy Availability Among Female and Male Elite Runners Competing at the 26th European Cross-Country Championships." *Nutrients* 13, no. 3 (March 2021): 873. https://www.mdpi.com/2072-6643/13/3/873.

Layman, Donald K. "Dietary Guidelines Should Reflect New Understandings about Adult Protein Needs." *Nutrition and Metabolism (Lond)*. 2009; 6: 12. Published online March 13, 2009. doi:10.1186/1743-7075-6-12.

Logue, Danielle M., Sharon M. Madigan, Anna Melin, Eamonn Delahunt, Mirjam M. Heinen, Sarah-Jane Mc Donnell, and Clare Corish. "Low Energy Availability in Athletes 2020: An Updated Narrative Review of Prevalence, Risk, Within-Day Energy Balance, Knowledge, and Impact on Sports Performance." *Nutrients* 12, no. 3 (March 20, 2020): 835. https://www.mdpi.com/2072-6643/12/3/835.

McKay, Alannah K. A., Peter Peeling, David B. Pyne, Nicolin Tee, Jamie Whitfield, Avish P. Sharma, Ida A. Heikura, and Louise M. Burke. "Six Days of Low Carbohydrate, Not Energy Availability, Alters the Iron and Immune Response to Exercise in Elite Athletes." *Medicine and Science in Sports and Exercise* 54, no. 3 (October 25, 2021): 377–87. https://pubmed.ncbi.nlm.nih.gov/34690285/.

Morehen, James C., Christopher Rosimus, Bryce P Cavanagh, Catherine Hambly, John R. Speakman, Kirsty J Elliot-Sale, Marcus P. Hannon, and James P. Morton. "Energy Expenditure of Female International Standard Soccer Players: A Doubly Labeled Water Investigation." *Medicine and Science in Sports and Exercise* 54, no. 5 (December 2021): 769–79. https://pubmed.ncbi.nlm.nih.gov/34974499/.

Moore, Daniel R., Jennifer Sygo, and James P. Morton. "Fuelling the Female Athlete: Carbohydrate and Protein Recommendations." *European Journal of Sport Science* 22, no. 5 (May 2021): 684–96. https://www.tandfonline.com/doi/abs/10.1080/17461391.2021.1922508?journalCode=tejs20.

National Institutes of Health. "Reducing Total Fat Intake May Have Small Effect on Risk of Breast Cancer, No Effect on Risk of Colorectal Cancer, Heart Disease, or Stroke." February 7, 2006. http://www.nih.gov/news-events/news-releases/news-womens-health-initiative-reducing-total-fat-intake-may-have-small-effect-risk-breast-cancer-no-effect-risk-colorectal-cancer-heart-disease-or-stroke.

"No Need to Avoid Healthy Omega-6 Fats." Harvard Health. August 20, 2019. https://www.health.harvard.edu/newsletter_article/no-need-to-avoid-healthy-omega-6-fats.

Rebić, Nemanja, Vladmir Ilić, and Igor Zlatović. "Effects of a Low Carbohydrate Diet on Sports Performance." *Trends in Sport Sciences* 28, no. 4 (2021): 249–258. http://tss.awf.poznan.pl/files/2021/Vol%2028%20no%204/1_Rebic_TSS_2021_284_249-258.pdf.

Schaal, Karine, Eve Tiollier, Yann Le Meur, Gretchen A. Casazza, and Christophe Hausswirth. "Elite Synchronized Swimmers Display Decreased Energy Availability during Intensified Training." *Scandinavian Journal of Medicine & Science in Sports* 27, no. 9 (July 1, 2016): 925–34. https://pubmed.ncbi.nlm.nih.gov/27367601/.

Siri-Tarino, P. W., Q. Sun, F. B. Hu, and R. M. Krauss. "Meta-Analysis of Prospective Cohort Studies Evaluating the Association of Saturated Fat with Cardiovascular Disease." *American Journal of Clinical Nutrition* 91, no. 3 (March 2010): 535–46. doi:10.3945/ajcn.2009.27725. Epub January 13, 2010.

"Synergistic Effect of Increased Total Protein Intake and Strength Training on Muscle Strength: A Dose-Response Meta-analysis of Randomized Controlled Trials." https://sportsmedicine-open.springeropen.com/articles/10.1186/s40798-022-00508-w.

Tagawa, Ryoichi, Daiki Watanabe, Kyoko Ito, Takeru Otsuyama, Kyosuke Nakayama, Chiaki Sanbongi, and Motohiko Miyachi. "Synergistic Effect of Increased Total Protein Intake and Strength Training on Muscle Strength: A Dose-Response Meta-Analysis of Randomized Controlled Trials." *Sports Medicine—Open* 8, no. 1 (September 4, 2022). https://sportsmedicine-open.springeropen.com/articles/10.1186/s40798-022-00508-w.

Torres-McGehee, Toni M., Dawn M. Emerson, Kelly Pritchett, E. Whitney G. Moore, Allison Smith, and Nancy A. Uriegas. "Energy Availability with or without Eating Disorder Risk in Collegiate Female Athletes and Performing Artists." *Journal of Athletic Training* 56, no. 9 (December 2020): 993–1002. https://www.ncbi.nlm.nih.gov/pmc/articles/PMC8448477.

"The 2022 Hormone Therapy Position Statement of The North American Menopause Society." Menopause 29, no. 7 (2022): 767–794.

Wasserfurth, Paulina, Jana Palmowski, Andreas Hahn, and Karsten Krüger. "Reasons for and Consequences of Low Energy Availability in Female and Male Athletes: Social Environment, Adaptations, and Prevention." *Sports Medicine—Open* 6, no. 1 (September 2020). https://sportsmedicine-open.springeropen.com/articles/10.1186/s40798-020-00275-6.

Weigle, D. S., P. A. Breen, C. C. Matthys, H. S. Callahan, K. E. Meeuws, V. R. Burden, and J. Q. Purnell. "A High-Protein Diet Induces Sustained Reductions in Appetite, Ad Libitum Caloric Intake, and Body Weight Despite Compensatory Changes in Diurnal Plasma Leptin and Ghrelin Concentrations." *American Journal of Clinical Nutrition* 82 (July 2005): 41–48.

Wohlgemuth, Kealey J., Luke R. Arieta, Gabrielle J. Brewer, Andrew Hoselton, Lacey M. Gould, and Abbie E. Smith-Ryan. "Sex Differences and Considerations for Female Specific Nutritional Strategies: A Narrative Review." *Journal of the International Society of Sports Nutrition* 18, no. 1 (January 2021). https://jissn.biomedcentral.com/articles/10.1186/s12970-021-00422-8.

Zafari, Mandana, Fereshteh Behmanesh, and Azar Agha Mohammadi. "Comparison of the Effect of Fish Oil and Ibuprofen on Treatment of Severe Pain in Primary Dysmenorrhea." *Caspian Journal of Internal Medicine* 2, no. 3 (January 2011): 279–82. https://www.ncbi.nlm.nih.gov/pmc/articles/PMC3770499/.

Chapter 11

Bellissimo, Moriah P., Dan Benardot, Walt Thompson, and Anita Nucci. "Relationship Between Within-day Energy Balance on Body Composition in Professional Cheerleaders." *The FASEB Journal* 31, no. 51 (April 2017): 795.2–795.2. https://faseb.onlinelibrary.wiley.com/doi/abs/10.1096/fasebj.31.1_supplement.795.2.

"International society of sports nutrition position stand: nutritional concerns of the female athlete." https://www.tandfonline.com/doi/full/10.1080/15502783.2023.2204066.

Kerksick, Chad M., Shawn M. Arent, Brad J. Schoenfeld, Jeffrey R. Stout, Bill Campbell, Colin Wilborn, Lem Taylor, et al. "International Society of Sports Nutrition Position Stand: Nutrient Timing."

Journal of the International Society of Sports Nutrition 14, no. 1 (January 2017). https://www.ncb.nlm.nih.gov/pmc/articles/PMC5596471/.

King, Andy, Joshua Rowe, and Louise M. Burke. "Carbohydrate Hydrogel Products Do Not Improve Performance or Gastrointestinal Distress during Moderate-Intensity Endurance Exercise." *International Journal of Sport Nutrition and Exercise Metabolism* 30, no. 5 (September 2020): 305–14. https://pubmed.ncbi.nlm.nih.gov/32707564/.

Schoenfeld, Brad J., Alan A. Aragon, Colin Wilborn, James Krieger, and Gul Tiryaki Sonmez. "Body Composition Changes Associated with Fasted versus Non-Fasted Aerobic Exercise." *Journal of the International Society of Sports Nutrition* 11, no. 1 (August 2014). https://jissn.biomedcentral.com/articles/10.1186/s12970-014-0054-7.

Sims, Stacy T., Chad M. Kerksick, Abbie E. Smith-Ryan, X. Janse De Jonge, Katie R. Hirsch, Shawn M. Arent, Susan Hewlings, et al. "International Society of Sports Nutrition Position Stand: Nutritional Concerns of the Female Athlete." *Journal of the International Society of Sports Nutrition* 20, no. 1 (May 24, 2023). https://www.tandfonline.com/doi/full/10.1080/15502783.2023.2204066.

Smith, J. W., D. D. Pascoe, D. H. Passe, B. C. Ruby, L. K. Stewart, L. B. Baker, and J. J. Zachwieja. "Curvilinear Dose–Response Relationship of Carbohydrate (0–120 g.h-1) and Performance." *Medicine and Science in Sports and Exercise* 45, no. 2 (2013): 336–41.

Stannard, Stephen R., Alexandra Buckley, Johann Edge, and Martin W. Thompson. "Adaptations to Skeletal Muscle with Endurance Exercise Training in the Acutely Fed versus Overnight-Fasted State." *Journal of Science and Medicine in Sport* 13, no. 4 (July 2010): 465–69. https://www.jsams.org/article/S1440-2440(10)00073-3/fulltext.

Stenqvist, Thomas Birkedal, Monica Klungland Torstveit, Jens Faber, and Anna Melin. "Impact of a 4-Week Intensified Endurance Training Intervention on Markers of Relative Energy Deficiency in Sport (RED-S) and Performance among Well-Trained Male Cyclists." *Frontiers in Endocrinology* 11 (September 2020). https://pubmed.ncbi.nlm.nih.gov/33101190.

Chapter 12

Almond, Christopher S. D., Andrew Y. Shin, Elizabeth B. Fortescue, Rebekah C. Mannix, David Wypij, Bryce A. Binstadt, Christine N. Duncan, David P. Olson, Ann E. Salerno, Jane W. Newburger, and David S. Greenes. "Hyponatremia among Runners in the Boston Marathon." *New England Journal of Medicine* 352 (April 14, 2005): 1550–56. doi:10.1056/NEJMoa043901.

Benson, Daniel. "Tayler Wiles 'Heart Broken' after Missing out on Olympic Games Selection." *Cycling News*. June 11, 2021. https://www.cyclingnews.com/news/tayler-wiles-heart-broken-after-missing-out-on-olympic-games-selection.

Gandy, Joan. "Water Intake: Validity of Population Assessment and Recommendations." *European Journal of Nutrition* 54, no. S2 (June 1, 2015): 11–16. https://www.ncbi.nlm.nih.gov/pmc/articles/PMC4473081.

Klous, Lisa, C.J. De Ruiter, S. Scherrer, Nicola Gerrett, and H.A.M. Daanen. "The (in)Dependency of Blood and Sweat Sodium, Chloride, Potassium, Ammonia, Lactate and Glucose Concentrations during Submaximal Exercise." *European Journal of Applied Physiology* 121, no. 3 (December 2020): 803–16. https://link.springer.com/article/10.1007/s00421-020-04562-8.

Sims, Stacy T., Nancy J. Rehrer, Melanie L. Bell, and James D. Cotter. "Preexercise Sodium Loading Aids Fluid Balance and Endurance for Women Exercising in the Heat." *Journal of Applied Physiology* 103, no. 2 (August 1, 2007): 534–41. https://doi.org/10.1152/japplphysiol.01203.2006.

Venkatasubramanian, Jayashree, Ao Mei, and Mrinalini C. Rao. "Ion Transport in the Small Intestine." *Current Opinion in Gastroenterology* 26, no. 2 (March 2010): 123–28. https://doi.org/10.1097/mog.0b013e3283358a45.

Wickham, Kate A., Devin G. McCarthy, Lawrence L. Spriet, and Stephen S. Cheung. "Sex Differences in the Physiological Responses to Exercise-Induced Dehydration: Consequences and Mechanisms." *Journal of Applied Physiology* 131, no. 2 (August 1, 2021): 504–10. https://journals.physiology.org/doi/full/10.1152/japplphysiol.00266.2021.

Chapter 13

Baker, Lindsay B. "Physiology of Sweat Gland Function: The Roles of Sweating and Sweat Composition in Human Health." *Temperature* 6, no. 3 (July 2019): 211–59. https://www.ncbi.nlm.nih.gov/pmc/articles/PMC6773238.

Barwood, Martin J., Jo Corbett, Heather Massey, Terry McMorris, Michael J. Tipton, and Christopher Wagstaff. "Acute Anxiety Predicts Components of the Cold Shock Response on Cold Water Immersion: Toward an Integrated Psychophysiological Model of Acute Cold Water Survival." *Frontiers in Psychology* 9, no. 510 (April 2018). https://www.ncbi.nlm.nih.gov/pmc/articles/PMC5904285.

Beidleman, Beth A., Paul B. Rock, Stephen R. Muza, Charles S. Fulco. Lindsay L. Gibson, Gary H. Kamimori, and Allen Cymerman. "Substrate Oxidation Is Altered in Women during Exercise upon Acute Altitude Exposure." *Medicine & Science in Sports & Exercise* 34, no. 3 (March 2002): 430–437. https://journals.lww.com/acsm-msse/Fulltext/2002/03000/Substrate_oxidation_is_altered_in_women_during.8.aspx.

Bernardi, Luciano, Annette Schneider, Luca Pomidori, Emily M. Paolucci, and Annalisa Cogo. "Hypoxic Ventilatory Response in Successful Extreme Altitude Climbers." *The European Respiratory Journal* 27, no. 1 (January 2006): 165–71. https://erj.ersjournals.com/content/27/1/165.

Braun, B., G. E. Butterfield, J. T. Mawson, S. Muza; B. S. Dominick, P. B. Rock, and L. G. Moore. "Women at Altitude: Substrate Oxidation during Steady-State Exercise at Sea Level and after Acclimatization to 4300 Meters Elevation 784." *Medicine and Science in Sports and Exercise* 29, no. 5 (May 1997): 136.

Drake, Christopher L., and Kenneth P. Wright. "Shift Work, Shift-Work Disorder, and Jet Lag." In *Elsevier EBooks*, 784–98, 2011. https://www.scribbr.com/citation/generator/folders/IXF7k7ZWIMqEHsjEyGtUp/lists/2tOhPuV7nF9X6MuWFYyPbU.

Fraenkel, Liana, Yuqing Zhang, Christine E. Chaisson, Stephen R. Evans, Peter W. F. Wilson, and David T. Felson. "The Association of Estrogen Replacement Therapy and the Raynaud Phenomenon in Postmenopausal Women." *Annals of Internal Medicine* 129, no. 3 (1998): 208–11. doi:10.7326/0003-4819-129-3-199808010-00009.

Georges, Thomas, Pierre Menu, Carolin Le Blanc, S. Ferréol, Marc Dauty, and Alban Fouasson-Chailloux. "Contribution of Hypoxic Exercise Testing to Predict High-Altitude Pathology: A Systematic Review." *Life* 12, no. 3 (March 2022): 377. https://www.mdpi.com/2075-1729/12/3/377/htm.

Kaikaew, Kasiphak, Johanna C. Van Den Beukel, Sebastian J. C. M. M. Neggers, Axel P. N. Themmen, Jenny A. Visser, and Aldo Grefhorst. "Sex Difference in Cold Perception and Shivering Onset upon Gradual Cold Exposure." *Journal of Thermal Biology* 77 (October 2018): 137–44. https://pubmed.ncbi.nlm.nih.gov/30196892.

Kegel, Magdalena. "Estrogen Likely Contributes to Cold-Induced Raynaud's in Women." Raynaud News, February 15, 2017. https://raynaudsnews.com/2017/02/15/estrogen-contributes-to-cold-induced-raynauds-reduced-blood-flow.

Kingma, Boris and Wouter van Marken Lichtenbelt. "Energy Consumption in Buildings and Female Thermal Demand." *Nature Climate Change* 5 (2015): 1054–56.

Kirby, Nathalie V., Samuel J. E. Lucas, and Rebekah A. I. Lucas. "Nine-, But Not Four-Days Heat Acclimation Improves Self-Paced Endurance Performance in Females." *Frontiers in Physiology* 10 (May 2019). https://www.frontiersin.org/articles/10.3389/fphys.2019.00539/full.

Madeira, Luciana Gonçalves, Michele Atalla Da Fonseca, Ivana Alice Teixeira Fonseca, Karina Pessoa Oliveira, Renata Lane De Freitas Passos, Christiano A. Machado-Moreira, and Luiz Oswaldo Carneiro Rodrigues. "Sex-Related Differences in Sweat Gland Cholinergic Sensitivity Exist Irrespective of Differences in Aerobic Capacity." *European Journal of Applied Physiology* 109, no. 1 (November 2009): 93–100. https://pubmed.ncbi.nlm.nih.gov/19902243.

Richalet, Jean-Paul, François Lhuissier, and Dominique Jean. "Ventilatory Response to Hypoxia and Tolerance to High Altitude in Women: Influence of Menstrual Cycle, Oral Contraception, and Menopause." *High Altitude Medicine & Biology* 21, no. 1 (March 1, 2020): 12–19. https://pubmed.ncbi.nlm.nih.gov/31855465.

San, Turhan, Senol Polat, Cemal Cingi, Görkem Eskiizmir, Fatih Oghan, and Burak Ömür Çakir. "Effects of High Altitude on Sleep and Respiratory System and Theirs Adaptations." *The Scientific World Journal* 2013 (January 1, 2013): 1–7. https://www.ncbi.nlm.nih.gov/pmc/articles/PMC3654241/.

Shevchuk, Nikolai A. "Adapted Cold Shower as a Potential Treatment for Depression." *Medical Hypotheses* 70, no. 5 (January 2008): 995–1001. https://pubmed.ncbi.nlm.nih.gov/17993252.

Velickovic, Ksenija, Hilda Anaid Lugo Leija, Ian Bloor, James Law, Harold S. Sacks, Michael Symonds, and Virginie Sottile. "Low Temperature Exposure Induces Browning of Bone Marrow Stem Cell Derived Adipocytes in Vitro." *Scientific Reports* 8, no. 1 (March 2018). https://www.nature.com/articles/s41598-018-23267-9.

Wickham, Kate A., and Lawrence L. Spriet. "No Longer Beeting around the Bush: A Review of Potential Sex Differences with Dietary Nitrate Supplementation." *Applied Physiology, Nutrition, and Metabolism* 44, no. 9 (September 1, 2019): 915–24. https://cdnsciencepub.com/doi/10.1139/apnm-2019-0063.

Chapter 14

Ansdell, Paul, Callum G. Brownstein, Jakob Škarabot, Kirsty M. Hicks, Glyn Howatson, Kevin Thomas, Sandra K. Hunter, and Stuart Goodall. "Sex Differences in Fatigability and Recovery Relative to the Intensity-Duration Relationship." *The Journal of Physiology* 597, no. 23 (October 2019): 5577–95. https://physoc.onlinelibrary.wiley.com/doi/epdf/10.1113/JP278699.

Armstrong, Stuart, Eloise S Till, Stephen Maloney, and Gregory A. Harris. "Compression Socks and Functional Recovery Following Marathon Running." *Journal of Strength and Conditioning Research* 29, no. 2 (February 2015): 528–33. https://pubmed.ncbi.nlm.nih.gov/25627452.

Bessman, Dale A. Hirsch, Adam Cooper, Sean P.A. Drummond, and Rachel R. Markwald. "Performance of Seven Consumer Sleep-Tracking Devices Compared with Polysomnography." *Sleep* 44, no. 5 (December 2020). https://pubmed.ncbi.nlm.nih.gov/33378539.

Botonis, Petros G., Nickos Koutouvakis, and Argyris G. Toubekis. "The Impact of Daytime Napping on Athletic Performance—A Narrative Review." *Scandinavian Journal of Medicine & Science in Sports* 31, no. 12 (October 2021): 2164–77. https://pubmed.ncbi.nlm.nih.gov/34559915.

Chinoy, Evan D., Joseph A Cuellar, Kirbie E Huwa, Jason Jameson, Catherine Watson, Sara C. Bergland, Christopher. "Diaphragmatic Breathing Exercises and Your Vagus Nerve." *Psychology Today.* May 16, 2017. https://www.psychologytoday.com/us/blog/the-athletes-way/201705/diaphragmatic-breathing-exercises-and-your-vagus-nerve.

Datta, Kamal, Manjari Tripathi, and Hruda Nanda Mallick. "*Yoga Nidra:* An Innovative Approach for Management of Chronic Insomnia- A Case Report." *Sleep Science and Practice* 1, no. 1 (April 2017). https://sleep.biomedcentral.com/articles/10.1186/s41606-017-0009-4.

Dupuy, O., Wafa Douzi, Dimitri Theurot, Laurent Bosquet, and Benoit Dugué. "An Evidence-Based Approach for Choosing Post-Exercise Recovery Techniques to Reduce Markers of Muscle Damage, Soreness, Fatigue, and Inflammation: A Systematic Review with Meta-Analysis." *Frontiers in Physiology* 9 (April 2018). https://pubmed.ncbi.nlm.nih.gov/29755363/.

Franklin, Nina C., Mohamed M. Ali, Austin T. Robinson, Edita Norkeviciute, and Shane A. Phillips. "Massage Therapy Restores Peripheral Vascular Function following Exertion." *Archives of Physical Medicine and Rehabilitation* 95, no. 6 (June 2014): 1127–34.

Peternelj, T. T. and J. S. Coombes. "Antioxidant Supplementation during Exercise Training: Beneficial or Detrimental?" *Sports Medicine* 41, no. 12 (December 1, 2011): 1043–69. doi:10.2165/11594400-000000000-00000.

Ristowa, Michael, Kim Zarsea, Andreas Oberbach, Nora Klöting, Marc Birringera, Michael Kiehntopf, Michael Stumboli, C. Ronald Kahn, and M. Blüherc. "Antioxidants Prevent Health-Promoting Effects of Physical Exercise in Humans." *Proceedings of the National Academy of Sciences USA* 106, no. 21 (May 26, 2009): 8665–70.

Sargent, Charli, Michele Lastella, Shona L. Halson, and Gregory D. Roach. "How Much Sleep Does an Elite Athlete Need?" *International Journal of Sports Physiology and Performance* 16, no. 12 (December 2021): 1746–57. https://journals.humankinetics.com/view/journals/ijspp/16/12/article-p1746.xml.

Schmitz, Boris, Hannah Niehues, L. Thorwesten, Andreas Klose, Michael Krüger, and Stefan-Martin Brand. "Sex Differences in High-Intensity Interval Training—Are HIIT Protocols Interchangeable between Females and Males?" *Frontiers in Physiology* 11 (January 2020). https://www.frontiersin.org/articles/10.3389/fphys.2020.00038/full.

Chapter 15

Badenhorst, Claire E., Kazushige Goto, Wendy J. O'Brien, and Stacy T. Sims. "Iron Status in Athletic Females, a Shift in Perspective on an Old Paradigm." *Journal of Sports Sciences* 39, no. 14 (February 2021): 1565–75. https://www.tandfonline.com/doi/full/10.1080/02640414.2021.1885782.

Bescós, R., F. A. Rodríguez, X. Iglesias, M. D. Ferrer, E. Iborra, and A. Pons. "Acute Administration of Inorganic Nitrate Reduces VO(2peak) in Endurance Athletes." *Medicine and Science in Sports and Exercise* 43, no. 10 (October 2011): 1979–86.

Dahlquist, Dylan T., Brad P. Dieter, and Michael S. Koehle. "Plausible Ergogenic Effects of Vitamin D on Athletic Performance and Recovery." *Journal of the International Society of Sports Nutrition* 2015, 12:33. doi:10.1186/s12970-015-0093-8.

DeNoon, Daniel. "Death Stalks Smokers in Beta-Carotene Study." *WebMD Health News* (November 30, 2004). http://www.webmd.com/smoking-cessation/news/20041130/death-stalks-smokers-in-beta-carotene-study.

Hamzeh, Yazan. "Should I Nap Right After My Workout?" Sleep Foundation (December 16, 2022). https://www.sleepfoundation.org/physical-activity/should-i-nap-right-after-my-workout.

Higgins, Madalyn, Azimeh Izadi, and Mojtaba Kaviani. "Antioxidants and Exercise Performance: With a Focus on Vitamin E and C Supplementation." *International Journal of Environmental Research and Public Health* 17, no. 22 (November 2020): 8452. https://www.ncbi.nlm.nih.gov/pmc/articles/PMC7697466.

Hoffman, J. R., N. A. Ratamess, A. D. Faigenbaum, R. Ross, J. Kang, J. R. Stout, and J. A. Wise. "Short-Duration Beta-Alanine Supplementation Increases Training Volume and Reduces Subjective Feelings of Fatigue in College Football Players." *Nutrition Research* 28 (2008): 31–35.

Hunt, Lindsey Alexander, Lily Hospers, James W. Smallcombe, Yorgi Mavros, and Ollie Jay. "Caffeine Alters Thermoregulatory Responses to Exercise in the Heat Only in Caffeine-Habituated Individuals: A Double-Blind Placebo-Controlled Trial." *Journal of Applied Physiology* 131, no. 4 (October 2021): 1300–1310. https://journals.physiology.org/doi/full/10.1152/japplphysiol.00172.2021.

"Iron." National Institutes of Health Office of Dietary Supplements. https://ods.od.nih.gov/factsheets/Iron-HealthProfessional/.

Kaviani, Mojtaba. "Antioxidants and Exercise Performance: With a Focus on Vitamin E and C Supplementation." *International Journal of Environmental Research and Public Health* 17, no. 22 (November 2020): 8452. https://www.ncbi.nlm.nih.gov/pmc/articles/PMC7697466.

Lansley, Katherine E., Paul G. Winyard, Stephen J. Bailey, Anni Vanhatalo, Daryl P. Wilkerson, Jamie R. Blackwell, and Andrew M. Jones. "Acute Dietary Nitrate Supplementation Improves Cycling Time Trial Performance." *Medicine and Science in Sports and Exercise* 43, no. 6 (June 2011): 1125–31.

Lansley, Katherine E., Paul G. Winyard, Stephen J. Bailey, Anni Vanhatalo, Daryl P. Wilkerson, Jamie R. Blackwell, F. J. DiMenna, M. Gilchrist, N. Benjamin, and Andrew M. Jones. "Dietary Nitrate Supplementation Reduces the O2 Cost of Walking and Running: A Placebo-Controlled Study." *Journal of Applied Physiology* 110, no. 3 (2011b): 591–600.

Lundberg, J. O., M. Carlström, F. J. Larsen, and E. Weitzberg. "Roles of Dietary Inorganic Nitrate in Cardiovascular Health and Disease." *Cardiovascular Research* 89, no. 3 (February 15, 2011): 525–32. Epub October 11, 2010.

Mason, Shaun, Adam J. Trewin, Lewan Parker, and Glenn D. Wadley. "Antioxidant Supplements and Endurance Exercise: Current Evidence and Mechanistic Insights." *Redox Biology* 35 (August 2020): 101471. https://www.sciencedirect.com/science/article/pii/S2213231719315447.

Moyer, V. A. "Vitamin D and Calcium to Prevent Fractures in Adults: US Preventive Services Task Force Recommendation Statement." *Annals of Internal Medicine* 158, no. 9 (May 7, 2013): 691–96.

Mursu, J., K. Robien, L. J. Harnack, K. Park, and D. R. Jacobs Jr. "Dietary Supplements and Mortality Rate in Older Women: The Iowa Women's Health Study." *Archives of Internal Medicine* 171, no. 18 (October 10, 2011): 1625–33. doi:10.1001/archinternmed.2011.445.

Nielsen, Forrest H., and Henry C. Lukaski. "Magnesium Research: Update on the Relationship between Magnesium and Exercise." *Magnesium Research* 19(3) (September 2006): 180–89.

Pasricha, S.-R., M. Low, J. Thompson, A. Farrell, and L.-M. De-Regil. "Iron Supplementation Benefits Physical Performance in Women of Reproductive Age: A Systematic Review and Meta-Analysis." *Journal of Nutrition* (2014). doi:10.3945/jn.113.189589.

Pedlar, Charles R., Carlo Brugnara, Georgie Bruinvels, and Richard Burden. "Iron Balance and Iron Supplementation for the Female Athlete: A Practical Approach." *European Journal of Sport Science* 18, no. 2 (December 2017): 295–305. https://www.tandfonline.com/doi/full/10.1080/17461391.2017.1416178.

Prentice, R. L., M. B. Pettinger, R. D. Jackson, J. Wactawski-Wende, A. Z. Lacroix, G. L. Anderson, R. T. Chlebowski, J. E. Manson, L. Van Horn, M. Z. Vitolins, M. Datta, E. S. LeBlanc, J. A. Cauley, and J. E. Rossouw. "Health Risks and Benefits from Calcium and Vitamin D Supplementation: Women's Health Initiative Clinical Trial and Cohort Study." *Osteoporosis International* 24, no. 2 (February 2013): 567–80.

Sale, C., B. Saunders, S. Hudson, J. A. Wise, R. C. Harris, and C. D. Sunderland. "Effect of β-alanine Plus Sodium Bicarbonate on High-Intensity Cycling Capacity." *Medicine and Science in Sports and Exercise* 43, no. 10 (October 2011): 1972–78. doi:10.1249/MSS.0b013e3182188501.

Trexler, Eric T., Abbie E. Smith-Ryan, Jeffrey R. Stout, Jay R. Hoffman, Colin D. Wilborn, Craig Sale, Richard B. Kreider, Ralf Jager, Conrad P. Earnest, Laurent Bannock, Bill Campbell, Douglas Kalman, Tim N. Ziegenfuss, and Jose Antonio. "International Society of Sports Nutrition Position Stand: Beta-Alanine." *Journal of the International Society of Sports Nutrition* 12, no. 30 (July 2015). doi:10.1186/s12970-015-0090-y.

Chapter 16

Blanchfield, A. W., J. Hardy, H. M. De Morree, W. Staiano, and S. M. Marcora. "Talking Yourself out of Exhaustion: The Effects of Self-Talk on Endurance Performance." *Medicine and Science in Sports and Exercise* 46, no. 5 (2014): 998–1007. doi:10.1249/MSS.0000000000000184.

Bowler, Amy-Lee, Jamie Whitfield, Liam E. Marshall, Vernon G. Coffey, Louise M. Burke, and Gregory R. Cox. "The Use of Continuous Glucose Monitors in Sport: Possible Applications and Considerations." *International Journal of Sport Nutrition and Exercise Metabolism* 33, no. 2 (March 1, 2023): 121–32. https://doi.org/10.1123/ijsnem.2022-0139.

"Concussion Trajectory in Female Athletes Prolonged When Specialty Care Delayed." Columbia Orthopedics, September 24, 2019. https://www.columbiaortho.org/news/concussion-trajectory-female-athletes-prolonged-when-specialty-care-delayed.

Covassin, Tracey, Ryan Moran, and R. J. Elbin. "Sex Differences in Reported Concussion Injury Rates and Time Loss from Participation: An Update of the National Collegiate Athletic Association Injury Surveillance Program from 2004–2005 through 2008–2009." *Journal of Athletic Training* 51, no. 3 (March 2016): 189–94. https://www.ncbi.nlm.nih.gov/pmc/articles/PMC4852524.

DeCasien, Alex R., Elisa Guma, Siyuan Liu, and Armin Raznahan. "Sex Differences in the Human Brain: A Roadmap for More Careful Analysis and Interpretation of a Biological Reality." *Biology of Sex Differences* 13, no. 1 (July 2022). https://bsd.biomedcentral.com/articles/10.1186/s13293-022-00448-w.

Edmonds, Molly. "Do Men and Women Have Different Brains?" HowStuffWorks.com (October 8, 2008). http://science.howstuffworks.com/life/inside-the-mind/human-brain/men-women-different-brains.htm.

Ingalhalikar, Madhura, Alex Smith, Drew Parker, Theodore D. Satterthwaite, Mark A. Elliott, Kosha Ruparel, Hakon Hakonarson, Raquel E. Gur, Ruben C. Gur, and Ragini Verma. "Sex Differences in the Structural Connectome of the Human Brain." *Proceedings of the National Academy of Sciences USA* 111, no. 2 (2013): 823–88.

Jovanovic, Hristina, J. Lundberg, Per Karlsson, Åsta Cerin, Tomoyuki Saijo, Andrea Varrone, Christer Halldin, and Anna-Lena Nordström. "Sex Differences in the Serotonin 1A Receptor and Serotonin Transporter Binding in the Human Brain Measured by PET." *NeuroImage* 39, no. 3 (February 2008): 1408–19. https://citeseerx.ist.psu.edu/document?repid=rep1&type=pdf&doi=0663c680041c548ba5556d7f36ddd1812a58e940.

Karolinska Institutet. "Sex Differences in the Brain's Serotonin System." www.sciencedaily.com/releases/2008/02/080213111043.htm (accessed December 21, 2015).

Koerte, Inga K., Vivian Schultz, Valerie J. Sydnor, David R. Howell, Jeffrey P. Guenette, Emily Dennis, Janna Kochsiek, et al. "Sex-Related Differences in the Effects of Sports-Related Concussion: A Review." *Journal of Neuroimaging* 30, no. 4 (June 2020): 387–409. https://onlinelibrary.wiley.com/doi/full/10.1111/jon.12726.

Lee, Tatia M.C., Che Hin Chetwyn Chan, Ada Leung, Peter T. Fox, and Jia-Hong Gao. "Sex-Related Differences in Neural Activity during Risk Taking: An FMRI Study." *Cerebral Cortex* 19, no. 6 (October 2008): 1303–12. https://www.ncbi.nlm.nih.gov/pmc/articles/PMC2677650/.

Lewis, Tanya. "How Men's Brains Are Wired Differently than Women's." *Scientific American*, December 2, 2013. https://www.scientificamerican.com/article/how-mens-brains-are-wired-differently-than-women.

Lotze, Martin, Martin Domin, F.H. Gerlach, Christian Gaser, Eileen Lueders, Carsten Oliver Schmidt, and Nicola Neumann. "Novel Findings from 2,838 Adult Brains on Sex Differences in Gray Matter Brain Volume." *Scientific Reports* 9, no. 1 (February 2019). https://www.nature.com/articles/s41598-018-38239-2.

Master, Christina L., Barry P. Katz, Kristy B. Arbogast, Michael McCrea, Thomas W. McAllister, Paul F. Pasquina, Michelle LaPradd, Wenxian Zhou, and Steven P. Broglio. "Differences in Sport-Related Concussion for Female and Male Athletes in Comparable Collegiate Sports: A Study from the NCAA-DoD Concussion Assessment, Research and Education (CARE) Consortium." *British Journal of Sports Medicine* 55, no. 24 (December 21, 2020): 1387–94. bjsports-2020-103316 DOI: 10.1136/bjsports-2020-103316. https://bjsm.bmj.com/content/55/24/1387.

Mosconi, Lisa, Valentina Berti, Jonathan P. Dyke, Eva Schelbaum, Steven Jett, Lacey Loughlin, Grace Jang, et al. "Menopause Impacts Human Brain Structure, Connectivity, Energy Metabolism, and Amyloid-Beta Deposition." *Scientific Reports* 11, no. 1 (June 2021). https://www.nature.com/articles/s41598-021-90084-y.pdf.

News-Medical.net. "Brain's Serotonin System Differs between Men and Women." February 14, 2008. http://www.news-medical.net/news/2008/02/14/35266.aspx.

Portugal, Eduardo Matta Mello, Poliane Gomes Torres Vasconcelos, Renata Martins De Souza, Eduardo Lattari, Renato Sobral Monteiro-Junior, Sergio Machado, and Andrea Camaz Deslandes. "Aging Process, Cognitive Decline and Alzheimer's Disease: Can Strength Training Modulate These Responses?" *CNS & Neurological Disorders-Drug Targets* 14, no. 9 (November 2015): 1209–13. https://www.ingentaconnect.com/content/ben/cnsnddt/2015/00000014/00000009/art00014.

Ranganathan, Vinoth K., Vlodek Siemionowa, Jing Z. Liu, Vinod Sahgal, and Guang H. Yue. "From Mental Power to Muscle Power—Gaining Strength by Using the Mind." *Neuropsychologia* 42 (2004): 944–56.

"Sex Differences in the Brain's Serotonin System." EurekAlert!, February 13, 2008. https://www.eurekalert.org/news-releases/661978.

Singh, Maria A. Fiatarone, Nicola Gates, Nidhi Saigal, Guy C. Wilson, Jacinda Meiklejohn, Henry Brodaty, Wen Wang, et al. "The Study of Mental and Resistance Training (SMART) Study—Resistance Training and/or Cognitive Training in Mild Cognitive Impairment: A Randomized, Double-Blind, Double-Sham Controlled Trial." *Journal of the American Medical Directors Association* 15, no. 12 (December 2014): 873–80.

"Women May Be at Higher Risk for Sports-Related Concussion Than Men." American Academy of Neurology, February 28, 2017. https://www.aan.com/PressRoom/Home/PressRelease/1529.

Wunderle, Kathryn, Kathleen M. Hoeger, Erin B. Wasserman, and Jeffrey J. Bazarian. "Menstrual Phase as Predictor of Outcome after Mild Traumatic Brain Injury in Women." *Journal of Head Trauma Rehabilitation* 29, no. 5 (September 2014): E1–8. https://www.ncbi.nlm.nih.gov/pmc/articles/PMC5237582.

Xin, Jiang, Yaoxue Zhang, Yan Tang, and Yuan Yang. "Brain Differences between Men and Women: Evidence from Deep Learning." *Frontiers in Neuroscience* 13 (March 2019). https://www.frontiersin.org/articles/10.3389/fnins.2019.00185/full.

Chapter 17

Bowler, Amy-Lee, Jamie Whitfield, Liam E. Marshall, Vernon G. Coffey, Louise M. Burke, and Gregory R. Cox. "The Use of Continuous Glucose Monitors in Sport: Possible Applications and Considerations." *International Journal of Sport Nutrition and Exercise Metabolism* 33, no. 2 (March 1, 2023): 121–32. https://doi.org/10.1123/ijsnem.2022-0139.

Kirby, Brett S., David Clark, Eric M. Bradley, and Brad W. Wilkins. "The Balance of Muscle Oxygen Supply and Demand Reveals Critical Metabolic Rate and Predicts Time to Exhaustion." *Journal of Applied Physiology* 130, no. 6 (June 1, 2021): 1915–27. https://doi.org/10.1152/japplphysiol.00058.2021.

ACKNOWLEDGMENTS

December 2014: I am sitting at my mom's house in the "other" Fairfax (VA), when I receive an email from one of the people I respect most, Selene Yeager: "Stac, I have a great idea . . . you know all the stuff you talk about regarding women? We need to put that out there in one fell swoop . . . can you Skype?" One Skype call later, Selene is putting thoughts to paper and paper to proposal. Without her, this book would just be a thought, in the back of my head that would come out as a series of ad hoc lectures and magazine articles. Not only did Selene push our thoughts to a publisher, she was the magic to take my science speak and translate it into easy-to-read and understandable language. Just when I thought I couldn't respect anyone more, I have found a new level for Selene, her craft, and most of all her friendship. Thank you for all that you do and continue to do!

Over the past 9 years, Selene and I have continued to challenge the dogma, and I think we might be winning! We see the conversations around the menstrual cycle, menopause, and puberty becoming more open and common, with policy change and incredible positive outcomes for female athletes. I have my hopes up that we have passed the tipping point and all of us are now riding the wave toward more equality across sport and gender. I thank you, the reader, for this; without a groundswell, we wouldn't be seeing this!

In a wider brushstroke of gratitude, I'd like to thank all my male coaches, academic instructors, and colleagues who have said that women are just "different" or

"Why do you want to study women when we don't know enough about men?", for pushing me to find the answers that you couldn't supply and to research and think outside the box. Without them, I would not have the distinction of being "that girl," the one who always asks, "Well, what about women?"

In a less general scope, I'd like to thank my kick-ass grandma and my mom for being who you both are: inquisitive, impressive, athletic, and genuine women. You are incredible role models, and I am honored to follow your footsteps. Thank you to Marcia Stefanick for pulling me into her realm of the Women's Health Initiative and teaching me that sex differences do, in fact, begin before birth. Thank you to my best friend and riding buddy, Ashley Fouts, for being the genuine you! Thank you to all my athletes, men and women, for asking the questions you do, and keeping me on my toes. Thank you to all the women who have asked, and now have, the answers to "Why does this happen, am I going crazy?" No, it's not your fitness—it's your physiology.

Most of all, thank you SNS and JESS for putting up with my early and late hours to edit and think and stress; without you both, I would be uniplanar.

INDEX

D

E

F

G

I

J

K

L

M

N

O

P

Q

R

S

T

X

Y

Z

ABOUT THE AUTHORS

Stacy Sims, MSc, PhD, is a forward-thinking international exercise physiologist and nutrition scientist who aims to revolutionize sport and exercise training and performance, especially for women. She has directed research programs at Stanford, Auckland University of Technology, and the University of Waikato in New Zealand, focusing on female athlete health and performance, pushing the dogma to improve research on all women.

As a retired elite athlete herself, Dr. Sims has extensive experience working with athletes at all levels: from beginning recreational athletes to Olympians and Tour de France–caliber cyclists. Her contributions to the international research environment and the sports nutrition industry have established a new niche in sports nutrition and established her reputation as the expert in sex differences in training, nutrition, and health. Dr. Sims is in high demand in the sports science, performance, and active women's universes for her "Women Are Not Small Men" lectures. She is a regularly featured speaker at professional and academic conferences and is on the advisory board of several high-impact companies.

Selene Yeager is a bestselling professional health and exercise science writer who lives what she writes as an NASM-certified personal trainer, Pn1 certified nutrition coach, off-road racer, and former All-American Ironman triathlete. She has authored, coauthored, and contributed to more than two dozen books, including *Next Level* (also with Dr. Stacy Sims), *Gravel!, The Bomb Doctor, Rusch to Glory,* and *The Bicycling Big Book of Cycling for Women.* Her work has appeared in numerous magazines and newspapers, including *Details, Shape, O, The Oprah Magazine, Men's Health, Marie Claire, Runner's World,* and *Cosmopolitan.* Yeager was nominated for a National Magazine Award for excellence in service journalism for her work in *Bicycling* magazine. These days you can find her helping active, performance-minded women who aren't willing to put their best years behind them through her work as host of the *Hit Play Not Pause* podcast and content manager at *Feisty Menopause.*

Also available from

STACY T. SIMS, PhD, with SELENE YEAGER

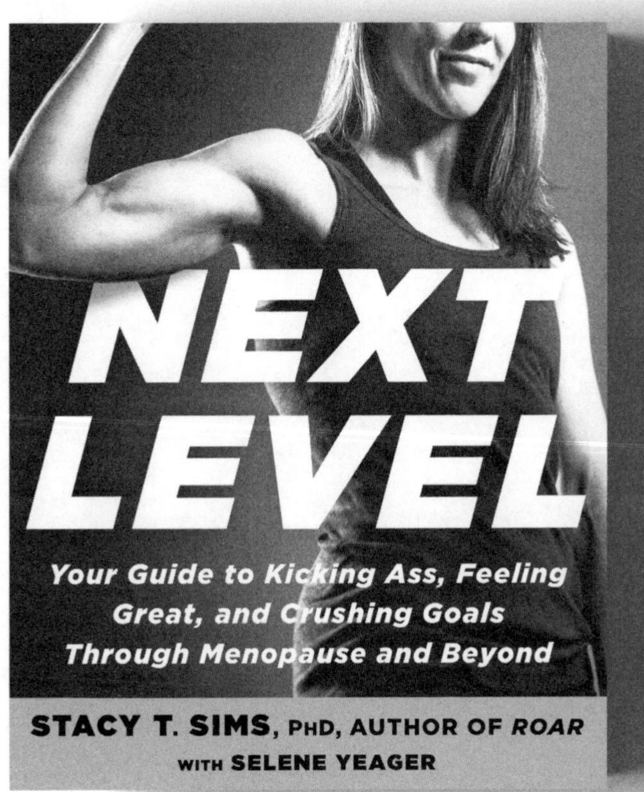

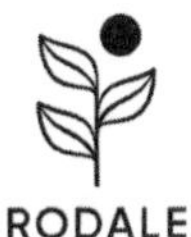

RODALE

Available wherever books are sold